Assemblages of Health

Cameron Duff

Assemblages of Health

Deleuze's Empiricism and the Ethology of Life

Springer

Cameron Duff
Social Sciences and Health Research Unit
Monash University
Caulfield East, VIC
Australia

This author wishes to thank Andrea Eckersley for permission to reproduce her painting ("Untitled # 5, 2008") on the cover of this book.

ISBN 978-94-017-7896-1 ISBN 978-94-017-8893-9 (eBook)
DOI 10.1007/978-94-017-8893-9
Springer Dordrecht Heidelberg New York London

Printed on acid-free paper

Springer is part of Springer Science+Business Media (www.springer.com)

Magic, magic, magic, the pair of them . . . like princelings in the dawn light

The environment enters into the nature of each thing.
– Alfred North Whitehead, *Modes of Thought*

In so far as the Cogito refers to a fractured I, an I split from end to end by the form of time which runs through it, it must be said that Ideas swarm in the fracture, constantly emerging on its edges, ceaselessly coming out and going back, being composed in a thousand different manners.
– Gilles Deleuze, *Difference and Repetition*

Whether we are individuals or groups, we are made up of lines and these lines are very varied in nature.
– Gilles Deleuze and Claire Parnet, *Dialogues*

Each line of life is related to a type of matter that is not merely an external environment, but in terms of which the living being manufactures a body, a form, for itself.
– Gilles Deleuze, *Bergsonism*

Preface

This book presents a study of health and illness derived in large measure from the writings of French philosopher Gilles Deleuze. It provides the first systematic assessment of the significance of Deleuze's thought for contemporary research in the health sciences, including work in public health, quality of life studies and human development. The book will introduce many of Deleuze's key ideas, exploring the application of his method, what he called "transcendental empiricism", to the analysis of select problems in the study of health and society. Of principal interest are the inventive accounts of subjectivity, embodiment and experience that Deleuze proposes, and the varied concepts that these accounts engender. In pursuing these interests, the book will confirm the need for a Deleuzian approach to research in the health and social sciences, along with the innovations in research practice that such an approach should inspire. Each task will entail a critical reading of several of Deleuze's most important concepts, including 'event', 'affect', 'relation', 'life', 'difference', 'immanence', 'becoming' and 'assemblage', in an effort to establish grounds for the more widespread adoption of Deleuze's ideas across the health and social sciences.

The book will focus on the treatment of subjectivity and the body such that the notion of 'human life' may be reframed in the health and social sciences. I argue that such a shift is critical given recent affirmations of the convergence of the human and the nonhuman in social, political and biological life (see Latour 2005). While for some, this convergence signals the need for a *posthuman* account of health and illness more alert to the imbrications of science, technology, politics and biology (Rose 2007: 1–8), I am just as interested in the implications of this 'decentring of the human' for research innovation in the health and social sciences. I aim to extend Deleuze's account of subjectivity and the body in order to sketch the most important implications of 'posthumanism' for thinking about health itself (see Wolfe 2010). The major problem the book seeks to confront, therefore, is the task of rethinking the ontological and epistemological status of health at a time when the 'human subject', to which the attribution of health necessarily refers, seems everywhere in retreat (Fox 2011). The book ventures to explain how health may be reframed in the absence of conventional ontological distinctions such as human/nonhuman, nature/culture and body/society. It asks what health may look like, and how it ought to be conceptualised, in the context of a posthuman, more-than-human, assemblage of spaces, forces and bodies. In addressing these questions, the book will present a number of case studies indicating how Deleuze's account of (human) life may afford fresh insights into enduring health problems such as addiction and mental illness.

I should note that problems concerning subjectivity and embodiment are central to a number of critical debates in the contemporary health sciences (Turner 2008). Of course, the very notion of a science devoted to health may be regarded as a peculiarly humanist enterprise, charged with the preservation of certain kinds of embodied existence to the neglect of others (Fox 2012: 2–7). The health sciences are certainly preoccupied with the body, with both its limitations and capacities, which combined with the demands of public health and the ministrations of clinical medicine effect a unique "government of the living" (Foucault 1997: 81). In Foucault's seminal reckoning, this 'governmentality' works to draw specific forces out of the body, installing a discipline of the flesh in the cultivation of its corporeal agency. Such insights have prompted a good deal of innovation across the health and social sciences (see Fox 2012; Petersen and Bunton 1997), although in analysing health problems scholars have sometimes exaggerated instances of domination and control at the expense of a more balanced assessment of the practices of resistance and self-fashioning central to Foucault's later writing. Recent examples of this tendency include debates regarding the rise of obesity and related health problems; the management of chronic health conditions such as diabetes, depression and HIV/AIDS; and attempts to reduce the use of alcohol and other drugs. Research in each domain typically endorses the 'governmentalities' expressed in the attempt to discipline certain kinds of subjects in an effort to preserve or restore particular kinds of embodied experience (Coveney 1998: 461–465). Health may, indeed, be usefully conceived in this fashion; as an exercise in endorsing specific forms of embodied experience in the interest of defending particular kinds of human life (Greco 2009).

Despite the impact of Foucault's work across the health and social sciences, scholars have often struggled with the methodological implications of his 'genealogy of the subject' for applied research (Turner 2008; Petersen and Bunton 1997). It may, in fact, be argued that the health and social sciences remain caught in the paradox of subjectivity; on the one hand committed to the study of meaning and individual experience, while increasingly aware of the 'illusion' of subjectivity, of its evanescent, mediated character (Law 2004; Mol 2002). The subject, like the body it seems, has lost the reassuring stability it once enjoyed. I argue throughout the book that the examination of human life presents an ontological problem, insofar as the 'subject' of the health and social sciences now evinces a bewildering ontological pluralism. This includes theories and perspectives that reject humanism altogether, treating it as a 'cultural fiction', to more moderate positions that regard 'human life' as a cultural and biological artefact supported within a web of social and 'natural' relations, through to traditional models which cling to the ideal of a sovereign entity endowed with inalienable rights and committed to their assertion and defence (Turner 2008).

Often this pluralism is treated as a convenient resource for the health and social sciences, affording diverse analytical strategies to suit diverse empirical challenges. Yet the antinomies that fracture human life cannot be dismissed so readily. The 'subject' of health cannot be both natural and artificial, body and society, without conceding an ontology of confusion that is forever revising the point at which nature and culture meet. Redrawing the boundaries between self and world may momentarily clarify the 'being' of human life, including those aspects which pertain to health and illness, but it usually serves to reintroduce a traditional subject, albeit within ever more onerous restrictions. Such moves retain the 'subject' and 'culture' as distinctive, reified things that shift and morph in their relations, retreating and advancing according to the predilections of observation and theoretical inclination. The health and social sciences have, in this way, settled for a fraught compromise, accepting both a 'natural' and a 'cultural' subject, a 'natural' and a 'cultural' body, forever arguing over the precise balance of this commingling, while ignoring the ontological tumult such a compromise entails (see Turner 2008: 1–5). The book rejects this fix, noting that the traditional subject cannot hold in the face of evidence confirming its historical and political contingency, just as the 'cultural' subject cannot account for the body without reducing it to artifice (Foucault 1983: 208). The subject, like the body, cannot be both nature and culture without confounding the very status of each. Human life must be explained, along with the full measure of its health.

I would add that the whole idea of health becomes hopelessly confused in this mix of bodies and worlds, subjects and cultures. Indeed, the 'cultural' subject that now rivals the 'traditional' subject in health and social science research opens up at least as many problems as it solves. For it asserts at the same time that health is a 'normal' property of a 'naturally' healthy body, just as it reflects the outcome of discrete structural interactions in the world. Yet how can health be both 'natural' and 'cultural'? Which aspects pertain to the 'nature' of health and which aspects concern its 'culture'? And how might the natural aspects of health be discerned among its cultural ramifications? Surely health must be denaturalised as soon as it is conceded that health is as much a function of historical, political and technological processes, as it is the expression of a hypostasised biology (Mol 2002: 56–60). The body, like the subject, becomes slippery and elusive in this commingling of forces, clinging to the assurances of the flesh as surely as it is distributed among the structures of a ubiquitous culture. So what does the health of a 'natural/cultural' body refer to; and what can it mean to describe such a body as healthy? Do such questions concern individual bodies; a particular set of salubrious practices; an especially conducive environment; an enviable genetic endowment; or do they concern all these things at once? The latter position merely confounds the ontological status of the embodied subject of health and illness, and the interactions which mediate it. It inevitably confounds causality and correlation in neglecting to consider whether the subject is a *party* to social and structural interactions, or *formed and modified* in them. Medical science usually endorses the first position along with the idea of a natural, healthy body, while the study of the 'social determinants of health' opts for the second, even as it retains a vestigial commitment to the 'natural' body of biomedicine (Fox 2012).

Foucault (1978) observed that the problem of determining the proper ontological status of the embodied subject haunts the human sciences because it renders uncertain the very object of their analysis. While each such science usually manages this matter internally, retreating to the certainties of long established disciplinary maxims, the epistemological challenges occasioned by the problem of 'human life' remain a source of enduring unease throughout the health and social sciences (Greco 2009; Rose 2007). This suggests that the time is ripe for a thoroughgoing reappraisal of the 'subject' of the health and social sciences in the interests of overturning the nature/culture, human/nonhuman dyads that bedevil so much contemporary work in these fields. The book proceeds from the conviction that Deleuze's philosophy provides the most coherent intellectual resources for this task.

The book will argue that Deleuze's transcendental empiricism furnishes a compelling basis for reorienting the study of 'human life', and the more specific investigation of the experience of healthy and ill subjects. Furthermore, Deleuze's empiricism offers a means of exploring the *territorialisation* of human life in ways that may revitalise accounts of the social dimensions of health. Abandoning the ontology of nature and culture, of nature *or* culture, Deleuze (1988: 104–122) prefers a "vital topology" of the "inside" and the "outside" in which the inside is always yet another fold of the outside, just as the outside is always a folding of the inside. Human life (the embodied subject) is involuted, "implicated" in this process of folding by which an "inside" (or interiority) like mind, consciousness or subjectivity is produced in a "differential synthesis" of an always present, always folded "outside" that includes the folds of habit, practice, sense data, food and water, other bodies, ideas and technologies (Deleuze 1994: 70–74). It follows that "the whole of the inside finds itself actively present on the outside" (Deleuze 1988: 119) such that subjectivity and embodiment ought to be regarded as *assemblages of the inside and the outside*, of forces and processes distributed in multiple, dynamic and recursive relations. Nature and culture, body and world, inside and outside can no longer be regarded as ontologically distinct and separable entities. As Alfred North Whitehead (1968: 21) observed in a sympathetic context, "we cannot define where a body begins and where external nature ends. . .exactness is out of the question. It can only be obtained by some trivial convention". Eschewing such conventions, Deleuze instead posits a pre-subjective, pre-individual field of forces, affects and percepts, of intensive and extensive singularities, out of which the assemblages which support or express human life are formed. Subjectivity is expressed in an assemblage, but cannot be reduced to any particular element, or set of elements, within it. The body is equally "multiple" assembled in the congeries of objects, actors and worlds (Mol 2002: 172).

The book contends that such logic presents a breakthrough in recent attempts to resolve the status of 'human life' in the health and social sciences (see Grosz 2011; Fox 2011). In developing this argument, the book will move from Deleuze's biophilosophy to consider those processes, events and relations that support the *vital expression of health in life*. This will involve an attempt to derive a 'developmental ethology' from Deleuze's writings, specifically his commentaries on Spinoza and Bergson. On the basis of these commentaries, I will emphasise the ethological composition of human life in order to identify the specific relations, affects and events that enable joyous, or healthy, encounters between bodies, and those that precipitate sad, or unhealthy, relations. The book will define health as a particular state of embodied subjectivity that is formed or produced in an assemblage of relations, affects and events. I will go on to argue that Deleuze's work provides a means of tracing the characteristic features of this assemblage, suggesting a basis for eliciting positive accounts of health by clarifying those relations, affects and events wherein a body's health is sustained or promoted. Having established a means of defining health in a more substantive way, the book will turn to consider the impact of various social and structural processes in mediating health outcomes in specific settings and populations. The purpose of this analysis is to advance a Deleuzian account of the social determinants of health, along with a novel causal analytics for studying them. Starting with those relations, affects and events that compose individual bodies, Deleuze's empiricism affords a method for discerning how broader social processes shape the everyday experience of health and illness. Transcendental empiricism should facilitate the identification of the specific individual processes that materially impact the health status of individuals and groups, including that bundle of relations, affects and events that constitute 'the social', as well as the more immediate relations typical of 'local' interactions (Fox 2011). The development of this argument will include the presentation of case studies designed to illustrate the innovations associated with the application of Deleuze's methods, as well as the most significant health policy implications that follow from their use.

Assemblages of Health is thus concerned to generate an account of health, subjectivity, embodiment and experience alert to the teeming heterogeneity of 'human life'. Taken from a Deleuzian perspective, health may be characterised as a discontinuous process of affective and relational becoming in which the *quality of life* is advanced in the provision of new affective sensitivities and new relational capacities. As Foucault (2001: 108) so cogently observed, this perspective remains in essence an ethical one. It supports a creative ethics of experience – of affects, relations and events, their encounters and resonances – equal to the vital expression of health. Yet this is not primarily an 'ethics of the self' akin to the one Foucault himself proposed. As I have noted, the traditional self all but disappears in Deleuze's mature philosophy, replaced by a 'swarm' of intensive singularities that coalesce in the assemblages that sustain (human) life. This is not to suggest an irredeemable antagonism between Foucault's and Deleuze's rival ethical postulates, only that the work of thinking through these postulates, and their various coherences and antinomies, has barely begun. *Assemblages of Health* contributes to this reckoning, finding in the quotidian logistics of Foucault's ethics a suggestive praxis for determining how Deleuze's ethological account of life and its becomings may be realised in an everyday pragmatics of health. The book is devoted to this life, to an ethics of the assemblage and the peculiar normativity proffered in it, along with the empiricism necessary for the practice of such an ethics. In this ethics lies the promise of an entirely new mode of health research, and a very different kind of life.

Caulfield East, VIC, Australia Cameron Duff

References

Coveney, J. 1998. The government and ethics of health promotion: The importance of Michel Foucault. *Health Education Research* 13(3): 459–468.

Deleuze, G. 1988. *Foucault*. London: The Athlone Press.

Deleuze, G. 1994. *Difference and repetition*. London: The Athlone Press.

Foucault, M. 1978. *The history of sexuality. Vol. 1: An introduction*. London: Penguin.

Foucault, M. 1983. Afterword: The subject and power. In *Michel Foucault: Beyond structuralism and hermeneutics,* 2nd ed, ed. H. Dreyfus and P. Rabinow. Chicago: University of Chicago Press.

Foucault, M. 1997. *Michel Foucault ethics: The essential works*, vol. 1, ed. Paul Rabinow. London: Allen Lane/Penguin.

Foucault, M. 2001. *Power: The essential works*, vol. 3, ed. James Faubion. London: Allen Lane/Penguin.

Fox, N. 2011. The ill-health assemblage: Beyond the body-with-organs. *Health Sociology Review* 20(4): 434–446.

Fox, N. 2012. *The body*. Cambridge: Polity Press.

Greco, M. 2009. Thinking beyond polemics: Approaching the health society through Foucault. *Oesterreichische Zeitschrift fuer Soziologie* 34(2): 13–27.

Grosz, E. 2011. *Becoming undone: Darwinian reflections on life, politics and art*. Durham: Duke University Press.

Latour, B. 2005. *Reassembling the social: An introduction to actor-network theory*. Oxford: Oxford University Press.

Law, J. 2004. *After method: Mess in social science research*. London: Routledge.

Mol, A. 2002. *The body multiple: Ontology in medical practice*. Durham: Duke University Press.

Petersen, A., and R. Bunton (eds.). 1997. *Foucault, health and medicine*. London: Routledge.

Rose, N. 2007. *The politics of life itself: Biomedicine, power, and subjectivity in the twenty-first century*. Princeton: Princeton University Press.

Turner, B. 2008. *The body & society: Explorations in social theory*, 3rd ed. London: Sage.

Whitehead, A. N. 1968. *Modes of thought*. London: Free Press.

Wolfe, C. 2010. *What is Posthumanism?* Minneapolis: University of Minnesota Press.

Acknowledgements

Already several, all writing enjoins a crowd of collaborators. Events and discussions, conversations long felt, comments overheard; a swarm of instigators and allies in the labour of thinking. This book was pieced together in and of these discussions. Lines and ideas cohering in recollection, struggle and volition, all converging in the presentation of an ethical study of health as it is lived in an assemblage of forces. Andrea Eckersley was present at the origin of most of these lines, already advancing, anticipating change, eager for the affects to come. The dividend has been a life lived together in the blooming discovery of a means of living it well. We share it now with our two boys, Amory and Aurelian, to whom the ensuing pages are dedicated at every turn. Without Andrea's lead, these pages may have had less of the force of thinking, feeling and knowing in them. Amory, Aurelian and I are grateful, always, for this lead. I hope the book is some consolation for the cost of its gestation.

On a train from Beacon in the summer of 2007, Lexi Neame coaxed from me a tepid iteration of the germinal ideas that led ultimately to the completion of the book. Her enthusiasm for the discussion, despite the meanderings of its content, left me with a renewed sense of the value of the ideas, and the importance of corralling them into a form that could be shared. The course of our discussion prompted a confidence that I could complete a book and that I had something meaningful to record. Doubtless, you will form your own judgement Lexi, regarding this confidence now you have the record to assess. Suzanne Fraser and Lenore Manderson were equally instrumental in encouraging me to commit to the writing of the book. Each has contributed greatly to the development of my thinking, doing much to correct obvious errors, and to temper any dubious affection for the occasional extravagances of Deleuze's style.

All the same, Ian Buchanan, Keith Robinson, Martin Wood, Hélène Frichot and Stephen Loo have taught me that proper attention to Deleuze's style is central to the discovery of how his thinking may advance the study of health. Much of the content of our discussions is echoed in the pages that follow. Naturally, I have sought to acknowledge this debt in each instance, but the real virtue of this generosity lies in the ways it has affected me in writing this book. Ian's observations regarding the character of Deleuze's empiricism; Keith's sense of the significance of Deleuze's treatment of affects and relations; Martin's sensitivity to the provenance of Deleuze's innovations in Bergson and Nietzsche; Hélène's commitment to 'thinking with' Deleuze; and Stephen's appreciation of the relevance of Deleuze's work for the social sciences; these contributions have profoundly shaped the preparation of this volume and the living, thinking and feeling that informs it. If Deleuze ultimately furnishes an empiricism of real experience, Ian, Keith, Martin, Hélène and Stephen have been singularly important in helping me to grasp this empiricism and the experiences it indexes. The book is immeasurably richer for these contributions.

Much of the writing of the book was supported by a generous 5 year career development fellowship from Monash University. It is impossible to imagine how the book may have been completed without this assistance and the congenial home that Monash has provided for the work of thinking and writing. Across the University, colleagues in the School of Psychology and Psychiatry and the School of Political and Social Inquiry have offered great encouragement in the development of the ideas and arguments presented in the chapters that follow. I should like to single out Alan Petersen, Mark Davis, Andrea Whittaker, Narelle Warren and Renata Kokanovic for special thanks. Elsewhere in Melbourne, Candice Boyd, Lauren Ban and David Moore have offered much advice at various points in the drafting of the chapters.

The empirical research canvased in Chaps. 4 and 5 was supported by grants from the Australian Housing and Urban Research Institute and the Social Sciences and Humanities Research Council in Canada. In the case of the former grant I should thank my co-investigators Keith Jacobs and Stephen Loo and in the latter case I must acknowledge Pat Erickson, David Marsh and Mark Asbridge. In Melbourne, Cameron Sugden provided about the most effective research assistance a scholar could ever hope for before wanderlust took him and his delightful partner on a sojourn as yet without pause. Much of the analysis in Chap. 4 was fleshed out over long conversations with Cam in the backyard of my home in Carlton and I miss him still. I should also thank my recent doctoral students, especially Ella Dilkes-Frayne, Aaron Hart, Rhys Robertson and Molly Bond, who have tolerated long expositions of the book's themes, adding probing questions and pointed corrections. I appreciate these contributions and look forward to long discussions to come. Finally I must thank Esther Otten and Hendrikje Tuerlings at Springer for their unfailing support, understanding and encouragement throughout the process of completing the book.

Sections of Chap. 3 originally appeared in the paper "Towards a Developmental Ethology: Exploring Deleuze's Contribution to the Study of Health and Human Development" published in 2010 in *Health,* volume 14(6):619–634. Sections of Chap. 5 originally appeared in the paper "Accounting for Context: Exploring the Role of Objects and Spaces in the Consumption of Alcohol and Other Drugs" published in 2012 in *Social and Cultural Geography,* volume 13(3):13–26.

Melbourne, August 2013 Cameron Duff

Contents

Chapter 1
Introduction

Few issues trouble contemplation quite like the paradox of health. It is at once the most natural of embodied states and yet remains forever vulnerable to the hostilities of an inclement environment. The formal study of health and its physical, social and political manifestations occupies huge swathes of the contemporary human sciences, demanding an ever increasing share of available research funding (Greco 2004). Public and private investment in the provision of health care grows too, albeit more reliably (Baum 2008). Recurrent investment in research, planning and policy development, infrastructure and service delivery illustrates what the sociologist Nikolas Rose (2001: 17–20) has called the "will to health" to describe one of the most distinctive features of contemporary Western life. In reviewing this "obligation" to be well, Rose (2001: 17) traces a shift in the ways health is conceived in modern societies from a problem of illness and dysfunction towards a dynamic and innately political process of "optimization". Exemplified in the promise of the genetic sciences; the emergence of population health and the identification of social and structural determinants of illness; the growing health literacy of a responsibilized and risk-averse population; as well as the everyday practice of self-help and the solicitations of the popular media, "optimization" reflects the various exhortations by which the modern individual is obliged to maximise his or her "biological destiny" (Rose 2001: 17). Comfortable in the assurances of organised health care, and confident that the risk of illness may be managed, the individual is *enjoined to be well*, while the promise of a life lived well takes on a kind of covenant of the governed (Foucault 2008: 227–230). It is against this backdrop of a profound shift in the meaning, practice and experience of health and illness that the present book ought to be situated.

The varied assessments of health and illness offered in the work of Michel Foucault, Nikolas Rose, Ulrich Beck, John Law and Annemarie Mol, among many others, suggest three enduring problems central to the concerns of this book. First, the obligations demanded by an emergent 'will to health' indicate the need for a substantive definition of health that goes beyond traditional understandings of "normal functioning" figured as the mere absence of disease (Blaxter 2004: 10). As the clinical advances associated with institutionalised

C. Duff, *Assemblages of Health: Deleuze's Empiricism and the Ethology of Life*,
DOI 10.1007/978-94-017-8893-9_1, © Springer Science+Business Media Dordrecht 2014

health care render more and more conditions liable to treatment (if not outright cure), the challenge of defining the over-arching purpose of health and wellbeing has grown (Tengland 2006). Monica Greco (2004: 3–5) stresses that judgments about health go well beyond the issue of "normality" and the extent to which ill individuals might be said to differ from normal, healthy ones. Health inevitably invites normative judgements too regarding the character of the 'ideal body' and the various goals, values and practices to which such a body must accord. Greco (2004: 1–3) adds that efforts to clarify the normative character of health are a feature of contemporary debates in many parts of the world, even though these efforts rarely generate the desired consensus. More commonly, attempts to define the normative aspects of health merely propose more or less agreeable synonyms such as wellbeing, quality of life, vitality, capability or resource (see Gorin and Arnold 2006). This only confounds an already elusive and ill-defined notion, one that is routinely regarded as a taken-for-grant given, even as it takes on ever more significant moral, political, ontological, ethical and aesthetic baggage. The book takes up the indeterminacy of health, offering a kind of health in indeterminacy.

The second preoccupation of the book involves the ontological and empirical distinctions that have long sustained health care research, planning and service delivery in the West. It is routinely noted that distinctions such as natural/artificial, biology/technology, inside/outside and subject/object are beginning to break down in the health and social sciences in ways that have significant and far reaching implications, not only for the way health itself is conceived, but also for the way in which 'human life' is positioned in research and practice (Mol 2002). Although efforts to revisit the foundational binaries that subtend research and practice in the health and social sciences have a long history, the 'subject', 'nature' and 'biology' each retain a privileged position despite the threats to their hegemony that are everywhere apparent in scientific innovation (Protevi 2009). Examples include the prospect of a human genetics finally susceptible to manipulation and correction (Rabinow and Rose 2006: 212–214), alongside studies of the social determinants of health that dismiss the very idea of a natural, acultural subject (Baum 2008). Each of these developments undermines the distinctions between nature and culture, biology and technology that have informed the health and social sciences since their inception. Each suggests the need for a *posthuman account of health and illness*, more alert to the multiple, overlapping and endemic imbrications of biology and technology, the human and the nonhuman in contemporary life. It is no doubt true that offering such an account in the absence of a reified subject and its sequestered biology offends the primary methodological conventions governing the health and social sciences, their broader moral and ethical purpose too (see Mol 2002: 160–170). And yet Bruno Latour (2003: 78) has recently claimed that "a strong distinction between humans and nonhumans is no longer required for research purposes" in the human sciences. *Assemblages of Health* examines the implications of this claim, exploring the prospects of a posthuman account of health and illness, along with the value of such an account for research innovation in the health and social sciences.

The third and final organising theme of the book builds on the second in presenting a critique of the social and structural determinants of health. Recent analysis of the social determinants extends and deepens earlier studies which described a 'social gradient' in health outcomes between poorer groups and those with higher social and economic status (see Dawson 2009 for a review). Research in subsequent decades, undertaken in both the developed and developing world, has identified diverse social, economic and political conditions and their role in shaping health inequalities (see Scriven and Garman 2007: 34–40). Notable examples of these social determinants include income distribution, housing security, availability of essential services such as health care, transport and income support, social exclusion, education and employment opportunities, as well as gender, class and sexuality (see Marmot 2005 for a review). Each of these factors has been implicated in chronic health problems such as heart disease, diabetes, obesity and alcohol misuse, leading researchers to argue for comprehensive public health interventions targeting the social determinants in an effort to improve health outcomes in particular populations (Baum 2008). However, one of the longstanding problems with this research has been the challenge of documenting clear causal links between specific social or structural processes and the generation of health inequalities in particular instances, groups or places (Duff 2011; Fox 2012). This problem recalls enduring debates in the social sciences regarding the links between structure and agency, the macro and the micro, yet it also introduces new challenges for applied research.

At issue is the identification of the specific mechanisms or processes by which macro-structural factors may be shown to mediate health outcomes in particular settings among particular groups at particular times. Philosophers of science such as Bruno Latour, Isabelle Stengers and Annemarie Mol insist that ideas like the social determinants of health rely on a dubious logic of 'social context' in order to assert the links between structure and place (Duff 2011). To the extent that the health sciences now take social contexts to include factors and processes as diverse as employment security, access to essential public services, norms and culture, gender and class, it is tempting to conclude that there is nothing outside context, and hence little in collective life that doesn't somehow mediate the health status of individuals and groups. This leaves social contexts seemingly everywhere and nowhere; everywhere involved in the organisation of interactions vital to the experience of health, and yet nowhere leaving a unique material trace, a domain that might be amenable to empirical inquiry. As a result, empirical assessments of the social determinants of health are increasingly bereft of novel insights, notwithstanding the delineation of social gradients in relation to an ever-increasing range of health problems and conditions (Marmot 2005). Even if one accepts the caveat that population health research is primarily concerned with quantifying risk and the probability of harm, the identification of associations between already complex social and structural phenomena does little to confirm how more direct causal relationships may be identified between social processes and the experience of health in discrete settings.

In the absence of a properly causal account of social context, amenable to application and analysis in a wide variety of settings, the whole notion of the social determinants of health risks being reduced to a rhetorical trope, useful for expanding the administrative purview of health and social policy but unhelpful as a guide for action in individual settings. For how is one to decide in a particular locale, at a particular time, how one should tackle social processes as diverse as employment trends, gender roles, cultural attitudes, economic fluctuations and poverty? Where should one's priorities lie? Where should one start? And how do the various social determinants already identified interact or compound one another such that the likely unintended consequences of proposed interventions might be assessed? In canvassing these issues, I am not seeking to undermine the broader aim of clarifying the social and structural aspects of health and wellbeing in particular settings. I am more concerned with the ethical, pragmatic and political implications of this work. The risk, illustrated so profoundly in recent analyses of the social determinants of health, is that the 'context' and 'structure' are installed as near monolithic constants in everyday life, impossible to ignore but equally resistant to remedial action. Indeed, recent assessments of the social determinants of health are so exhaustive that one is left wondering whether the task confronting health and social policy has simply become too daunting. The gap between 'structure' and 'locale', 'politics' and 'place' seems wider than ever, while there is little support in recent studies for determining how specific structural factors might be tackled at the local level, where presumably health is actually experienced as an inescapable fact of daily life. It is equally unclear how broad structural interventions, such as changes in employment, housing or welfare arrangements, actually impact specific health outcomes in particular settings. Arguably a more useful course for analysis is to devise a method for identifying how select local and non-local actors, entities and processes come to participate in, or otherwise meditate health related phenomena in particular places at particular times. This suggests the need to move away from the habit of differentiating particular health problems, conditions or phenomena from their putative social contexts.

The notion that health problems are mediated in a social context – the primary theoretical condition of all analysis of the social determinants of health – effects an ontological, epistemological and experiential disjuncture between the health status of individual bodies (or populations) and the settings, contexts or environments these bodies may be said to inhabit. This is a logic which presupposes health problems and their contexts as discrete axioms. The reading of Deleuze's methods provided in this book establishes an alternative logic to guide research into the social, political and economic dimensions of health. Modelled after the assemblage, I will argue that health cannot be methodologically, ontologically or epistemologically distinguished from particular experiential, social, political, economic or cultural factors, processes or 'determinants'. There is, in this sense, no social aspect of health distinguishable from economic or political ones in anything other than a particular species of epidemiological analysis. In what Deleuze (1994) calls "actual" or "real experience", biological, material, affective, social, semiotic, political and economic forces necessarily cohere in the articulation of an assemblage of health. As such, one should never speak of the social or political context of a particular health condition because this logic prematurely differentiates forces, processes or bodies without having first established the epistemological basis for this separation. To identify, for example, the social context of HIV/AIDS in a particular setting, or the social dimension of a rise in the prevalence of obesity, proceeds from the assumption that particular factors held to be separate in experience may nonetheless be connected in analysis. "Assemblage thinking" establishes an alternative method for analysing social contexts (Marcus and Saka 2006: 102–104), suggesting a critique of the social determinants of health that will be applied later in the book to case studies investigating the experience of recovery from mental illness and the most effective way of responding to problems associated with the use of alcohol and other drugs.

Assemblages of Health thus proceeds from the conviction that the need to establish a robust, substantive account of health, alert to the challenge of revoking the hegemony of the 'subject', 'nature' and 'biology', and capable of accommodating an array of social and structural phenomena, is among the most pressing tasks confronting the contemporary health and social sciences. Two broad trends may be observed in the ways these sciences have hitherto tackled this 'posthuman' challenge (see Clough and Halley 2007). The first, common to public health and the applied health sciences, has been to adopt a largely acritical and atheoretical course, treating health as a 'natural fact' of the 'normal' body (Mol 2002). This approach installs illness as the primary research problem, and disparities in the 'social epidemiology' of illness as the phenomenon most in need of explanation (Sen 2006: 23–25). To the extent that health is considered in a more positive sense, it is largely treated as a product of social, biological and individual factors. Health, in this respect, is presented as the inevitable outcome of a propitious environment, supportive public policy or a favourable genetic endowment. What this outcome looks like in its substantive, lived reality is rarely countenanced (see Fox 2012). For example, the World Health Organisation (1986: 1) defines health as a "state of complete physical, mental, and social well-being. . .a resource for everyday life, not the objective of living". Yet health is merely instrumentalized in this definition, converted into a resource rather than an end in itself such that the "objective of living" is cast outside the scientific realm into the domain of private affairs. As a result, theoretical reflection on the positive features of health is largely neglected in favour of the analysis of factors known to generate *health inequalities* in particular populations. Even the practice of health promotion is less concerned with the substantive content of health than the task of combating the structural determinants of illness by augmenting various 'protective factors' known to be associated with health, no matter how ill-defined (see Fertman and Allensworth 2010: 4–12). While it is curious that the field of health promotion should remain indifferent to the character of its primary objective, this attitude is common across the applied health sciences.

A very different stance can be observed in other parts of the health and social sciences. Contrary to the preoccupations of public health, a more critical approach has emerged in contemporaneous debates in anthropology, sociology and political science regarding "biopolitics" and the emergence of "biopower" (Rabinow and Rose 2006). This countervailing impulse treats health as the contingent object of various social, cultural, political and economic forces engaged in the extraction of "biovalue" from a 'docile' population (Foucault 2008; Latour 2002). Far more interested than public health in the theoretical and political implications of 'biopower' – and thus more sensitive to the need to move beyond the biology/technology and human/nonhuman dyads that structure so much work in the human sciences – the study of biopower nonetheless shares with public health an abiding indifference to the positive and substantive character of health (see Rose 2007: 22–23). It is no exaggeration to argue that scholars interested in biopolitics are apt to regard any attempt to furnish such a definition as yet another instantiation of biopower appropriating the brute forces of the material body. Rose's (2001) account of 'optimization' exemplifies this suspicion, a suspicion shared in much recent commentary on biopower, which seems uniformly more interested in interrogating the instruments of social control than proposing a (post)human account of wellbeing. And so the task of describing a more substantive account of health goes unresolved.

I argue throughout this book that the development of a more substantive account of health is crucial not only for the promotion of research innovation in the health sciences, but also for the design of interventions into the very "politics of life itself" that so many contemporary scholars have espoused (Rabinow and Rose 2006: 195–201). I would add that the 'will to health' should not be condemned too lightly for it no doubt presents great opportunities for life and for health. After all, no one should wish for a return to Victorian medicine no matter how insidious the organs of biopolitics turn out to be. All the same, the 'will to health' requires some kind of ethical orientation if it is to avoid the trap of biovalue so elegantly chronicled in recent analysis (see Rose 2007 for a review). Otherwise, health is left without a *normative foundation*, inviting the substitution of economic, political and social alternatives in the selection of values to guide research and practice. Among the inventory of intellectual resources available for the design of such foundations, only Gilles Deleuze can provide a normativity that is not at the same time a morality; an ethics that is not a set of edicts. The rest of this book is devoted to the analysis of Deleuze's ethics and its potential for the founding of a "minor science" of health and illness (Alliez 2004: 46–51). This is a science concerned to trace the affects, relations and events of a body's becomings, rather than the stable identities, the substances, laws and axioms, which stand as natural objects for all "royal sciences" (Deleuze and Guattari 1987: 364–369). A *minor science* of health must, therefore, abandon the reified body of biomedicine, along with its ineluctable biology, in favour of the empirical study of bodies in their posthuman assembling, in their becoming well or ill (see also Fox 2011: 434–440). First some justification of this course seems warranted.

1.1 Why Deleuze? Why Now?

If the problem of normativity is inevitably introduced in any attempt to define health, then the task of providing a robust normative foundation for health research, analysis and debate seems unavoidable. The fact that this task has been avoided for so long in the health and social sciences is unquestionably attributable to their enduring unease with the very notion of the normative. It is important that I address this unease before turning to outline the kinds of normative positions that might be derived from Deleuze's mature philosophy. Too redolent of the grand ambitions of high modernity, and too easily distorted in the pragmatic interventions of politics and markets, the normative lingers in the historical imagination of the human sciences as a spectre of past failures, a reminder of the folly of all 'totalising' discourses (Foucault 1972). Elsewhere, faltering interest in the normative is more a function of benign neglect than deliberate hostility. In any event, the distaste for the normative evident across the health and social sciences is arguably traceable to a deeper and more enduring suspicion of metaphysics. The rejection of metaphysics is among the signature commitments of the contemporary human sciences, the social sciences in particular, central both to their scepticism and their peculiar brand of "social realism" (De Landa 2006: 1–3). One of the most powerfully effective examples of this distaste has been the relentless extirpation of all essentialisms from the methods and analytics employed in the social sciences. While one should hardly feel any regret at the passing of these hopeless caricatures, the animosity with which this task has been prosecuted has engendered a range of unexpected challenges for the social sciences, challenges that increasingly bedevil the health sciences too. Chief among them has been a growing uncertainty about the status of the *objects* of the health and social sciences, including the 'body' and the 'subject', even 'human life' itself.

While it perhaps exaggerates the point, each of the health and social sciences has gravitated towards one or another uniform response to this uncertainty (see Mol 2002: 9–17). On the one hand, the health sciences have generally elected for the sureties of positivism and the guarantee of a "rational, cognitive" subject free to survey the contents of an external reality populated by stable, knowable objects (Protevi 2009: 3–4). As such, the healthy body is regarded as a discrete, stable entity, amenable to observation and analysis. The health sciences have not been inured, however, from the withering critique of positivism levelled in various feminist, post-colonial and poststructuralist treatments, leading in places to a kind of 'soft' constructivism and an interest in the social and structural mediation of health and illness (see Fox 2012). The acceptance of a simultaneously 'natural' and 'cultural' subject, exemplified in studies of the social and structural determinants of health, evinces both an *a priori* commitment to the 'natural body', just as it confirms the *structuration* of the body in diverse social, political and economic processes (Turner 2008: 173–177). The ontological contradictions opened up by this settlement have led scholars to consider the effects of scientific analysis on the objects (and bodies) of health research, occasioning a cautious rethinking of some of the deeper nostrums of positivist inquiry (Rose 2007: 11–15). Elsewhere, the rejection of positivism has been complete and the commitment to various iterations of constructivism more enthusiastic. Indeed, in much of the social sciences the constructivist claim that science participates in the articulation of a reality it purportedly only describes has gained widespread traction. It follows that the subject of the health sciences may be regarded as a product of the very attempt to "know" that subject (Law 2004: 71–79). This position all but rejects the idea of an "objective reality", anterior to knowledge, demolishing one of the surest foundations of normative speculation (Mol 2002: 9–12).

All of this has made the presentation of normative claims in the health and social sciences more difficult. In an obstinate commitment to empirical inquiry, the health sciences have accepted the contention that claims about the way the world ought to be must never be derived from observations about the way the world actually is. The health sciences have thus settled for the remediation of the threats to health and the classification of the etiology of illness and disease. If the health sciences are wont to offer normative advice it is largely in keeping with this broader commitment to the proper functioning of the human organism, rather than in an effort to determine what the goals of life ought to be. Meanwhile, the social sciences, latterly suspicious of grand designs for life, reject normativity on more political and aesthetic grounds, although the outcome is the same. While contemporary cultures are everywhere obsessed with health – a development noted across the human sciences – the merits of prolonging life, or otherwise 'optimizing' the physiological and psychological functioning of the organism, are regarded as either too self evident to require clarification, or too subjective, too private for science to encroach upon. Health, like happiness, it seems is a private affair, and even in the attempt to engender a science of health and wellbeing, the reasons why it might be better to be healthy, better to be happy, are as elusive as they have ever been (Fox 2012; Mol 2002; Rose 2007). And so, the health sciences remain committed to the optimization of the organism without really knowing why, while a critical social science attempts to ascribe normative ambitions to this effort, mostly because it claims the search for norms exceeds the proper bounds of a scientific enterprise it is no longer sure it believes in.

This is an unsustainable antinomy. Health, as Foucault (1978) so ably demonstrated is always, already normative, and any attempt to deny this normativity serves merely to disguise it, or remove it from critical scrutiny. Ironically, Foucault himself forcefully rejected the task of formulating normative positions, arguing that critique is better served unmasking the effects of power than adding to them. This position is by now so widely accepted across the health and social sciences that a reluctance to interrogate or even consider the normative dimensions of health has become almost orthodox (Greco 2004). I understand that the health sciences routinely generate statements regarding the 'rules' by which a healthy life might be lived (Gorin and Arnold 2006: 3–10). And yet these are not properly speaking *normative injunctions* for while they may well establish *what* one might (or even should) do, they almost never establish *why* such advice should be followed. Insisting, for example, that one exercise for 30 min a day, consume five serves of vegetables, avoid excessive alcohol use, or refrain from smoking, among any number of admonitions levelled in the contemporary health sciences, does little to confirm why such a life is *ethically, logically or aesthetically* better or preferable to another (Metzl and Kirkland 2010). This serves merely to establish norms that remain vulnerable to revision given the paucity of their normative foundations and the relentless advance of empirical inquiry. It also leaves the health sciences susceptible to explaining any failure to observe the strict fiat of their injunctions as a simple problem of ignorance, or a lack of 'health literacy', when rival explanations abound, most of them bearing a more normative hue. I would add that this is the main reason why the health sciences have yet to secure the consensus (or *compliance*) they crave. Having long rejected the conceit of social engineering, the social sciences are likewise reluctant to countenance a return to normative affirmation. And so, the study of health and illness is mostly confined to a logic of the normal with little recourse to that of the normative.

Deleuze presents an elegant way out of this stalemate, proffering a means of establishing normative foundations for the analysis of health without at the same time installing a set of contingent interests as proxy for the concerns of a neutral subject (Patton 2000). Deleuze achieves this by substituting a metaphysics of process, of difference, for the more familiar metaphysics of substance. This yields a processual basis for normative reflection, replacing the substantive moral certitudes common to traditional normative analysis (Smith 2003: 307). I argue throughout this book that Deleuze's philosophy of difference – and the normative ethics that follow from it – provides a basis for responding to the three primary problems noted above concerning the need for a positive definition of health, sensitive to the convergence of the human and the nonhuman, and alert to the array of social and structural entities that mediate health outcomes in particular places at particular times. If the terms with which Deleuze advances his philosophy are as yet unfamiliar, the various concepts furnished in his immanent philosophy of difference provide robust support for analyses of the everyday experience of health and illness, and the myriad affects, relations and events by which such states are determined (Fox 2011). The book will draw on this support in presenting normative grounds for the development of novel empirical and theoretical assessments of health. What's more, the empirical analysis provided in later chapters should confirm the value of persevering with Deleuze's thought at a juncture where the health sciences are at best indifferent to social theory, while the social sciences seem almost to suffer from a surfeit of it (Mansfield 2000: 1–15). With these goals in mind, *Assemblages of Health* will confirm the need for a Deleuzian intervention in the health and social sciences, spelling out the various conceptual and practical problems this approach should help to resolve, as well as the limits of such forays. I will devote the rest of this chapter to a brief review of Deleuze's intellectual project, canvassing the ways I intend to use Deleuze's concepts in the analysis of health and illness to follow. I will also provide an overview of the book's principal arguments, and the concerns of the individual chapters.

1.2 Thinking with Deleuze

Deleuze is rare among post-war continental philosophers for his enduring commitment to metaphysics (De Landa 2002). In a late accounting of his intellectual project, Deleuze (2001) confirmed his life-long interest in the creation of an immanent philosophy capable of accommodating the forces of life, its desires and becomings (see also Grosz 2011). Central to such a metaphysics, and to Deleuze's peculiar form of empiricism, is an effort to explain (human) life, which Deleuze (1994) regards as the primary 'abstraction' upon which metaphysics since Plato has been founded. Metaphysics traditionally conceives of the human subject as a unified or 'transcendental' entity, responsible for the various 'syntheses' by which the bare qualia of sensate experience are transformed into substantive ways of knowing the world (Audi 1995). The transcendental subject, secure in the substance of its identity, is thus both the source (or 'subject') of metaphysical inquiry, as well as the primary 'object' of this speculation (see also Foucault 1972: 375–377). Yet for Deleuze, the abstractions of subjectivity that all traditional metaphysics rely upon cannot explain experience, life, thought or knowledge, but must themselves be explained (Deleuze and Parnet 1987: vii). The subject cannot simply be abstracted from experience in order to secure some enduring foundation for metaphysical speculation, for this leaves the subject external to life, a transcendental entity whose origins, inexplicably, lie elsewhere. While the latter explanation fits neatly with more traditional metaphysical approaches, Deleuze remained committed throughout his life to a properly *empirical* account of (human) life, consistent with the "radical empiricism" inaugurated by Hume, Bergson, Nietzsche and Whitehead. It follows that the primary task is to explain the subject's emergence from within the flux of experience, what Deleuze poetically described as the "concrete richness of the sensible" (Deleuze and Parnet 1987: 54). The subject that emerges in this flux is a product of the sensible, rather than the measure of its organisation (Alliez 2004: 89).

Deleuze's search for a metaphysics of the sensible, capable of accounting for the genetic conditions of "actual experience" and the means of the subject's emergence within it, gives rise to a series of novel conceptualisations (like 'actual' and 'virtual', 'differentiation' and 'individuation', 'intensive' and 'extensive') that together comprise "transcendental empiricism" (Alliez 2004: 103–106). Importantly, the treatment of these concepts lends itself both to metaphysical reflection, as well as concrete empirical inquiry. It is also true, however, that existing commentaries on Deleuze's empiricism tend to emphasise the speculative metaphysics that underpin it (see Bryant 2008), at the expense of a more thoroughgoing assessment of the uniquely *empirical implications* of Deleuze's thought. Hence, the reading of various concepts associated with a transcendental empiricism offered below (and in greater detail in Chap. 2) will mostly eschew metaphysical exegesis in favour of a more detailed assessment of the *methodological promise* of Deleuze's work (see also Bell 2009: 2–18). In setting this course, I am not attempting to argue that Deleuze's empiricism may simply be shorn of its metaphysical properties. I am more interested in the ways Deleuze's methods and concepts may be applied in the health and social sciences, in a context where, as I have noted, metaphysical conceits are mostly frowned upon. This calls for a critical, creative reading of Deleuze's 'ontology of the sensible', concerned both with "bringing forward something new and useful" (Buchanan 2011: 8) in this ontology, along with the fidelity of the concepts presented therein.

To this end, it is important that I briefly clarify the way I intend to approach Deleuze's thought in the course of reviewing his metaphysics. In a sense, I am prepared to risk the loss of some measure of metaphysical rigor in order to gain what I hope will be no small measure of methodological insight. This argument proceeds from the contention that Deleuze offers a novel 'life science', a *biophilosophy,* capable of illuminating the everyday experience of health and illness for both individuals and groups (see also Ansell Pearson 1999: 209–218; Grosz 2011: 33–39). However, my purpose is less concerned with getting Deleuze 'right' than with the dedicated and pragmatic application of his concepts. The goal is to extract particular "tendencies" present in Deleuze's concepts, and then put them to work in the analysis of select health problems, to "take them as far as they can go" (Massumi 2010: 12). I would stress that the most fecund of Deleuze's commitments, certainly the one that exhibits the most prolific 'tendencies' in Massumi's sense, is the notion of immanence that subtends Deleuze's empiricism and the account of (human) life presented therein (see de Beistegui 2010). Further discussion of Deleuze's immanence should also clarify the way concepts such as 'intensive' and 'extensive', 'virtual' and 'actual', 'difference' and 'individuation' function in support of a transcendental empiricism.

The commitment to immanence is a singular illustration of Deleuze's "empiricist conversion"; his insistence that the task of "believing in this world, in this life" is perhaps the most important philosophical, political, ethical and aesthetic challenge of "our" time (Deleuze and Guattari 1994: 75). Such a conversion conjures an immanent world, an immanent life, no longer reliant on transcendental phenomena such as God, Reason, Man or Nature to explain its origins, manifestations and diversities. For Deleuze, the empiricist conversion inaugurates a search for the genetic conditions of experience sufficient to explain the diversity of life. The 'sufficient causes' that explain life are always immanent to life itself, and should never be attributed to some transcendental entity or process like God, Reason or Being. If the world cannot ultimately be predicated on a 'higher realm', then the task for philosophy is to *explain the world in life*, in immanence, by way of the "actual" means by which it is generated or produced (Deleuze 1994). Deleuze's own explanation of (human) life involves the positing of a transcendental field of pre-subjective, pre-individual singularities (including affects, percepts, signs, events and relations) that enable the individuations of life, matter and sense. The description of this field as 'transcendental' may at first blush appear almost perverse, yet as Miguel de Beistegui (2010: 14) helpfully notes the "transcendental is here opposed to the transcendent insofar as it does not presuppose a consciousness, but escapes all determinations of the subject". The transcendental field which supports all life, exceeds (or is 'transcendental' to) the individual, manifest forms of this life, understood in terms of the actual bodies, species, ideas and entities that comprise it (see Baugh 1992; Rolli 2009). Such a field is immanence itself, establishing the genetic conditions in which life emerges, including the life of the individuated subject.

So what comprises this transcendental field? *Haecceities*, intensities, singularities, the virtual: all that is "real without being actual, ideal without being abstract"

(Deleuze 1994: 208). Such terminology almost inevitably occludes as much as it clarifies, so it is perhaps helpful to observe that Deleuze is primarily interested in salvaging the principle of difference from the reifications of identity, the ceaseless return of the same. Deleuze's virtual field guarantees difference precisely because it is transcendental to the specific (or actual) forms of individuated life, of determinate matter. The virtual is not simply expressed in the actual, such that the condition is manifested in the conditioned. To misunderstand the virtual in this way is to reduce immanence to mere potential or possibility, suggesting that all matter, all life, is prefigured in some underlying set of essences or identities that simply await their expression, their actualisation, in life. Difference, conceived in this guise, is inevitably subordinated to identity, as 'difference from' some prior and always transcendent identity, transcendent precisely because its origins cannot be explained in the world but must be grounded outside it in God, Reason or Being (Deleuze 1994: 35–39). Deleuze however, seeks to invert this logic, positing difference and differentiation as the genetic conditions by which individual forms emerge and settle into entities capable of being identified as such (Shaviro 2009: 34–36). There can be no external condition, no transcendental cause in the Kantian sense, only 'sufficient reasons' immanent to life itself. Human life, the embodied subject, to return at length to my earlier concerns, must therefore be explained in the manner of immanent life, or the genetic conditions of their actual emergence. Given Deleuze's refusal to ground the subject in the principle of identity (Bell 2009), the subject must be explained *in its emergence* in an immanent process of differentiation or individuation, which never settles into stable forms of identity, but is forever individuating, differing from itself.

And so, human life may be regarded as a product of differentiation by which diverse elements are combined (or folded) in a process of individuation without pause. Differentiation entails diverse intensive processes which draw together innumerable differences folded inside and outside the body; both a subject and a world (Deleuze 1994: 245–250). That said, these intensive processes are typically obscured in the extensive properties they generate. As Deleuze (1994) stresses, common sense invariably dictates that one regard the body in its extension as primary, thereby reducing difference to mere change over time, leaving the body in its enduring essence unaltered. Yet this does little to explain the emergence of the body or the processes by which a body extended in space and time is actually produced. The body cannot be the cause of the body, both cause and effect, and so the genetic conditions of its emergence must be sought elsewhere, in the virtual, the intensive, in "different/ciation" (Patton 1994: xi). Parsing these distinctions in terms more directly relevant to the concerns of this book, Dan Smith and John Protevi (2008: 3–4) describe the embodied subject as a product of three distinctive but overlapping or conjunctive syntheses. These syntheses collect, assemble or contract pre-individual singularities like affects, habits, utterances, mannerisms, percepts, relations, desires, expressions, events, ideas, concepts or signs, giving extensive form to the intensive multiplicities by which the body and subjectivity emerge (see also Rolli 2009: 29–32; Shaviro 2009: 32–35). These singularities are said to be 'pre-individual' because they do not properly 'belong' to any one individual body (or subject), but are instead the very genetic elements out of which embodied subjects are individuated. Smith and Protevi (2008: 3–4) thus speak of the 'serial' syntheses of habits, affects, percepts, energy sources and utterances (or *haecceities*) that give a distinctive form to the body, as well as the syntheses that transpire between haecceities within the individuating body (like the syntheses that correspond in and between the distinct organs of sense perception), and the serial syntheses that emerge between individuating bodies in their capacity to affect and be affected by one another. These three syntheses "fold in on themselves" in the generation of an intensive and extensive "site of self awareness" constitutive of a body, a life (Smith and Protevi 2008: 4). The body emerges in a multiplicity of dynamic singularities (affects, events and relations) that later settle into the more familiar guise of material extension. Yet as Deleuze (1994: 245–250) insists, and this really is the most important of Deleuze's insights in relation to the body and subjectivity, the extensive relations that comprise the body never simply displace the more genetic and intensive relations by which the body is actualised. The intensive and the extensive are forever involved (or implicated) in the ceaseless individuations by which a body differs from itself over time. The principle of difference must, for this reason, replace the principle of identity in the way the body is approached as an object for the health and social sciences.

Deleuze's biophilosophy has important implications for the conceptualisation of subjectivity (or the 'self') too, emphasising the figure of differentiation at the expense of the more common notion of identity or substance (Boundas 1994: 113–115). Like the body, subjectivity cannot be regarded as a stable, singular entity, but must be reconceived as an assemblage of individuating singularities, which are constantly folded and refolded in the genetic organisation of an awareness of self; an autopoietic process of perspective, apperception, memory and duration (Rolli 2009: 48–50). It follows that "individuality is not a characteristic of the Self but, on the contrary, forms and sustains the system of the dissolved Self" (Deleuze 1994: 254). As such, subjectivity is disjunctive, intensive and genetic, a "task" waiting to be "fulfilled" (Boundas 1994: 103–105). It is constantly produced and reproduced in a "developing experience" capable of supporting "subjectivation effects" (Rolli 2009: 40). Subjectivity is produced (or *effectuated*) in experience, in the serial organisation of affects, percepts, habits and sensations by which the syntheses of consciousness are derived (Deleuze 1991). The self, in its manufactured unity, is a genetic effect of various intensive and extensive processes, which is not the same as calling the subject a fiction, or an illusion, but rather describes the actual conditions, or sufficient causes, necessary to explain the subject in experience (Deleuze 1994).

It follows of course that the subject is not the same thing at all times, and so cannot provide a stable basis for the attribution of a substantive identity necessary for the generation of metaphysical claims about it. Only the doxa of common sense obscures this genetic, empirical reality; only "the habit of saying 'I'" (Deleuze 1991: x). As Deleuze (1991: x) adds, "isn't this the answer to the question 'what are we'? We are habits, nothing but habits…there is no more striking answer to the problem of the self". This observation orients the development of a transcendental empiricism in that Deleuze (1994) is concerned to identify the actual conditions of emergence peculiar to habits, understood as the morphogenetic expression of embodied subjectivity. If subjectivity is produced or expressed in a transcendental field of intensive and extensive singularities, then a truly transcendental empiricism is required to trace the actualisation of these singularities in bodies, and in subjects. A more conventional empiricism might be capable of mapping those actualisations which are the *product* of a virtual field, but only a transcendental empiricism is equal to the genetic conditions of their *emergence* in a field of experience (Rolli 2009). In any case, the subject is real because it produces real effects, it is the product of real events, even if they are sometimes real without being actual. This invitation to the virtual is the primary call of a transcendental empiricism (Baugh 1993; Bell 2009).

The virtual, to be clear, can be regarded as an intensive field of force relations, including diverse affects, percepts, qualities, sensations, ideas, expressions, habits and energy sources. Empiricism becomes transcendental to the extent that it is able to account for the genetic conditions of these qualities or forces, and their actualisation in particular bodies and/or states-of-affairs (Rolli 2009: 37–39). Given that "we know intensity only as already developed within an extensity, and as covered over by qualities", Deleuze (1994: 223) is compelled to devise an empiricism capable of transcending, or exceeding, the familiar empirical qualities of observable, actualised entities, thereby reaching the intensive conditions of their production. This move preserves difference by making identity the contingent and unstable achievement of intensive, differential processes. There is, as such, no stable subject in life, only a series of restless, morphogenetic processes of subjectivation by which subjects are created, transformed, modified and eliminated. These differential, intensive processes are fundamental to Deleuze's metaphysics, and the distinctive conceptualisations of subjectivity and embodiment presented within it (Bryant 2008).

In other words, the subject cannot be said to bear a substantive essence, and so it cannot be said to be *naturally* or *essentially* healthy, stable or moral (Fox 2011: 434–437). Of course, subjects and bodies are often healthy, stable and moral, but the problem for philosophy, for science and for art as Deleuze understands them is to *explain the actual experiences, events and relations by which bodies become healthy or moral*, rather than to take these qualities as presuppositions for the organisation of a "science of the subject" (Foucault 1983: 214). The great innovation occasioned by Deleuze's work is the provision of an empirical basis for the study of health and illness, whereby neither health nor illness are taken to be stable, knowable properties of individual bodies, but are rather seen as intensive processes of individuation and becoming. Deleuze's empiricism provides a means of documenting the actual conditions of human life (the embodied subject) within a virtual field, as well as that subset of relations, affects and events by which health is actualised in a given assemblage of bodies, affects, habits, percepts and objects. This course should finally provide a basis for responding to the three great problems identified at the outset of this chapter, and the epistemological, ontological and methodological aporia associated with them. As such, the application of Deleuze's empiricism in later chapters will first consider a substantive definition of health, as Chap. 3 in particular will demonstrate. This definition will then enable the design in Chaps. 4 and 5 of empirical investigations of health and illness that do not presuppose the human/nonhuman, natural/artificial, biology/technology dyads that confound so much contemporary research in the human sciences (Latour 2003: 77–80). Moving beyond these dyads should also shed light on the various nonhuman or structural actors that participate in the formation and reformation of assemblages of health and illness. Deleuze's empiricism will, in these ways, provide conceptual support for the development of a *normative account of health*, along with a novel ethics conceived as an intervention into the very individuations of (human) life itself.

1.3 The Normative Deleuze

The satisfaction of these goals will ultimately depend on the utility of Deleuze's idiosyncratic understanding of norms. Deleuze's metaphysics, along with the empiricism that emerges from it, may be construed as normative to the extent that it satisfies the two criteria by which normativity is typically assessed (see Jun 2011). First, Deleuze advances a series of *ontological claims about the nature of reality* and the kinds of entities that might reasonably be claimed to comprise it. These claims concern the characteristic features of the pre-subjective, 'transcendental field' described above, and the intensive and extensive forces that populate this field (De Landa 2002: 2–3). Yet more importantly, Deleuze also offers a range of *normative, ethical and aesthetic arguments* concerning the political and experiential implications of his ontological speculations. Deleuze grounds these arguments in a series of claims about the nature of power or force (Jun 2011: 95–97). Deleuze contends that power can be taken to be normative (or can be shown to produce normative effects) whenever it supports the emergence of the 'new', and whenever it promotes the creativity necessary to produce novelty. Normativity, as such, provides the measure of life extended to its limits, at the reach of its "power of acting" (Deleuze 1992: 256).

In one of the few commentaries to assess such claims on their own terms, Paul Patton (2000: 2–3) observes that Deleuze's normativity is primarily concerned to determine the means of "deterritorialising" identity, essence, system, organisation or truth. By "deterritorialisation" Deleuze and Guattari (1987: 15) simply mean any discrete political, affective, ethical or aesthetic practice by which assemblages of bodies, systems, matter or life are transformed (or deterritorialised) so as to permit more movement, more creativity, novel conceptual developments, new styles of life, new forms of organisation, and so on. Any practice that transforms (or "counter-actualises") the virtual and intensive forces (affects, percepts, events or sensations) that express assemblages may be taken to be normative to the extent that it pushes the very force of life to the "limit of its power of acting" (Deleuze 1992: 256–258). This power of acting – understood as the force effected in a body in its composition in an assemblage of intensive and extensive parts – is a body's "natural right" (Deleuze 1992: 257). Spinoza argued that the pursuit of this right, in its expression to the fullest extent possible, is a law of nature. Deleuze (1992: 258–262) transforms this law into a "norm of power", which becomes normative precisely to the extent that it establishes a set of ethical obligations by which a given body may reach the limit of its power of acting "in such a way as to be affected by joy". Only in the expression of such norms, affects and powers may human life (the assembled or embodied subject) "become reasonable, strong and free" (Deleuze 1992: 262).

Patton (2000: 83–85) notes the extent to which Deleuze's account of freedom differs from the liberal tradition, which treats freedom as an absolute moral category capable of yielding ethical and political criteria for assessing events, institutions or practices in terms of the 'degrees of liberty' they avail. Such absolutist criteria cannot be found in Deleuze's work; yet something potentially more useful for the satisfaction of this book's aims can. Deleuze (1994: 193–195) argues that freedom should be understood as the capacity subjects obtain to affect or transform themselves, or more correctly, the constitutive properties of the assemblages within which they are expressed. Freedom demands a critical, reflexive awareness in order that one might "get free of oneself" in pursuing the limits of one's powers (Deleuze 1988: 96). In his commentary on Foucault, Deleuze notes that freedom involves "folding" or bending the individual force relations that comprise the subject. Folding entails "a relation which force has with itself, a power to affect itself, an affect of self on self" (Deleuze 1988: 101). The ethics of such a practice is further illuminated in Foucault's (1984: 50) own notion of a limit-attitude, figured as "a philosophical life in which the critique of what we are is at one and the same time the historical analysis of the limits that are imposed on us and an experiment with the possibility of going beyond them". Unlike Foucault, however, Deleuze (2001) does not demur from clarifying what the normative goals of such an attitude should be; namely the creation of "lines of flight" in the maximisation of a body's powers, the forces of life.

Deleuze's normativity, and the becomings it supports, has two principal features. First, it requires the rejection of the various objects and categories of 'the subject' as determined by a majoritarian consensus. That is to say that the 'relation which force has with itself' is normative to the extent that the folding of force deterritorialises all assemblages of subjective identity associated with, for example, sex, gender, age, class, status and ability. The creation of "smooth" spaces in which alternatives to such identities can flourish, extends or maximises the body's powers of acting as new forces, new powers and new affects are folded into the body (see Jun 2011: 96–99). Secondly, becoming "reasonable, strong and free" requires the transformation of select social, political, economic and cultural assemblages in an effort to establish "material conditions" sufficient to extend the powers of a "society" of bodies, and not merely the individual ethical subject (Patton 2000: 101–103). Both Patton (2008) and Jun (2011) find in this formulation a compelling logic for rethinking social justice, inequality, the problem of rights and the nature of democracy. The issue, however, is not to invent a 'universal subject' which stands for the interests of all, but rather to transform social, material and political conditions in ways that maximise the powers of acting, or forces of life, of a wider collective of bodies. This finally, suggests a strikingly novel way of defining or conceptualising health (see also Fox 2011). Health may, indeed, be characterised in more Deleuzian terms as a *differential process of becoming reasonable, strong and free*, where freedom is understood not in some totalising way synonymous with a prevailing moral order, but rather as a specific moment of rupture or transformation in which something new emerges in an active expression of creativity and invention. Health may thus be construed in normative terms as the effect (or force) of those deterritorialisations which advance a body ever closer to the limit of its power of acting, to the extent of its immanent life.

Such is the normativity that one finds in Deleuze's mature philosophy, committed to the liberation of difference from the confines of identity, and suggestive of a radical analytics for rethinking the experience of health and illness in diverse contexts. In an earlier section, I noted that recent work in the health and social sciences has sought to define health in ways consonant with the idea of growth, development, change, empowerment, functionality and transcendence (see Arnold and Breen 2006: 7–17). This approach moves beyond the physiological functioning of the organism to consider the experience of subjective wellbeing, or 'quality of life', however defined. A feature of this approach has been the selection of proxies for assessing wellbeing, such as 'functionality', 'empowerment', 'wholeness', 'life potential' and 'goodness of fit', each of which seem ultimately to concern the subject's *capacity for freedom* (Sen 1999: 2–5). The conundrum is that recent efforts to more closely align health, freedom and development mostly evade the problem of deciding how health ought to be conceptualised and/or empirically investigated in terms of freedom or empowerment. Nowhere in this literature is it clear how notions like wellbeing, empowerment, functionality or development actually constitute a practice of freedom commensurate with the experience of health and wellbeing. At worst, contemporary writings fall into a kind of voluntarism, positing freedom as an innate human right attributable to the simple expression of will or choice (see Rose 2007). Otherwise, freedom is regarded as a social and relational achievement, sustained within amenable economic, cultural and/or political contexts (see Sen 1999: 282–285). In any event, freedom has become yet another unhelpful synonym for health, unsatisfactory either as a basis for establishing a substantive understanding of health, or as a normative foundation to guide health care planning, research and service delivery.

Assemblages of Health argues that the normative account of freedom presented in Deleuze's ethics suggests a means of overcoming these two problems. Sympathetic to his goal of extending the power of (human) life to its limits, my assessment of Deleuze's ethics in later chapters will seek to clarify how the idea of maximising a body's power of acting may be applied to contemporary thinking about health and illness. My goal is to furnish a normative account of health capable of guiding the *everyday practice* of health and development in accordance with a body's "natural right" (Deleuze 1992: 257). However, this will not entail a universal normativity concerned to discipline life in the preservation of some timeworn set of moral postulates. Instead, I will strive to articulate a 'heterogenetic' normativity sensitive to the effulgence of life in the elaboration of difference and the promise of creativity. Of course, it is critical that notions like 'life', 'difference', 'freedom' and 'creativity' do not fall into easy cliché at the expense of a proper accounting of their pragmatic force. In accordance with Deleuze's empiricism, I intend to demonstrate how the normative claims presented in his empiricism may be applied to analysis of some of the most significant and enduring problems in the health and social sciences. I will do this by indicating how concepts such as 'life', 'creativity', 'freedom' and 'difference' may support the development of novel strategies for the promotion of health in "real experience" (Deleuze 1994: 68–69). These are the principal goals of *Assemblages of Health* and each will serve as enduring preoccupations for the chapters to follow.

1.4 Outline of the Book

Assemblages of Health proposes to review Deleuze's empiricism in order to indicate how his concepts may be employed in the study of health and illness. As I have noted, the book will identify three key problems in the health and social sciences that the adoption of Deleuze's methods should help to resolve. My principal goal is to provide a normative definition of health capable of accounting for the means by which bodies become well (or ill). This effort should, in turn, reveal more of the human and nonhuman actors, objects, affects, events and relations involved in the expression or modulation of health and illness. Third, I aim to establish a novel method of investigating the social and structural forces active in the experience of health and illness. In addressing these problems, the book will also consider case studies designed to illustrate how Deleuze's methods may be applied to the study of health and illness. The presentation of case studies will also provide an opportunity to review the specific intellectual and methodological innovations associated with Deleuze's thought. The first case study will explore recent research regarding recovery from mental illness, with a focus on the role of place and social inclusion. I will then introduce qualitative data collected in Melbourne, Australia among individuals recovering from mental illness. Drawing on Deleuze's empiricism, I will describe how recovery obtains in particular relations, affects and events, in particular places (or territories). I will then indicate how this analysis may inspire novel 'place-based' mental health initiatives. The second case study will yield a Deleuzian account of the use of alcohol and other drugs (AOD). My goal is to articulate a posthuman ethics of consumption and responsibility, more sensitive to the array of human and nonhuman forces active in AOD use. The analysis offered in each case study will also serve to illustrate the contours of a minor science of health and illness.

Chapter 2 will continue to introduce the broad features of Deleuze's philosophy, identifying and assessing the key features of transcendental empiricism. I will also reflect more directly on the ways Deleuze's empiricism may be applied to research in the health and social sciences, touching on contemporary debates in public health, the sociology of health and illness, medical anthropology, geography and related fields. I will argue that Deleuze's empiricism is subtended by three primary concepts; relations, affects and events. Each of these concepts explicates the various "pre-individual singularities" that Deleuze (2004) regards as constitutive of life on specific planes or territories. The chapter will go on to contend that the application of transcendental empiricism within the health and social sciences hinges on the distinctive account of *human life* (the embodied subject) described in Deleuze's work. Far from abandoning the subject as some critics argue, Deleuze provides a compelling account of the production or emergence of subjectivity within an assemblage of forces. I will argue that this logic presents a breakthrough in recent attempts to reframe the study of (posthuman) life in contemporary health research. The development of my thesis will first involve a brief account of the broad scope of Deleuze's empiricism, before advancing a fuller discussion of relations, affects and events. The purpose of this review will be to derive *specific methodological principles* for the analysis of relations, affects and events in discrete settings, territories or contexts. The chapter will close with a discussion of the application of transcendental empiricism to the study of select problems in the study of health and illness as a way of further illustrating the promise of a minor science of health. In so doing, the chapter will also point to the more detailed analyses to follow in the two case studies.

Chapter 3 will formally commence the work of applying Deleuze's ideas to the study of health and illness. The chapter contends that Deleuze's work furnishes a host of novel ontological and epistemological resources for such study, ushering in new methods and establishing novel objects of inquiry. I will focus on deepening and extending the analysis of 'human life' introduced in earlier chapters, highlighting Deleuze's contributions to the study of health and human development and its varied courses and processes. In considering this contribution, the chapter will introduce the notion of a "developmental ethology". On the basis of this innovation I will argue that health and human development may be characterised as a discontinuous process of affective and relational encounters. I will then argue that health is advanced or promoted in the provision of new affective sensitivities and new relational capacities. Drawing on Deleuze's (1992) account of Spinoza's ethics, the extension of a body's affective sensitivities will be characterised in terms of the modification of that body's power of acting, or the enhancement of its "scope of activity". On the basis of this analysis, the chapter will go on to argue that one of the most important achievements of Deleuze's ethology is the grounds it provides for establishing a positive definition of health. Such a definition moves beyond the construal of health as the absence of disease to encompass the very forces of life. The chapter will next contrast Deleuze's ethology with more conventional accounts of health and human development, focusing on Amartya Sen's 'capabilities' model. In comparing the two models, I will argue that a developmental ethology has the advantage of offering a more viable explanation of the ways developmental capacities (affects, relations and forces) are acquired, cultivated or maintained.

Chapter 4 introduces the first of two case studies, assessing recent debates regarding the nature of recovery from mental illness and the most effective means of its promotion. In so doing, the chapter will continue to assess the contributions Deleuze's work may make to critical analysis of the social determinants of health. I will argue that Deleuze's account of matter, affect and force provides a basis for identifying the specific mechanisms by which social and structural processes mediate (mental) health outcomes in specific settings. I will then use the conceptual resources furnished in Deleuze's empiricism to identify the human and nonhuman forces active in a body's recovery from mental illness. In developing this inquiry, the chapter will first review existing accounts of recovery, focusing on the role of social inclusion, community participation and 'place attachment'. I will then examine recent studies of therapeutic landscapes, enabling environments and restorative places (see Duff 2011) to clarify the various social, material and affective forces active in the promotion of mental health. This analysis should extend and refine the positive definition of health established in earlier chapters. Drawing on Deleuze's empiricism, the chapter will introduce a conceptual logic of recovery grounded in the analysis of sense, signs, learning and becoming. I will argue that recovery involves a process of becoming sensitive to the social, material and affective signs of one's 'becoming well' within an assemblage of human and nonhuman forces. The chapter will apply this logic to analysis of the role of social inclusion and place attachment in recovery in order to begin to sketch novel 'place-based' responses to mental health problems.

Chapter 5 addresses the major implications of Deleuze's empiricism for the analysis of problems associated with the misuse of alcohol and other drugs (AOD), what might be characterised as 'dangerous consumption'. I will focus, in particular, on the problem of theorising and analysing AOD use in relation to the molecular, the ethological and the affective. The chapter argues that Deleuze's characterisation of the assemblage introduces new ways of thinking about consumption, and new ways of approaching key problems in the analysis of AOD use such as responsibility, addiction, agency, harm and context. It is not the case, as critics of Deleuze sometimes argue, that his posthuman ontology does away with the problems of ethics and responsibility, yet it does introduce new ways of conceiving of the ethical. The chapter proposes to draw from Deleuze's work in sketching a theory of alcohol and other drug consumption 'beyond the subject', before assessing how such a theory may lead to a new affective ethics of responsibility. The chapter will also assess the major policy implications of such a theory, focusing on the development of novel place-based alcohol and drug prevention and harm reduction strategies.

Chapter 6 will work towards a fuller account of the character and orientation of Deleuze's ethics. This will require the identification and assessment of an *immanent ethics* concerned with extending a body's power of acting. The chapter will examine how the forces of life may be 'folded' or 'reterritorialised' in an everyday practice of health and wellbeing. This will entail an ethics of the body, of the assemblage, and of life, which convert the very constitution of the assemblage into an ethical concern. Central to this task will be the identification of immanent criteria for the modification of assemblages in the interest of transforming life and promoting health (see Fox 2012: 66–70). Reflecting the substantive account of health proposed in earlier chapters, Chap. 6 will align the ethical practice of health with the objective of becoming "reasonable, strong and free". Such endeavour ought to entail the concrete affirmation of life and a commitment to the lived expression of its forces. In an effort to further indicate how Deleuze's ethics might avail effective strategies for the everyday promotion of health, I will next examine Foucault's cognate 'aesthetics of existence'. Foucault's ethics will avail a more pragmatic organising principle for the articulation of a Deleuzian ethics of health. The sixth chapter will thus complete the task initiated here in the first chapter of presenting the rudiments of a Deleuzian minor science of health, and the normative and ethical innovations associated with it.

The concluding chapter will review the key arguments advanced in earlier chapters, summarising the distinctive contribution Deleuze's ideas have for scholars, students and policy makers in public health, the sociology of health and illness, human development, quality of life studies and related fields. The chapter will also assess the book's overarching goal of fostering more widespread critical engagement with Deleuze's work in the interests of facilitating a Deleuzian 'life science'. In canvassing these themes, the final chapter will provide substance for the book's broader and more ambitious articulation of alternative pragmatic and epistemological grounds for the development of health promotion policies and programs. Arguing that all existing public health strategies impose distinctive ethical obligations on their subjects, the concluding chapter will consider how public health programming may be transformed in order to incorporate new ethical considerations more cognisant of the molecular, the relational and the affective. I will focus once again on the issues of mental illness, and the use and misuse of alcohol and other drugs to sketch a more ethical approach to health promotion. Arguing for an ethics of the assemblage, I will seek to indicate how a variety of human and nonhuman forces may be enrolled in the promotion of health and the mitigation of illness. This should further clarify the contours of a more posthuman approach to health initiated here in the first chapter. All of this depends, of course, on Deleuze's idiosyncratic account of life, empiricism, difference and becoming, the basic features of which I shall now turn to consider.

References

Alliez, E. 2004. *The signature of the world: What is Deleuze and Guattari's philosophy?* London: Continuum.

Ansell Pearson, K. 1999. *Germinal life: The difference and repetition of Gilles Deleuze*. London: Routledge.

Arnold, J., and L. Breen. 2006. Images of health. In *Health promotion in practice*, ed. S. Gorin and J. Arnold, 3–20. London: Wiley.

Audi, R. (ed.). 1995. *The Cambridge dictionary of philosophy*. Cambridge: Cambridge University Press.

Baugh, B. 1992. Transcendental empiricism: Deleuze's response to Hegel. *Man and World* 25(2): 133–148.

Baugh, B. 1993. Deleuze and empiricism. *Journal of the British Society for Phenomenology* 24(1): 15–31.

Baum, F. 2008. *The new public health*, 3rd ed. Melbourne: Oxford University Press.

Bell, J. 2009. *Deleuze's Hume: Philosophy, culture and the Scottish enlightenment*. Edinburgh: Edinburgh University Press.

Blaxter, M. 2004. *Health: Key concepts*. London: Wiley.

Boundas, C. 1994. Deleuze: Serialization and subject-formation. In *Gilles Deleuze and the theatre of philosophy*, ed. C. Boundas and D. Olkowski. London: Routledge.

Bryant, L. 2008. *Difference and givenness: Deleuze's transcendental empiricism and the ontology of immanence*. Evanston: Northwestern University Press.

Buchanan, I. 2011. Desire and ethics. *Deleuze Studies* 5(S1): 7–20.

Clough, P., and J. Halley (eds.). 2007. *The affective turn: Theorizing the social*. Durham: Duke University Press.

Dawson, A. (ed.). 2009. *The philosophy of public health*. London: Ashgate.

De Beistegui, M. 2010. *Immanence: Deleuze and philosophy*. Edinburgh: Edinburgh University Press.

De Landa, M. 2002. *Intensive science and virtual philosophy*. London: Continuum.

De Landa, M. 2006. *A new philosophy of society: Assemblage theory and social complexity*. London: Continuum.

Deleuze, G. 1988. *Foucault*. London: The Athlone Press.

Deleuze, G. 1991. *Empiricism and Subjectivity: An Essay on Hume's Theory of Human Nature*. Trans. C. Boundas. Columbia: Columbia University Press.

Deleuze, G. 1992. *Expressionism in Philosophy: Spinoza*. Trans. Martin Joughin. New York: Zone Books.

Deleuze, G. 1994. *Difference and repetition*. London: The Athlone Press.

Deleuze, G. 2001. *Pure Immanence: Essays on a Life*. Trans. Anne Boyman. New York: Zone Books.

Deleuze, G. 2004. *Desert Islands and Other Texts (1953–1974)*. Trans. Mike Taormina. New York: Semiotext(e).

Deleuze, G., and F. Guattari. 1987. *A Thousand Plateaus: Capitalism and Schizophrenia*. Trans. Brian Massumi. Minnesota: University of Minnesota Press.

Deleuze, G., and F. Guattari. 1994. *What is philosophy?* London: Verso.

Deleuze, G., and C. Parnet. 1987. *Dialogues*. London: Athlone Press.

Duff, C. 2011. Networks, resources and agencies: On the character and production of enabling places. *Health and Place* 17(1): 149–156.

Fertman, C., and D. Allensworth (eds.). 2010. *Health promotion programs: From theory to practice*. San Francisco: Jossey-Bass Publishers.

Foucault, M. 1972. *The order of things: An archaeology of the human sciences*. London: Tavistock.

Foucault, M. 1978. *The history of sexuality. Vol. 1: An introduction*. London: Penguin.

Foucault, M. 1983. Afterword: The subject and power. In *Michel Foucault: Beyond structuralism and hermeneutics*, 2nd ed, ed. H. Dreyfus and P. Rabinow. Chicago: University of Chicago Press.

Foucault, M. 1984. *The Foucault reader*, ed. Paul Rabinow. London: Penguin.

Foucault, M. 2008. *The birth of biopolitics: Lectures at the College De France, 1978–1979*. London: Palgrave MacMillan.

Fox, N. 2011. The ill-health assemblage: Beyond the body-with-organs. *Health Sociology Review* 20(4): 434–446.

Fox, N. 2012. *The body*. Cambridge: Polity Press.

Gorin, S., and J. Arnold (eds.). 2006. *Health promotion in practice*. London: Wiley.
Greco, M. 2004. The politics of indeterminacy and the right to health. *Theory, Culture and Society* 21(6): 1–22.
Grosz, E. 2011. *Becoming undone: Darwinian reflections on life, politics and art*. Durham: Duke University Press.
Jun, N. 2011. Deleuze, values, and normativity. In *Deleuze and ethics*, ed. N. Jun and D. Smith, 89–107. Edinburgh: Edinburgh University Press.
Latour, B. 2002. The body, cyborgs and the politics of incarnation. In *The body*, ed. S. Sweeney and I. Hodder. Cambridge: Cambridge University Press.
Latour, B. 2003. A strong distinction between humans and non-humans is no longer required for research purposes: A debate between Bruno Latour and Steve Fuller. *History of the Human Sciences* 16(2): 77–99.
Law, J. 2004. *After method: Mess in social science research*. London: Routledge.
Mansfield, N. 2000. *Subjectivity: Theories of the self from Freud to Haraway*. Sydney: Allen and Unwin.
Marcus, G., and E. Saka. 2006. Assemblage. *Theory, Culture & Society* 23(2–3): 101–106.
Marmot, M. 2005. *The status syndrome: How social standing affects our health and longevity*. London: Holt Paperbacks.
Massumi, B. 2010. What concepts do: Preface to the Chinese translation of a thousand plateaus. *Deleuze Studies* 4(1): 1–15.
Metzl, J., and A. Kirkland (eds.). 2010. *Against health: How health became the new morality*. New York: New York University Press.
Mol, A. 2002. *The body multiple: Ontology in medical practice*. Durham: Duke University Press.
Patton, P. 1994. Translator's preface. In *Difference and repetition*, ed. G. Deleuze, xi–xiv. London: The Athlone Press.
Patton, P. 2000. *Deleuze and the political*. London: Routledge.
Patton, P. 2008. Becoming democratic. In *Deleuze and politics*, ed. I. Buchanan and N. Thoburn, 178–195. Edinburgh: Edinburgh University Press.
Protevi, J. 2009. *Political affect: Connecting the social and the somatic*. Minneapolis: University of Minnesota Press.
Rabinow, P., and N. Rose. 2006. Biopower today. *BioSocieties* 1(2): 195–214.
Rolli, M. 2009. Deleuze on intensity differentials and the being of the sensible. *Deleuze Studies* 3(1): 26–53.
Rose, N. 2001. The politics of life itself. *Theory, Culture & Society* 18(6): 1–30.
Rose, N. 2007. *The politics of life itself: Biomedicine, power, and subjectivity in the twenty-first century*. Princeton: Princeton University Press.
Scriven, A., and S. Garman (eds.). 2007. *Public health: Social context and action*. London: Open University Press.
Sen, A. 1999. *Development as freedom*. Oxford: Oxford University Press.
Sen, A. 2006. Why health equity? In *Public health, ethics and equity*, ed. S. Anand, F. Peter, and A. Sen. Oxford: Oxford University Press.
Shaviro, S. 2009. *Without criteria: Kant, Whitehead, Deleuze and Aesthetics*. Cambridge: The MIT Press.
Smith, D. 2003. Deleuze and the liberal tradition: normativity, freedom and judgement. Economy and Society 32(2): 299–324.
Smith, D., and J. Protevi. 2008. Gilles Deleuze. In *The Stanford encyclopedia of philosophy*, ed. E. Zalta. http://plato.stanford.edu/archives/fall2008/entries/deleuze/. Accessed 18 Nov 2011.
Tengland, P. 2006. The goals of health work: Quality of life, health and welfare. *Medicine, Health Care and Philosophy* 9(2): 155–167.
Turner, B. 2008. *The body & society: Explorations in social theory*, 3rd ed. London: Sage.
World Health Organisation. 1986. *The Ottawa charter for health promotion*. Geneva: WHO.

Chapter 2
The Concrete Richness of the Sensible

The full measure of Deleuze's contribution to the contemporary human sciences is still too remote for the reckoning. Commonly a Deleuzian thread may be observed, yet rarely is his "proper name" invoked (Deleuze and Guattari 1987: 37). Doubtless, the cause of this uneven reception lies in the provocations that abound in Deleuze's thought, both alone and in his collaborations with Felix Guattari, unsettling debates in diverse fields and opening up new problems for analysis (Alliez 2004: 105–107). Deleuze's influence is discernible in much recent innovation in the health and social sciences, including investigations of the body, movement and sensation (Massumi 2002); examinations of affect and emotion (Pile 2010); the social study of science and technology (Jensen and Rödje 2010); the proposal of 'non-representational' accounts of everyday life (Thrift 2007); and the study of health and human development (Fox 2011). Yet in each case Deleuze's contribution is elusive, sometimes acknowledged and sustained and other times evanescent and implied (Viveiros de Castro 2010). Unlike the more fulsome reception enjoyed by Foucault's work (Turner 2008), Deleuze's oeuvre presents something of a mystery for health and social scientists, full of promise and yet fraught with unfamiliar challenges. The present chapter explores some of these challenges in assessing the prospects of a minor science of health and illness modelled on Deleuze's idiosyncratic empiricism.

I am particularly interested in the kinds of research innovation that this minor science may entail. In addressing this question, I aim to confront what is arguably the most pervasive trend in the reception of Deleuze's ideas in the health and social sciences; namely, the selective appropriation of Deleuze's concepts and their redeployment as "tools" in the analysis of discrete social, cultural and health related problems (Buchanan 1997b: 482–484). While the co-option of Deleuze's work as a kind of conceptual 'tool-box' was famously endorsed by the thinker himself (Bouchard 1980: 208), the adoption of this technique in the health and social sciences has often had the perverse effect of limiting wider engagement with Deleuze's mature philosophy. While the deployment of concepts such as 'affect', 'assemblage', 'desire', 'becoming' and the 'body without organs' has opened up a range of innovative new lines of inquiry (Fox 2012: 63–69), this innovation has

C. Duff, *Assemblages of Health: Deleuze's Empiricism and the Ethology of Life*,
DOI 10.1007/978-94-017-8893-9_2, © Springer Science+Business Media Dordrecht 2014

largely been at the expense of clarifying what a distinctly Deleuzian health science might consist of. For a thinker who remained throughout his career committed to the realisation of a distinctive philosophical 'system', the habit of selectively applying concepts in the course of analyses often unrelated to themes that Deleuze himself considered arguably obscures the deeper and more systematic thrust of Deleuze's project. Taken as a whole, Deleuze's work furnishes a distinctive "ontology of the sensible"; a unique method or "pragmatics" capable of "determining the conditions of real experience" (Alliez 2004: 103–112). It is the argument of this chapter that the most effective means of characterising this method, and assessing its value in the renovation of health science inquiry, is to focus on what Deleuze meant by "transcendental empiricism".

Of course, the challenge in clarifying Deleuze's empiricism is that its character must be pieced together from the diverse treatments it receives throughout the thinker's oeuvre. Nowhere is this method plainly characterised – at least in a way that might be familiar to health or social scientists – with Deleuze's varying accounts of transcendental empiricism as often allusive and discordant, as they are instructive (Hayden 1995: 283–285). It is also true that existing commentaries on Deleuze's empiricism tend to emphasise the speculative metaphysics that underpin his method (Bryant 2008). In sketching the key features of Deleuze's metaphysics, most commentators ignore the *empirical implications* of Deleuze's thought and the novel methods this work might avail for the interrogation of 'real experience'. Given such oversights, I will focus here on the *methodological promise* of transcendental empiricism. In setting this course, I aim to follow Deleuze's lead in the conduct of philosophical commentary. In *Difference and Repetition*, Deleuze (1994: xxi) argues that "a commentary should act as a veritable double, and bear the maximal modification appropriate to a double". Bearing in mind comments Deleuze (1995: 136) offers elsewhere regarding the role of concepts in the pragmatic work of philosophy, Deleuze's remark in the preface to *Difference and Repetition* has been taken to suggest that the reception of his thought should emphasise the deployment of concepts in the articulation of novel problems, rather than the hermeneutic task of deciphering what such concepts might mean or represent (see Smith 2010: 58–59).

The exposition of Deleuze's empiricism offered below must, therefore, be understood in relation to the distinctive problem I have set for myself. In attempting to determine how Deleuze's empiricism may be more *systematically adapted* to the analysis of health and illness, I am primarily interested in identifying the key concepts that comprise this empiricism, and the most methodologically sound means of deploying them. Given Deleuze's exhortations regarding the differential relations that compose concepts, I also want to problematise the practice noted above of selectively deploying individual concepts with little regard for the specific concept-problem-assemblage from which they are drawn. As such, I will treat Deleuze's empiricism as *a discrete methodology*, capable of inspiring research designs more sensitive to "what we are doing" (Deleuze 1991: 133). This, I wager, is an empiricism capable of leading the health sciences more deeply into the "concrete richness of the sensible" (Deleuze and Parnet 1987: 54); into "real experience" in all its complexity. There are significant efforts underway in various cognate disciplines to achieve this intimacy (see Bonta 2009; De Landa 2006; Dewsbury 2011; Manning 2009; Pile 2010), much of which draws explicitly from Deleuze's writings. The present chapter adds to this innovation by fleshing out the characteristic features of Deleuze's empiricism, and then indicating how this empiricism may be mobilised in the design of novel studies of health.

More directly, Deleuze's empiricism furnishes three operant concepts – relation, affect and event – useful for the analysis of health and illness. Each of these concepts explicates the 'pre-individual singularities' central to Deleuze's account of (human) life, and the habits, experiences, practices and beliefs these singularities express. Privileging the analysis of relations, affects and events may offend critics who find in Deleuze's writings a "flat ontology" opposed to all metaphysical hierarchies (De Landa 2002: 153). Certainly, my approach risks de-emphasising concepts like sensation, difference and the virtual that have a key place in Deleuze's metaphysics. However, I would stress that when considered in relation to the problem at hand, the elevation of relations, affects and events affords a means of clarifying the methodological significance of Deleuze's thought, and its relevance for research innovation in the health and social sciences. It is further the case that these three concepts provide an effective orientation to the conceptual plenitude of a transcendental empiricism (Baugh 1992: 137–141). The development of my argument will first require a brief sketch of the reception of Deleuze's ideas in the health and social sciences. The purpose of this review is twofold; first it is important that I canvas the various debates Deleuze's work has provoked in the health and social sciences as a prelude to a more thoroughgoing assessment of the ways Deleuze's empiricism may be further applied in these fields. This review should, in turn, provide a fuller genealogy of the three primary problems upon which the book is based (see Chap. 1). Following this review, I will outline the broad scope of Deleuze's empiricism, before turning to a longer discussion of relations, affects and events. Rather than offer a comprehensive exegetical summary of these concepts, I propose to identify *select methodological principles* for the analysis of relations, affects and events in discrete milieus. The chapter will close with a brief discussion of how Deleuze's methods may be further adopted across the health and social sciences as a way of introducing the analysis to follow in the two case studies.

2.1 Deleuze's Reception in the Health and Social Sciences

Deleuze's reception in the health and social sciences has generally featured as part of a broader engagement with the philosophers, ideas and problems associated with the poststructuralist turn in continental philosophy (Jensen and Rödje 2010). This intellectual context is significant in that Deleuze's work is often considered in relation to thinkers like Foucault, Derrida, Bourdieu, Lyotard, Virilio and Baudrillard, with whom Deleuze no doubt shares certain ontological and epistemological commitments. This includes the rejection of all ontological 'essences' such as the 'subject', 'life', 'being', 'gender' and 'identity', and an interest in the workings of power, language, discourse and desire (see Williams 2005 for a review). Perhaps the key feature of all poststructuralist philosophies is the refusal to posit the 'subject' as a necessary condition for philosophical reflection (Colwell 1997: 18). Neither 'self', 'subjectivity', 'consciousness', 'mind' nor 'reason' can provide a stable foundation for thought, nor should they be regarded as 'transcendental' entities somehow removed from the world of interaction, language and practice (Deleuze 2001). Like Foucault and Derrida, Deleuze is interested in the ways the subject is *produced in thought and practice*, and the broader consequences of this production for philosophy and politics. Unlike Foucault and Derrida though, Deleuze's writings have not inspired the work of commentary and exegesis necessary to fashion a "Deleuze effect" in the health and social sciences (Brown 2010). Although this is beginning to change, the translational work required to establish how Deleuze's ideas may be more comprehensively applied in these fields has yet to advance very far (Jensen and Rödje 2010). Indeed, it is fair to say that the nuances of Deleuze's philosophy are often overlooked in the health and social sciences in favour of a more generic set of arguments held to be common to all poststructuralist thinkers (see Mansfield 2000).

This is not true of course of all scholars in the health and social sciences. In the social sciences in particular, Deleuze's work has been routinely cited in the search for novel tools to guide research innovation (Brown 2010). In social and human geography for example, Deleuze's work has been central to the development of "non-representational theory" (Thrift 2007), and the corresponding attempt to yield a more pragmatic and relational understanding of place, scale, boundedness, belonging, movement, experience, territory and dwelling (see Anderson and Harrison 2010; Marston et al. 2005). Ben Anderson, Paul Harrison, Sallie Marston, Nigel Thrift and John Dewsbury, among others, have adopted key Deleuzian concepts such as affect, event, becoming and assemblage in an effort to explain the relational coproduction of places, subjects and contexts. This work rejects the *a priori* supposition of territories and populations, spaces and bodies, which then interact in the course of experience and habitation (Harrison 2000: 501–506). In contrast, geographers aligned with non-representational theory have taken up Deleuze's work in the hope of deriving more productive ontological suppositions to ground their research. Subsequent studies have tended to focus on processes of *production or emergence*, like those associated with place-making and the experience of belonging or attachment to place (Thrift 1999). Other scholars have focused on the topologies of place expressed in practices of mobility and movement (Cresswell 2010). Further interest has been expressed in the experience of "affective atmospheres" and their role in 'figuring' the array of activities, practices and/or interactions permissible within space (Anderson 2009). Others have explored the de/territorialisation of (human) life and the transmission of properties, qualities, affects and capacities between bodies and spaces (Jones 2009). These studies makes selective use of Deleuze's ideas in an attempt to free geography from a materialist ontology in favour of a more affective or 'vitalist' rendering of the topologies of place, self and world (see Dewsbury 2011; Thrift 2007 for a review).

Deleuze's distinctive reworkings of affect and intensity have also been central to the reception of his ideas in educational settings. Scholars in education and related disciplines have been drawn to Deleuze's work in an effort to anticipate the establishment of what are often called 'affective pedagogies' (Semetsky 2004, 2010; Hickey-Moody 2007; Probyn 2004; Zembylas 2007). This scholarship conceives of education and learning as intensive processes of affective and material production, in which forces, sensations and intensities are transmitted between bodies in ways that transform their distinctive capacities. In this respect, learning must not be reduced to a linear cognitive process whereby knowledge is simply transferred from one competent body to another in the process of acquiring such competencies. Rather, learning needs to be reconceived as a dynamic, intensive and rhizomatic *practice*, in which bodies are folded into and out of discrete assemblages of signs, affects, technologies, subjects and ideas. Learning is less cognitive than affective in this sense, insofar as bodies learn as their capacities for affecting and being affected are transformed by the array of entities they encounter.

Anna Hickey-Moody (2009) has developed these kinds of arguments in a series of studies of the ways discrete pedagogical modalities work to transform the materiality of bodies, signs and texts. Noting important differences in the affective and pedagogical effects of literature, sound and movement, and the ways each are positioned as distinctive learning modalities, Hickey-Moody goes on to explore novel affective strategies for transforming 'bodies of learning' in discrete communities of practice. Michalinos Zembylas (2007) pursues a similar course in his analysis of 'emotional intelligence' and 'emotion management' in education settings. Zembylas (2007: 19–20) shares with Hickey-Moody (2009), Probyn (2004) and Semetsky (2010) an interest in reconceptualising teaching and learning as practices or technologies for the production of "intensities" that connect and reconnect bodies in novel ways; to other human bodies, to bodies of practice, to ideas, to forces, to "lines of flight" and so on. Bogue (2004: 330–234) takes a slightly different view in presenting teaching and learning as an "apprenticeship in signs". This approach draws from Deleuze's book on Proust to present a model of learning based on the exposition of formal and informal signs, including non-linguistic or non-discursive signs such as memories, images, visual and aesthetic production, micro-perceptions, imagination and desires.

Similar intellectual concerns have inspired interest in Deleuze's work among sociologists and anthropologists, as well as scholars in cultural studies, media and communication studies (see Brown 2010; De Landa 2006; Fuglsang and Sørensen 2006; Jensen and Rödje 2010; Massumi 2002). Sociologists and anthropologists have tended to regard Deleuze's oeuvre as one resource among many furnished in contemporary poststructuralist debates. This is especially apparent in recent sociologies of the body, in which Deleuze's work has been read in relation to Foucault's and Bourdieu's writings, in particular, typically in an effort to escape the essentialism of the body and the antinomies of structure and agency (see Bogard 1998; Fox 2012 for a review). Scott Lash (1984), Ian Buchanan (1997b), Nick Fox (2012),

Bryan Turner (2008), Peta Malins (2004), Lisa Blackman and Mike Featherstone (2010), among others, have found much of interest in Deleuze's account of a (posthuman) body assembled in the folding and refolding of matter, life, signs, objects, technologies, habits and events. In refiguring (human) life in terms of the assemblage, Deleuze's work has assisted sociologists and anthropologists to trace the myriad activities by which the body differs from itself in relation to the varied affects, events and encounters it experiences. The body loses any sense of orderly identity in this treatment, replaced by a system of disjunctive becomings whereby bodies are forever assembled anew as novel objects, affects and forces are folded within them, just as others are lost to the assemblage as its relations unfold (Hughes 2011: 1–5). Conceiving of the body in this way effectively distributes the body within and among the myriad objects, structures and agencies that constitute a social territory, field or 'context' (see Duff 2007). This is a body between structure and agency reducible to neither yet clearly assembled out of elements of each. It also follows that the various 'segmentations' (Deleuze and Parnet 1987) or 'dividing practices' (Foucault 1983) by which bodies are conventionally distinguished – such as gender, sex, race, class, age, occupation and/or ability – should themselves be regarded as effects of this folding or assembling of bodies, and not as essential characteristics of a natural or transcendental body/subject (Bains 2002; Fox 2012).

The idea of a body assembled in a panoply of material and force relations has held special appeal for scholars in science and technology studies (STS), and for successive generations of feminist thinkers. The theoretical and epistemological innovations associated with STS – and with actor-network-theory more directly – are heavily indebted to Deleuze's ontological investments, even if this debt is only occasionally acknowledged (see Albertson and Diken 2006: 240; Jensen and Rödje 2010: 1–2). Nonetheless, STS relies on the key Deleuzian contention of a body assembled in its relations with the objects and technologies that dominate its social milieu (Law 2009). Sociologists, anthropologists and historians have been particularly drawn to the ways STS marshals this characterisation to describe the production and transformation of 'actors' in discrete networks of objects, actants, processes and associations. Further inspiration has been drawn from Deleuze's treatment of the body's de/territorialisations and the ways technologies 'reterritorialise' the body's component parts, advancing their (nonhuman) becomings. Examples include the hand made "prehensile" as it is reterritorialised by object-tools that it may "brandish or propel"; or the way the stirrup modifies the material, social and affective relations "amalgamating" human and horse, transforming the related technologies of travel, conquest and war-craft (Deleuze and Parnet 1987: 104–105). Recent sociologies of the body are thus indebted to Deleuze's *historicisation* of technology, and his conviction that the tool is a "variable machine assemblage" which effects a "certain relationship of vicinity with man, animals and things" (Deleuze and Parnet 1987: 104). Drawing on this insight, scholars of science and technology have taken the tool to be central to the ongoing transmission of action, and the wider distribution of agency between bodies (see Latour 2005: 46–50).

STS, however, follows Deleuze in radically opening the category of the actor to include humans as well as objects, tools, plans, logics and processes (Latour 2005: 64–70). The principle of absolute symmetry that underscores this move might appear to dismiss the distinctive agentic capacities of *human* actors (Sismondo 2010: 89–90), even though the intention is to extend agency beyond humans to better account for the actions and capacities that nonhuman entities exhibit. STS scholars John Law (2009), Bruno Latour (2005) and Annemarie Mol (2002) have drawn from Deleuze's account of bodies and assemblages to reject the notion that actors possess innate capacities, which are then realised or expressed in particular situations. In fine Deleuzian fashion, these authors stress that action is the product of specific network associations that spatially and temporally link one actor with another (Latour 2005: 206–208). This position is further reliant on Deleuze's (1992) reading of Spinoza and his conviction that the greater the array of relations a body is able to maintain, the greater the array of actions, capacities or affects that body will be capable of (Bell 2009: 4–5). It follows that agency, as STS scholars understand it, is a function of the slow development of network relations such that each actor's agentic capacities differ according to the character of these relations (Latour 2005). Consistent with Deleuze's ethological conception of bodies, research in STS confirms the function of affects and relations as conduits or mechanisms for the production, distribution and utilisation of agency (see also Armstrong 1997: 44–48). Successive waves of STS scholars have developed these themes in detailed empirical studies of settings and problems as diverse as urban drug use (Vitellone 2010); the experience of place and social inclusion (Duff 2011); ethnographies of scientific practice (Law 2004); the organisation of 'for profit' enterprises (Lee and Hassard 1999); and the embedding of information and communication technologies in contemporary social and political life (Avgerou et al. 2004). All bear the trace of Deleuze's conceptual invention, even if scholars like Annemarie Mol, Bruno Latour and John Law have emerged as far more successful social scientists.

The account of bodies, tools and assemblages derived from Deleuze's work and pressed into the service of a novel sociology of science and technology has also inspired feminist critics of science, including Isabelle Stengers (2011), Karen Barad (2007), Jane Bennett (2010) and Donna Haraway (1997). All have contributed important accounts of the gendered character of technology utilisation, and the work technologies 'perform' in the production and reproduction of sexual difference. Beyond the study of science and technology, a number of feminist thinkers have adopted Deleuze's ideas in an attempt to counter the politics of sexual identity (see Colebrook and Buchanan 2000). Claire Colebrook (2002), Rosi Braidotti (1994), Elizabeth Grosz (2005), Moira Gatens (2000), Donna Haraway (1997) and Paola Marrati (2006) have found productive resources in Deleuze's thought for the project of advancing feminist thinking in the absence of a recognisable, self-identical subject. Borrowing from Deleuze and Guattari's (1987) discussion of nomadology, Rosi Braidotti (1994) for example, develops the idea of the nomad in relation to the more specific problem of gendered and sexual difference. Braidotti suggests that the practice of 'becoming other' that lies at the heart of all attempts to disrupt configurations of sex and gender may be further facilitated by the practice of what she calls a 'nomadic ethics'. This is an ethics of nomadic wanderings beyond the established dictates of sexual identity, reassembling bodies, technologies, habits, affects and texts in ways that transform identity, reaffirm difference and destabilize sex and gender. Elizabeth Grosz (1994) has long shared Braidotti's interest in developing a novel 'post-identity' ethics beyond 'sex' and 'gender'. In a sustained engagement with the work of Deleuze and Guattari, Grosz (2008: ix) has sought to develop an ontology of sexual difference capable of accounting for the composition of "matter, force, nature, and the real", and the subsequent development of a novel "politics of difference". Endorsing Deleuze's commitment to the *indeterminacy* of difference, Grosz (2011) proposes a model for thinking through the experience of sex and gender, without at the same time reifying the differences that punctuate this experience in the preservation of essential sexual categories. Such a gesture clears the way for an ethics of becoming that retains an *ontology* of difference in its attempts to destabilize sex and gender, and so 'reconfigure' bodies and subjects.

Elsewhere, Moira Gatens (2000), Claire Colebrook (2002) and Paolo Marrati (2006) have conceived of this kind of 'politico-ethical' activity in explicitly affective and aesthetic terms. Each of these thinkers presents the politics of sexual difference as a dynamic intervention into the *ethological composition* of bodies and subjectivities, designed in every instance to transform the ways bodies may affect and be affected by the bodies/subjects/worlds they encounter (Gatens 2000: 71–72). This approach further dispenses with the dualisms that sustain identity politics (such as heterosexual/homosexual, male/female and man/woman), arguing instead for a "politics of becoming" counter to the "politics of production" that sustains "bi-sexed organisation" (Marrati 2006: 321). Escaping these "dualistic machines" requires an active and experimental ethics capable of transforming sexual identities in the elaboration of novel forms of (human) life (Marrati 2006: 321–322; Gatens 2000: 70–72; Colebrook 2002: 9–14). Ethics, so conceived, is ethological insofar as it is concerned with the composition of bodies and affects, practices and encounters, and with the ways each may be transformed in the interests of increasing a body's power of acting. Binary identities like male/female and gay/straight limit a body's power of acting by regulating the field of affects and encounters such a body may legitimately experience. "Overcoding" a body in this way limits its capacity to affect (or be affected by) particular kinds of bodies and encounters (Deleuze and Guattari 1987: 8–9). An affective politics of difference, along the lines endorsed by Braidotti, Grosz, Gatens, Colebrook and Marrati, challenges this overcoding by opening bodies up to a "process of contagion" that radically increases the differential elements at work within them (Marrati 2006: 321). The politics of difference that emerges in this reading of Deleuze's work is central to his enduring appeal among contemporary feminist thinkers (see Grosz 2008: 2–4). It is also critical to the wider reception of his thought in anthropology, political science, history, gender studies, geography, cultural studies and sociology. In each instance, Deleuze has provided tools for thinking afresh, revitalising old debates and opening up new lines of inquiry.

Within the health sciences themselves however, Deleuze's impact is more difficult to assess. It is only in the last 10–15 years that scholars have sought to develop Deleuze's ideas in the analysis of discrete health problems. This engagement has largely taken place in the sociology of health and illness, cultural studies, medical geography, disability studies and medical anthropology (Fox 2012: 63–75). Much of this work has assessed the philosophical significance of Deleuze's ideas, rather than addressing the practical and empirical implications of his thought for scholars working in health related disciplines. Indeed, early engagement with Deleuze's work exhibited a decidedly exegetical focus as scholars sought to position Deleuze's thought in novel contexts (see Fox 1993). More recently, this translational work has given way to a more concerted effort to 'think with' Deleuze in the investigation of select health problems. This is especially evident in the sociology of health and illness, where scholars have explored the implications of Deleuze's work for analysis of the lived experience of health and the design of novel health care interventions. Marc Roberts (2005), Dean Mitchell (1996), Anna Hickey-Moody (2009), Peta Malins (2004), John Fitzgerald (1997), Nick Fox (2011), Ian Tucker (2010), Petra Kuppers and James Overboe (2009), among others, have developed Deleuze's ideas in the study of varied health problems including addiction; the provision of health care for people recovering from mental illness; the adoption of 'enhancement technologies' such as cosmetic surgery; the experience of intellectual disability; the emergence of a logic of health care 'consumers'; and the treatment of people living with HIV/AIDS.

I offer a more extensive review of the adoption of Deleuze's thought in the contemporary health sciences in Chap. 3 where my goal will be to identify how and where Deleuze's methods may be further developed in these fields. Yet before I introduce these methods it should prove useful to briefly summarise the major intellectual contributions elaborated in the literature reviewed above. As I noted in the introduction to this chapter, the purpose of this summary is twofold. First, it should clarify the objects, methods and analytics of a minor science of health and illness. Second, it ought to afford a more explicit genealogy of the three problems identified in the Preface and again in Chap. 1 as justifications for this minor science, thus anticipating the empirical analysis to follow in the two case studies.

Central to the research reviewed above is the sympathetic endorsement of Deleuze's rejection of all dualisms, structures, identities and essences, and the subsequent development of a logic of relations, multiplicities or *assemblages* (see Bonta 2009; Fox 2012: Patton 2000; Rajchman 2000; Smith 2012). Reviewing the application of this logic in the contemporary social sciences, Marcus and Saka (2006: 102–104) argue that the assemblage has generally been mobilised to replace the more traditional notion of social structure. In contrast to the putative rigidities of structure, and the reifications of social context, the idea of the assemblage emphasises processes of emergence, heterogeneity, instability and flux. Whereas structure is typically understood to be resistant to change, the assemblage foregrounds the ways "heterogeneous elements" are organised in the formation of social, symbolic, economic and political "scaffolding" that "orders" interaction, 'meaning' and practice (Marcus and Saka 2006: 102). This suggests that the objects of social science inquiry cannot be regarded as static entities bearing some invariant essence, but must instead be examined in the context of their contingent becomings.

A commitment to this 'relational logic' is a feature of most engagements with Deleuze's work in the health and social sciences, including those studies reviewed above. Across these studies, the idea of the assemblage provides a means of suspending traditional ontological categories – such as 'subject', 'identity', 'essence', 'experience', 'object' and 'world' – to permit more refined analyses of the relations, affects and events by which these categories are assembled. "Assemblage thinking" thus provides the basis for a novel methodology of great promise for scholars right across the health and social sciences (Anderson et al. 2012; Brown 2010; De Landa 2006; Viveiros de Castro 2010). *This suggests, finally, that the assemblage ought to be the principal focus of any attempt to establish a Deleuzian health science.* What's more, the research reviewed above provides a range of insights regarding the primary research problems such a science should concern itself with. First, recent appropriations of Deleuze's thought in the health and social sciences suggest the importance of abandoning the differentiation of subjects and objects, humans and nonhumans, body and society in favour of a 'symmetrical' ontology capable of explaining the manner of these entities production and convergence. All bodies are composed in an assemblage of matter, technology, affect and force, such that to somehow untangle these entities and their effects is not only empirically taxing but also ontologically unreliable (De Landa 2006: 47–50). Such is the primary epistemological claim, incidentally, of actor-network theory (Latour 2005). Like actor-network theory, Deleuze's empiricism suggests the folly of abstracting (human) life from the web of affects, relations and events in which it is enmeshed. It follows that there can be no reasonable epistemological differentiation of subjects and objects, bodies and contexts, with any such distinction remaining an artefact of thought and not a reliable property of the "given" (Deleuze 2001: 25–27).

This suggests, more directly, the importance of studying the means of the assemblage's formation in the conduct of a Deleuzian health science. If the need to overturn the dualities of subject and object, the human and the nonhuman, is the first great methodological investment of such a science, then the second pertains to the merits of considering the divergent actors, entities, bodies, affects, forces and signs active in assemblages of health. As the discussion of Deleuze's empiricism below will make plain, the work of identifying and assessing the constituent features of the assemblage is itself an empirical task. While this task invites some innovation in the characterisation of the empirical, it lends itself nonetheless to routine social science inquiry. As I argued in Chap. 1, the notion of the social and structural determinants of health presents a useful test of this claim. Rather than present social and political factors, like educational disadvantage, poverty and income inequality, as *brute structural determinants* of health in any given setting, a more Deleuzian account suggests focusing instead on identifying the various assemblages by which these outcomes are enacted or expressed. The case studies presented in Chaps. 4 and 5 will flesh this argument out, although the point for now is that the various entities at work in assemblages of health can each be identified by way of the effects they generate (and the concrete relations they establish) between diverse bodies. The work of 'distal' structural actors like policy, taxation arrangements, income distribution, racism and stigma may, for example, be traced in individual settings via the effects they engender in bodies. This argument is very close to Bruno Latour's (2005: 1–6) description of actor-network-theory and its "tracings" of the effects of the "social" in local networks. Whatever the source, the point is not to posit some distal cast of structural actors which somehow mediates health outcomes in discrete settings. The properly empirical task is to document the array of bodies, technologies, affects and events 'involved' in local assemblages of health, and the work each does to either promote or diminish health. This suggests that health ought to be regarded as a *property of the assemblage* and not of any one individual body.

Furnishing an appropriately Deleuzian conceptualisation of health is thus the third principal research task indicated in the literature reviewed above. If the body cannot feasibly be removed from its context or environment – such that health must instead be regarded as a property of the assemblages in which bodies are expressed – then the problem of defining health becomes at once more complicated, but also potentially more productive (Fox 2011: 434–436). In the previous chapter I argued that the primary reason the health sciences have so far resisted providing a substantive definition of health is that these sciences are generally more interested in illness. Attempts to establish a positive definition of health mostly end up eliding capacity, function, empowerment or, more notoriously, wellbeing (Arnold and Breen 2006). Thinking of health in terms of the assemblage suggests the need to include a wider array of actors, objects, bodies and processes in this evaluation. I also suggested in Chap. 1 that health may profitably be defined in normative terms as a lived transition in a body's perfection, or its power of acting. Although I barely hinted at the complex status of such a body, thinking now in terms of the assemblage indicates the importance of regarding a body's power of acting as the function of innumerable bodies, both human and nonhuman, acting together. I should also reiterate the argument made earlier that only Deleuze can provide the conceptual tools necessary for the *empirical investigation* of these kinds of claims. It is important that I properly characterise Deleuze's empiricism before assessing its methodological promise.

2.2 The Challenge of a *Transcendental* Empiricism

Late in his career, Deleuze (Deleuze and Parnet 1987: vii) offered the following simple account of his intellectual project: "I have always felt that I am an empiricist, that is, a pluralist". This enigmatic remark betrays the complexity of Deleuze's thought, his interests and preoccupations, even as it highlights the characteristic thrust of his immanent philosophy. Deleuze proposes a decidedly inventive empiricism, deeply antagonistic to the foundational assumptions of traditional empirical inquiry. Empiricism is normally understood as a theory of the relationship between experience, sense impressions and knowledge, in which all knowledge is said to derive from sense impressions without recourse to *a priori* ideas (Audi 1995). While Deleuze (1991) endorses this rejection of *a priori* or innate ideas, he takes issue with the empiricist supposition of a natural 'subject' of experience. For Deleuze (1991, 1994), the subject of empiricism stands itself as an innate idea in that this subject ostensibly comes to experience 'fully formed' and then constructs ideas on the basis of this experience. This might explain the generation of knowledge, ideas and understanding, yet it fails to account for the character of subjectivity itself, its formation and orientations. What's more, traditional empiricisms impute an organisation to the subject – a systematic ordering of capacities – without explaining how this organisation emerges. Deleuze (1991: 89) argues that this leaves the subject of empiricism forever outside experience; the custodian of the ideas, impressions and knowledge derived from experience without itself being the product of these experiences. In countering the transcendental foundations of all idealist and rationalist epistemologies, empiricism merely shifts this transcendental ground, leaving the mystery of subjectivity intact. Deleuze's own response to this epistemological aporia involves the search for a "superior empiricism" (Baugh 1992).

Subjectivity should, in this respect, be understood as the distinctive problem for which a *transcendental* empiricism serves as a provisional solution (Boundas 1994: 113–115). This "higher" empiricism affords "a new conception of subjectivity" (Rajchman 2000: 9), alert to the mechanisms of the subject's *formation* within a "transcendental field" (Deleuze 2001: 25–27). Buchanan (1997b: 484–485) adds that "the problem of the subject's formation" must remain central to any attempt to fashion a Deleuzian social science. This is not to suggest that subjectivity is the only problem to which Deleuze's empiricism is drawn, but rather that his empiricism entails a thoroughgoing *reconceptualization of the subject* and its emergent ontology. Subjectivity is indeed a problem for Deleuze insofar as it is typically treated as a necessary abstraction in the work of securing reliable foundations for metaphysical and ontological inquiry. Deleuze insists that far from explaining the world, the abstract "must itself be explained" (Deleuze and Parnet 1987: vii–x); particularly an abstraction as entrenched as subjectivity (Bell 2009). However, in problematising the subject, transcendental empiricism does not 'abandon' or 'eliminate' subjectivity, but rather seeks to account for its emergence from within the "flux of the sensible" (Deleuze 1991: 87). And it does this, I would argue, in conceptualising *relations, affects and events* in very specific ways, always emphasising their collocation in assemblages of matter and force (see De Landa 2006: 47–50; Grosz 2011). The importance of relations in the development of a transcendental empiricism is surely uncontroversial given the explicit treatment of this concept in Deleuze's own accounts of his method (see Deleuze and Parnet 1987: 55–59). Deleuze is concerned, most directly, with the *externality* of relations; with the distinctive ontological status of relations separate from the relata or terms that relations conjoin (Rajchman 2000). Deleuze (2001) notes that few empiricists have granted such ontological security to relations, preferring the more secure foundations of substances, things and worlds. Yet in privileging the analysis of relations,

Deleuze foregrounds the importance of events and affects, in that a relation is always a product of an encounter, understood as the event that contains the encounter and the affects that encounters produce (see Buchanan 1997b: 490–491). Indeed, relations *presuppose* an encounter between subjects, bodies and worlds, and the affective modulations these encounters inspire.

To privilege relations in the characterisation of transcendental empiricism is thus to highlight the event of the encounter that relations instantiate, and the affective becomings that these encounters support (Deleuze and Guattari 1987: 283–285). Put another way, relations always produce affective responses in the various human and nonhuman bodies subject to the event of their encounter. This arguably explains why Deleuze and Parnet (1987: 54–66) are so careful to emphasise the significance of relations, affects and events in the discussion of empiricism in their *Dialogues*. The interrogation of relations, affects and events ought, for these reasons, to be central to any assessment of Deleuze's empiricism. Further consideration of these concepts will also clarify Deleuze's account of (human) life, and his treatment of the formal properties of the assemblage. With these goals in mind, my analysis of Deleuze's empiricism will proceed in three related sections: the first will explore Deleuze's reading of Hume and his account of relations, belief and practice. The second section will consider Deleuze's reading of Spinoza and the problem of affects and encounters, while the third will review Deleuze's treatment of the event and its implications for a theory of the subject, touching on Deleuze's reading of Whitehead. The final sections will draw these accounts together in describing how the key methodological features of Deleuze's empiricism may be applied in the study of health and illness. Throughout, the goal will be to establish a novel methodology for the interrogation of assemblages of health and the varying subjectivities they sustain.

2.2.1 What Is a Relation?

Deleuze's most important study of relations and relationality is furnished in his reading of the Scottish philosopher David Hume. This analysis also provides a series of revealing insights into Deleuze's conception of subjectivity. Deleuze (1991) finds in Hume a means of explaining the *emergence* of subjectivity within the flux of contingent experience, what Hume calls the "given". What is 'given' in experience is "the flux of the sensible, a collection of impressions and images, or a set of perceptions ... the totality of that which appears" (Deleuze 1991: 87). However, this flux cannot explain the subject, because subjectivity should be understood as a "synthesis" of these "impressions and images" rather than their source. As such, the proper question for philosophy is "how is the subject constituted in the given?" (Deleuze 1991: 87). How, in other words, does the distinctive ontological bearing of subjectivity emerge from the collection of impressions, images and perceptions that comprise the 'sensible'? Deleuze's analysis takes on a uniquely transcendental element as he begins to inquire after the ways a subject constituted in the given is able to *transcend* the given. Deleuze insists upon this transcendental element in order to account for change and invention. For without the capacity to transcend the given the subject is trapped in repetition, in the pre-determined structures of the 'real'. Indeed, denying the subject's capacity to manipulate, modify or transcend the given amounts to a "denigration of the richness and diversity of the life of the world" (Hayden 1995: 285). To clarify matters then, Deleuze's approach is empirical in that it seeks to explain the immanent constitution of subjectivity, impressions, experience and sensations without recourse to *a priori* ideas (see Colwell 1997: 18–20). Yet it is also transcendental in its attempt to map the ways subjects strive to transcend the given and "affirm more than they know" (Boundas 1991: 15). Deleuze (1991: 87) describes this idea of a subject constituted in the given but also able to transcend the given, as the "absolute essence of empiricism". He adds that it was Hume who discovered this transcendental aspect in his affirmation of the externality of relations.

The problem of relations arises in Hume's discussion of the subject and the more specific issue of how the mind acquires a nature. Hume argues that the flux of sensation cannot account for the structures of mind, given the arbitrary character of experience. Experience has no meaning in and of itself, and so nothing in the stream of consciousness is capable of forming the knowledge, ideas and understanding necessary for the emergence of subjectivity. As a disjunctive collection of perceptions and sense impressions, the mind does not "have a nature" and it is "not yet a subject" (Deleuze 1991: 22–24). For Hume, the concatenation of impressions present in experience only takes on the systematic guise of subjectivity as a result of the manifold *affections of the imagination*. Imagination serves to collect impressions in such a way that the ideas, sensations and impressions derived from experience affect one another in various ways, lending a certain vividness to these impressions. Affects "give the mind its qualities" consistent with what Hume calls the "principles of association" (Deleuze 1991: 24–26). These principles affect the imagination by ordering the diverse impressions present in the mind into more systematic relations of *contiguity, resemblance and causality*. In regulating the mind's "easy passage from one idea to another", the principles of association impose "constancy on the imagination" such that ideas are linked or related to one another in reliable and consistent ways (Deleuze 1991: 25). These principles produce relations between different sense impressions and affect different elements in the mind: contiguity affects the mind's senses; resemblance regulates the transitions of the imagination; and causality affects the mind's sense of time in the assessment of cause and effect.

More specifically, the senses present impressions in the mind that are contiguous in both a temporal and affective sense, such that sense-objects take on diverse sensory and ontological identities on the basis of the proximity (or contiguity) of these impressions. Resemblance proceeds by way of reflection and analogy, in that every impression "calls up" another impression, either from memory or from contemporaneous perception, to clarify the nature and affective tone of the initial impression (Deleuze 1991: 25). Causality is the most significant of the principles of association because the impression of cause and effect, and its confirmation in experience, serves as the foundation for all purposive action, understood as the capacity to make plans and to form beliefs about the world (Deleuze 2001: 39–41). Taken together, the principles of association "elect, choose, designate and invite certain impressions of sensation among others; and having done this, constitute impressions of reflection in connection with these elected impressions" (Deleuze 1991: 113). The selection of impressions and their subsequent organisation in the repose of reflection subsequently "provides the subject with its necessary form" (Deleuze 1991: 104). In this way, the principles of association give rise to the defining characteristic of subjectivity; the capacity to form relations between sense impressions in the course of directed reflection. Subjectivity is an *emergent property* of such relations, an "impression of reflection and nothing else" (Deleuze 1991: 113).

Critically, however, the relations conceived in the mind according to the principles of association remain forever "external to their terms" (Deleuze 1991: 99). The importance of the externality of relations in Deleuze's reading of Hume cannot be overstated, serving ultimately to resolve one of empiricism's most enduring theoretical impasses. If all knowledge is said to derive from the given of experience, then how is one to account for change and invention? If all that exists is already given to the subject, then all that exists is effectively reduced to stasis. The assertion of the externality of relations reintroduces invention and dynamism into this epistemological gridlock, revealing the ways subjects invent or create relations between impressions in making sense of the world. Deleuze's argument relies on the differentiation of two broad categories of impressions in the mind; "the impressions or ideas of terms, and the impressions or ideas of relations" (Deleuze 2004: 163). Most empiricists have contested the significance of the latter, if not denied them altogether, and yet for Deleuze the capacity to form relations between disparate impressions stands as the characteristic achievement of subjectivity. For Deleuze, as for Hume, relations are in no way *determined* by their terms, by the sense-objects or impressions that relations effectively conjoin. To argue that relations are determined by their relata is to argue that these terms contain within themselves the universe of potential associations to which they might be put. This places relations and their terms within an "organic unity" (Hayden 1995: 285), effectively foreclosing difference and the creation of novel relations between disparate impressions. Indeed, if relations are determined by their terms "there is nothing to distinguish the term from the relation" (Hayden 1995: 285) and the ontological significance of relations is lost.

Deleuze (1991: 101) insists that relations bear their own unique ontological status for the simple reason that "ideas do not account for the nature of the operations that we perform on them and especially of the relations that we establish among them". This explains the emergence of novel relations (and novel understandings of these relations) in that the externality of relations ensures that sense-objects may be associated in unpredictable ways. It follows that the formation of relations between diverse sense-impressions, and the new forms of understanding that these relations support, is an innately creative process insofar as relations are always *made or invented* rather than discovered (Deleuze and Parnet 1987: 55–56). Subjectivity ought, therefore, to be understood as the capacity to take the sense impressions derived from experience and combine them in novel ways in the creation of new understandings. The creation of novel understandings (what Hume calls belief) is the transcendental component of Deleuze's empiricism. It clarifies how a subject constituted in the given is able, through the practice of sense-making, to transcend the given. This process calls attention to the importance of belief, habit and invention in Hume's account of the practical constitution of subjectivity (Deleuze 1991: 115).

In recasting subjectivity in terms of belief and invention, Hume emphasises the role of practice, habit and creativity in the production of knowledge. This move leads Deleuze (1991) to stress subjectivity's dual provenance in relations of ideas and impressions, and of practice and invention. Such processes begin with the development of relations in and between sense-impressions and their slow reification in habits. This also highlights the "circumstances, actions and passions" (Deleuze 1991: 130) which give rise to impressions, and the actions by which relations are forged between these impressions. This, for Deleuze (1991), is the very definition of habit; the insistent regularity with which the mind travels predictably from one idea to another. Yet the regularity of practice and relations, and their manifestation in habit, also permits the formation of durable beliefs about the world. What is interesting for Hume is not the extent to which beliefs may withstand objective verification, but that they support so much purposive action. Belief describes the means by which one "infer(s) one part of nature from another which is not given" (Deleuze 1991: 86). It determines one's capacity to "transcend experience and to transfer the past to the future" (Deleuze 1991: 71). Each of these capacities – to draw inferences about the world that exceed our experience of it, and to use our experience to make predictions about the future – are indispensable, almost by definition, for the planning of purposive action, from the incidental to the transformative. Beliefs are always contingent, in this sense, in that subjects form beliefs for a "specific, practical purpose, determined by a need, interest or passion" (Goodchild 1996: 14). Beliefs emerge in response to particular circumstances and hold for so long as they support action and/or understanding in relation to these circumstances. This is why Deleuze (1991: 86) regards the formation of relations, habits and beliefs to be innately creative processes, for each reveals the "dual power of subjectivity: to believe and to invent".

The model of subjectivity that emerges in Deleuze's reading of Hume inaugurates his broader effort to establish a "superior" or transcendental empiricism. The subject of such an empiricism remains a *process of differentiation* rather than an *a priori* ground or foundation (Buchanan 1997b). This is a subject of relations and beliefs, embedded in practice and habit, not a form awaiting its content. It is, more importantly, a subject of knowledge, ideas and beliefs, constituted in the nexus of associations that characterises all relations, all reflection and all imagination. Nonetheless, the emphasis on ideas, impressions and relations reveals a shortcoming in Deleuze's reading of Hume, in that it is not entirely clear what role embodiment plays in the accretions of subjectivity. For all the discussion of habit and practice, Deleuze's reworking of Hume's empiricism appears to present subjectivity as an emergent effect of mind, and the organisation of sensations and impressions in particular. Even the practice of habit appears to refer to the habit of associating particular impressions or ideas in the mind, and the way these relations give rise to coherent beliefs about the world. The body here stands as a mere container for the senses, with all the real work of subjectivity taking place elsewhere. Yet in Deleuze's mature philosophy one finds a compelling account of subjectivity conceived both in the relational connections of the mind *and* in the practical and affective relations of the body (Boundas 1994; Colwell 1997). In his collaborations with Felix Guattari and Claire Parnet, for example, Deleuze builds on his earlier study of relations to clarify both the corporeal dimensions of the subject, as well as the formal properties of the assemblage. This work presents subjectivity as an assemblage (or "non-homogenous set") of diverse relations of "sympathy, symbiosis" (Deleuze and Parnet 1987: 52–54). Sympathy is subsequently described as a process of "assembling" that establishes "agreements of convenience between bodies of all kinds . . . physical, biological, psychic, social, verbal" (Deleuze and Parnet 1987: 54). Subjectivity is thus construed as an assemblage composed in relations of sympathy between bodies, both human and nonhuman. This notion of a body assembled or composed in its relations receives further elaboration in Deleuze's reading of Baruch Spinoza, adding a properly corporeal dimension to his transcendental empiricism.

2.2.2 *What Is an Affect?*

The significance of Spinoza's legacy in the articulation of Deleuze's philosophy is almost without parallel (see Grosz 2011; Hardt 1993). Deleuze (1992: 11) regarded Spinoza as the "prince of philosophers" for his unyielding commitment to the creation of a "plane of immanence" to express both his ethics and his philosophy. All that exists in the world is, for Spinoza, a series of modifications (or modes) of an immanent substance expressed in a distinctive attribute or set of attributes (Friedman 1978: 67–75). This substance (or world) – and the infinite modes and attributes that are its expressions – remains immanent to itself as it were, free of any transcendental condition such as God, truth or soul (Deleuze 1988a). This plane of immanence serves, for Deleuze, as an important philosophical template for the development of a "superior empiricism". It provides, in particular, a means of escaping the transcendental hold of consciousness, reason, morality and justice (Buchanan 1997b: 494). Eschewing all such transcendental motifs, Deleuze (1988a) adopts Spinoza's account of the immanent constitution of 'experience', 'being' and 'embodiment' in order to rethink subjectivity, the body, relations and ethics. Deleuze (1988a: 17) ground this effort in Spinoza's unique model of philosophy; *a philosophy of the body*, of encounters and relations, ideas and affects, ethics and ethology.

For Deleuze (1992: 257), Spinoza utterly transforms philosophy in asking not what a body is, but rather "what can a body do?" This displacement enables Spinoza to recast the analysis of experience, corporeality and ontology in radical ways

(Marrati 2006). Rather than conceiving of individuals in organic terms according to a taxonomy of species or genera – such that one might conclude that all members of a species share some fundamental homology – Spinoza is concerned with the distinctiveness of *individual bodies* and the manifold affects and relations that comprise their characteristic structure. Hence, to ask what a body can do is to ask what particular relations a body is capable of "composing" with other bodies, both human and nonhuman. It is to ask what particular affects determine that body in its capacity to affect and be affected by other bodies (Deleuze 1992: 254–257). This approach defines individual bodies in terms of their "capacities" rather than their "functions" (Buchanan 1997a: 75), drawing attention to the differences that distinguish one body from another, even those of the same species. By way of example, Deleuze (1988a: 124) notes that in terms of affects and relations, a draft horse has more in common with an ox than a racehorse; "this is because the racehorse and the (draft) horse do not have the same affects nor the same capacity for being affected". This classification of individual bodies or animals according to their distinctive affects and relations is called "ethology" (see Deleuze 1988a: 125).

More directly, ethology is the "study of the relations of speed and slowness, of the capacities for affecting and being affected that characterise each thing. For each thing these relations and capacities have an amplitude, thresholds (maximum and minimum) and variations or transformations that are peculiar to them" (Deleuze 1988a: 125). The ethology advanced in Spinoza's *Ethics* provides a compelling model for Deleuze's investigations of subjectivity, the body and experience. Following Spinoza, Deleuze (1992: 201–204) notes that individual bodies are composed of an "indefinite" number of "extensive parts" connected in various "characteristic relations". The "complex body" is "permanently open to its surroundings" (Gatens 2000: 61) in that the extensive parts that make up the complex body are constantly entering into differential relations with other 'simple' bodies. Spinoza provides the example of the digestive system to characterise the way the body enters into relations with other bodies – in this instance particular foodstuffs – that are then "decomposed" or digested according to the work of simple bodies (the mouth, the oesophagus, the stomach) subsumed within the body proper. The complex body necessarily enters into relations with myriad simple bodies in order to preserve those associations which "maintain the individual in its existence" (Gatens 2000: 62).

The extensive parts that make up the complex body routinely pass through relations of 'composition' and 'decomposition' as certain parts of this complex body are lost while others are added. These parts are themselves organised in *kinetic* relations of "motion and rest, of slowness and speed" (Deleuze 1988a: 123). These relations determine the distinctive manner in which the body's extensive parts are connected or composed. They are also unique to each body and so determine its individuality or identity. Yet this individuality extends to the unique combination of affects and sensations that inhabit individual bodies. Spinoza observed that the body is characterised by *dynamic* capacities to affect and be affected by other bodies, both complex and simple. Affects are an emergent effect of the body's manifold encounters, with each encounter transforming the nature of the body's characteristic relations, and hence its manifest capacities (Deleuze 1992: 217). Relations between bodies are, in this way, "inseparable from the capacity to be affected" (Deleuze 1992: 218). Given the dynamic character of these relations (and the encounters which support them) the body's "capacity to be affected does not remain fixed at all times and from all viewpoints" (Deleuze 1992: 222). Determined in each instance anew by its relations and its affects, the body is defined by its 'continuous variations', its becoming other from itself, rather than its continuities (Deleuze 1978: np).

It is for this reason that Deleuze insists that we do not know what a body can do, because we cannot know in advance what distinctive affects and relations a complex body might become capable of. The range of affective capacities that determine the individuality of the body is itself the product of the "very great number" of relations that compose that body (Deleuze 1992: 218). It follows, moreover, that all complex bodies differ from one another by a matter of degrees according to their capacities to affect and be affected by other bodies, and by their capacities to enter into relations both simple and complex with these bodies. This produces a "new conception of the embodied individual" whereby the analysis of affects and relations displaces the study of structure and functions (Deleuze 1992: 257). This new conception also requires that one consider individual bodies in terms of their "power of acting", where this power stands as *an index* of the body's capacity to enter into diverse relations and experience diverse affects (Deleuze 1992: 256). Such power grows as a body becomes more capable of entering into novel relations with other bodies, and thus more capable of affecting and being affected by other bodies. As Spinoza (cited in Deleuze 1992: 256–257) concludes, a body may be considered more capable or more powerful than another, when it might be said of that body that it is "more capable than others of doing many things at once, or being acted on in many ways at once, (and) its mind is more capable of perceiving many things at once. . .more capable of understanding distinctly". This suggests, moreover, that the body's "power of action (is) the same as (its) capacity to be affected" (Deleuze 1992: 225). It naturally follows of course, that the obverse is also true in terms of the body's relative loss of power.

This finally reveals something of the *nature* of affect in terms of its transitions and effects. Spinoza understands affect as a modulation or quantum of a body's power of action; or its capacity to affect the diverse bodies, both human and nonhuman, that it encounters. This power determines a body's capacity to affect the world, to manipulate the circumstances or conditions of its environment, and to shape the behaviour and/or actions of other bodies. Affects distinguish how far a body's power extends into the world as it strives to "organise its encounters" (Deleuze 1992: 261). Spinoza employs two distinctive definitions of affect in an attempt to capture the diverse character of these encounters. Drawing on semantic distinctions available in Latin – affectio and affectus – Spinoza notes that affect describes both the particular state of a body at any specific moment, as well as its passage or transition from one affective state to another, and thus from one quantum of power to another. And so "*affectio* refers to a state of the affected body and implies the presence of the affecting body, whereas the *affectus* refers to the passage from one state to another, taking into account the correlative variations of the affecting bodies" (Deleuze 1988a: 49). In each instance, the states and transitions that affects produce in the body are accompanied by ideas or impressions in the mind, which indicate the character or quality of these corporeal shifts (Deleuze 1992: 220). This is one aspect of Spinoza's *parallelism*; the doctrine that the "order of actions and passions of our body is, by nature, at one with the order of actions and passions of the mind" (Spinoza cited in Deleuze 1992: 256). This parallelism applies to affect no less than any other of the mind/body's various activities or processes (see Lloyd 2001: 44–45).

Experienced at once in the body and in the mind, affectio captures something of the lived experience of affect as feeling or emotion in describing the ways encounters produce affects that are typically understood as temporal feeling states. Spinoza's real innovation however, lies in the introduction of the notion of affectus and the argument that affects involve both a particular feeling state and a transition in the body's power or capacities. Affect is more than a feeling or an emotion; it is also a potential for action, a dispositional orientation to the world. In each sense (affectio and affectus), affects are inevitable by-products of encounters in the world, in that every encounter transforms the body's affective capacities. Spinoza argues that two kinds of encounters – and the affects they give rise to – must be distinguished (Deleuze 1992: 239). First, Spinoza describes encounters in which diverse bodies, human and nonhuman, meet in such a way that the characteristic relations of each body combine in ways that enhance or otherwise facilitate the power of acting of each body. These encounters are good or useful for each body in that they 'agree' with each body's essence or 'nature', thus producing the affects of joy. In experiencing joy, the body quite literally takes on new extensive parts that enhance its power or range of actions in the world. Joy is intensely useful in this regard.

Naturally, the body also experiences encounters that involve a diminution in its power of acting and so produce the affects of sadness. These encounters involve combinations of bodies and their attendant parts and relations that serve to undermine, decompose or even destroy one or another of the constituent relations that define each body. Deleuze variously draws the example of a poison or an unwelcome social interaction to illustrate this kind of 'bad' encounter. A poison is any substance that when ingested or "encountered" by the body serves to disrupt or even destroy one or another of that body's characteristic or "essential" relations (Deleuze 1988a: 22). Arsenic, for example, works to decompose the characteristic relations of the blood leading in acute instances to organ failure (another disruption of the body's characteristic relations) and death (Marks 1998). Though obviously less extreme, an encounter with an enemy or disliked social acquaintance works similarly to disrupt or decompose the body's relations in that it involves a diminution or immobilising of these extensive parts. This tends to diminish a body's power of acting in its own right, yet it also entails a very distinctive *occupation* of this power. Every bad encounter entails a "concentration" of the body's power of action in an attempt to "invest the trace" of the offending body and so "reject" or expel that body (Deleuze 1978: np). Such 'investment' leaves one not only affected by sadness, but also immobilised in one's forces in that all of this power is caught up in the attempt to be rid of the affects associated with the unwelcome encounter. This is the reason why Spinoza argues that encounters tend to involve a shift in a body's "perfection" or "force of existing" in that good encounters involve the transfer of power from the affecting body to the affected body and so invest that body with joy and an increase in its power of acting, while "bad" encounters involve a decrease in the power of the affected body and so invest that body with sadness (Deleuze 1988a: 50). Good encounters take a body closer to its maximum power of acting and closer to perfection in its force of existence. The effort to increase one's good encounters and the array of joyful affects generated therein, while also attempting to minimise one's bad encounters with their debilitating sorrows, is the cornerstone of Spinoza's ethics.

Deleuze's study of Spinoza thus builds on his earlier reading of Hume in the ongoing refinement of a superior empiricism. No doubt, the subject and subjectivity disappear from Deleuze's reading of Spinoza, even if the characteristic concerns that frame these questions do not. In place of the study of subjectivity common to his earlier work on Hume, Deleuze favours the more explicitly Spinozist theme of the body and its encounters. This approach insists that "we know nothing about a body until we know what it can do . . . what its affects are, how they can or cannot enter into composition with other affects, with the affects of another body" (Deleuze and Guattari 1987: 257). The problem of subjectivity is thus transformed into a problem of the body and its affects, relations and encounters. Organised in kinetic and dynamic relations, the body emerges as an *assemblage* of diverse simple bodies connected in extensive parts and composed in recursive encounters. The body, in this way, attains an individuality that is also a characteristic subjectivity. This is an embodied subjectivity, a situated subjectivity that is always, already a multiplicity or assemblage. And so, to Hume's account of the accretions of subjectivity in the association of ideas and relations, reflection and belief, Deleuze adds Spinoza's assessment of the ethological composition of the body in its affects and relations. This is a subject of connections and relations in the mind and of affects and relations in the flesh, all constituted in the manifold encounters of immanent experience. Such a formulation finally hints at the significance of the *event of the encounter* in Deleuze's ontology, opening up a further dimension to a transcendental empiricism.

2.2.3 *What Is an Event?*

Deleuze's account of the event serves primarily to clarify the vexed status of 'immanence' and the 'virtual' in the development of a transcendental empiricism (Marks 1998; Shaviro 2009). Consistent with his treatment of relations and affects, Deleuze's notion of the event elucidates the 'pre-individual singularities' that compose bodies, subjects and things on specific planes or territories. This, perhaps, is the meaning of Deleuze's (2001: 31) gnomic observation that "a life contains only virtuals. It is made up of virtualities, events, singularities". Later in the same essay, Deleuze adds that "events or singularities give to the plane all their virtuality, just as the plane of immanence gives virtual events their full reality". As such, the "immanent event is actualized in a state of things. . .an object and a subject to which it attributes itself" (Deleuze 2001: 31). Despite their abstruseness, these passages capture the key dimensions of Deleuze's understanding of the event, while alluding to the intellectual lineage of his thinking. In gesturing to the way events are "actualized" in specific 'states of things', Deleuze acknowledges the debt his thinking owes to the Stoics and their distinction between events understood as the 'things that happen' to material bodies, expressed in a particular state of affairs, and the incorporeal transformations, or singularities, that accompany the 'pure event' (Patton 2006: 110–112). As Deleuze (1993: 79–82) notes elsewhere, an event "does not just mean that 'a man has been run over'" or that "a concert is being performed tonight". Events also generate discrete *incorporeal* transformations among the bodies assembled therein. An example Deleuze returns to often concerns the incorporeal transformations 'incarnated' in the sentencing of an individual at the culmination of a criminal trial, whereby the accused is transformed into a convict in a "pure, instantaneous act or incorporeal attribute" (Deleuze and Guattari 1987: 80). The trial, as an event, involves both the specific states of affairs observable in the comingling of bodies within and outside the courtroom, and the *incorporeal transformations* rendered in such bodies by the event of the trial and its attendant judgements (see Marks 1998).

This incorporeal dimension is central to Deleuze's assertion of the ontological primacy of events over essences or substances. Indeed, the incorporeal transformations rendered in the event betray the transitive character of all states of affairs, bodies, substances and entities (see Williams 2008). All bodies (human and nonhuman) are forever becoming, or differing from themselves, according to the events they experience, without ever settling into the ontological security of the substantive. The world is thus comprised of "happenings rather than things, verbs rather than nouns, processes rather than substances" such that becoming ought to be construed as the "deepest dimension of being" (Shaviro 2009: 16–17). It follows, for example, that events don't happen to individual subjects, or put another way, it is not the subject that experiences the event, but rather it is the event that produces the effects of subjectivation in terms of the intensive and extensive individuations all events unleash (see Patton 2006; Robinson 2009). One of the most significant examples of the individuations immanent to the event concerns perception, understood in relation to the diverse perspectives, or points of view, that each event instantiates (Rolli 2009). Deleuze argues that it is wrong to assume that there exists an enduring subject who comes to the event and then gleans a sense or perspective on it. The event, more accurately, releases 'micro-perceptions' (affects and becomings) which enter into relations with bodies in ways that *produce perception* in the comingling of affects and percepts in the event (Deleuze and Guattari 1987: 252–254). Consistent with Deleuze's reading of Hume, perception, established as a point of view onto the event, is composed in innumerable micro-perceptions, intensities and impressions that coalesce in the production of subjectivity, "an impression of reflection and nothing else" (Deleuze 1991: 113, also Rolli 2009: 28–36). Constituted in relations of reflection, it is proper to assert that each event redoubles these processes of reflection such that each event enacts or promotes a *moment of subjectivation* that differs from itself in its repetition (or 'synthesis') from one event to another. The event is "intensive" in this respect. Its "genetic elements" concern the pre-individual singularities or intensities that enable the subjectivation of bodies in the event (Rolli 2009: 29). This is what Deleuze means by the 'pure event'. The pure event is nothing but a series of intensive processes ('magnitudes' or 'singularities') by which affects, percepts, sensations and qualities circulate on a given plane. These intensive qualities are actualised in the event in a series of "extensive" properties, or "persistent objects" (subjects, bodies and spaces), which give the event a recognisable identity as a discrete state of affairs (Rolli 2009: 28–29).

"Sense" provides a further illustration of the transition from the intensive to the extensive within the event. Deleuze's account of sense emphasises the processes or mechanisms by which events generate, produce or express sense, understood as a distinctive form of "significance" or "the way in which meaning matters or makes things matter" (Williams 2008: 3). Deleuze (1990) returns to the Stoic philosophers in order to explain the *production* of sense, noting that the Stoics were the first to reject defining sense purely as an effect of the various representations of events generated in language. For the Stoics, as for Deleuze, the sense or *meaning* of the event is irreducible to the various statements and propositions which purport to express this meaning. Propositions are merely the means by which events are 'actualised' in a specific state of affairs. Yet the pure event always exceeds its actualisations insofar as events are always too intensive, too "aliquid", for the full array of haecceities (affects, percepts, gestures, signs) assembled therein to be captured in the various propositions taken to describe the event (Deleuze 1990: 16–19). Indeed, statements invariably select certain of these haecceities, actualising them in language and thus prefiguring the array of meanings that might reasonably be ascribed to events. Deleuze rejects all representational or denotative accounts of sense for missing the *illocutionary force* of the propositions by which these representations are conveyed. Deleuze (1990: 19) argues instead that sense subsists in the *expressed* of the proposition, understood as "an incorporeal, complex and irreducible entity, at the surface of things, a pure event". The moment of expression conveys the movement from the intensive, 'pure event' and its haecceities, affects and percepts, to the realisation of an extensive state of affairs to which all propositions properly refer. Deleuze (1990: 21–22) thus concludes that while "sense does not exist outside the proposition which expresses it", sense nonetheless remains "the attribute of the thing or state of affairs". Sense is always in the world, both intensive and extensive.

Deleuze's analysis of the relationship between bodies, things, events and sense is further elaborated in his reading of Whitehead. Deleuze's (1993) brief discussion of Whitehead is especially useful for teasing out the implications of "event-thinking" (Fraser 2006) for the wider renovation of subjectivity inaugurated in the search for a transcendental empiricism. Following Whitehead, Deleuze's discussion of the event clarifies the means by which bodies and subjects are incarnated or transformed in relations of becoming according to the specific events they participate in. Whitehead regarded events and becomings as ontologically prior to being, such that the world, subjectivity, experience and nature ought to be reconceived in terms of processes rather than substances (Shaviro 2009: 17). As I have noted, events are always prior to the subjects, objects and entities that experience them, with the event providing the mechanism or process of the subject's becoming. Deleuze (1993: 79) goes on to identify four components or conditions of the event in Whitehead's work; "extensions, intensities, individuals or prehensions, and, finally, eternal objects or 'ingressions'".

'Extension' concerns the variety of extended 'series' that compose individual events, linking them one to another in a potentially infinite chain of antecedent incidents and precursors. Events are, in this sense, never determinate or self-contained in that events always unfold or extend in a series of spatial and temporal movements reaching back into a recursive past and forward into a future shaped by the event's "activity" (Shaviro 2009). James Williams (nd: 4) cites by way of example an injury leading to the contraction of tetanus and ultimately death, asking "where are we to situate the event" described in this scenario. Is the event instantiated in the moment of the original injury? Does it extend forward to the subsequent tetanus infection and the moment of death? What of the prior "refusal of an immunisation booster injection", or the events which led to the "deep fear of needles" that inspired such refusal (Williams nd: 4)? The point is that the spatial and temporal boundaries of an event can never be fixed, given the complexity of the relations that comprise each event and the consequences they unleash. Deleuze (1993: 77), for this reason, describes the event as "an infinite series that contains neither a final term nor a limit". While this contention may risk trapping all of life in one vast, interconnected web of events, without distinction or separation, Deleuze (1993: 80) insists that events have unique "intensive" features that distinguish individual series of events. Intensive features include "height, intensity, timbre of a sound, a tint, a value, a saturation of colour" that are unique to their distinctive actualisation in events. By way of example, Deleuze (1993: 80) reflects on the particular features apprehended in the experience of a concert, such as the "inner qualities" associated with the score, instruments, performers and audience response. These qualities are unique to the moment of their creation, even though they inevitably refer to other series, other events, such as the composition of the score, the training of performers, or the history of the venue.

Attention to the unique, intensive features of the event underscores Deleuze's (1993: 77–79) treatment of the third 'condition' of the event; "the individual". The 'intensive' properties of events are always unique inasmuch as they are new or unprecedented. The event may for this reason be described as a process or mechanism for the production of novelty. Deleuze, following Whitehead, understands novelty to be innately creative and individualising in that events always assemble, mobilise or contain entities, bodies and subjects in ways that render each as *distinctive kinds of individuals* in the moment of their expression in the event.

Such a process turns on Whitehead's notion of prehension. Whitehead's neologism reflects his wider interest in exploring how entities, objects and subjects encounter or affect one another in ways that exceed conscious perception (Shaviro 2009). Perception is, in fact, a very specialised and sophisticated form of prehension, although Whitehead is as interested in the ways stones, plants, stars and animals experience prehensions. All events involve a "nexus" (or convergence) of prehensions, reflecting the array of entities present in the event, and the ways these entities prehend one another. Given that this 'nexus of prehensions' is unique to each event, it follows that the individual, as a distinctive "concrescence" or assemblage of prehensions, is also unique to each event (Deleuze 1993: 77–79). It may be said, therefore, that individuals, whether human or nonhuman, differ from event to event as their prehensions differ, sometimes in subtle, imperceptible ways, sometimes in more profound and significant ways (Shaviro 2009: 28–32). This transformation ensures the distinctiveness of individual events as events take on meaning for the entities so assembled consistent with the unique prehensions they experience in these events.

Whitehead argues further that all events involve the incarnation (or actualisation) of specific "eternal objects" such as colours, sounds, sensations, figures, feelings and abstractions (Deleuze 1993: 79). Eternal objects like red, a circle, musical notes, the sensation of hardness, anger or love exist for Whitehead as "potentialities" that exceed (or outlive) their realisation in particular events (or "actual occasions"). This means that the colour red, for example, may never be exhausted, may never cease to exist, even if, in some unhappy circumstance, all actualisations of red were somehow to disappear. Anger too ought to be regarded as a distinctive, intensive quality that differs from its extensive actualisation in individual bodies. Eternal objects thus help to give individual events a distinctiveness, a definiteness, that serves to further distinguish one series of events from another. Such objects are indispensible features of the event even if they remain incorporeal, ideal or immaterial, "real without being actual" (Deleuze 1988b: 96). Perhaps health too might be regarded as an eternal object that endures at some remove from the individual actualisations (or expressions) of health in individual circumstances. I will develop this idea in later chapters in discussing how the manifold haecceities (affects, bodies, perfects, signs) at play within the event may be manipulated (or counter-actualised) in the work of composing or expressing a distinctive assemblage of health.

2.3 On the Uses of a Transcendental Empiricism

Addressing the utility of empiricism in one of his final essays, Deleuze (2001) described transcendental empiricism as an affirmative exploration of the immanent plenitude of "life" and the swarming multiplicities (the affects and sensations) that invest this life. Life for Deleuze (2001: 29–32) is defined by the relations and associations that are its characteristic modes of composition and becoming. Life is a process, a force of differential and intensive relations, rather than an essence or identity. As such, I have sought throughout this chapter to locate relations and relationality at the epistemological and ontological centre of Deleuze's empiricism. For this is an empiricism that entails "thinking with AND, instead of thinking IS, instead of thinking for IS" (Deleuze and Parnet 1987: 57). Deleuze's empiricism establishes a mode of thinking that eschews the thought or interrogation of static being (the "what is" of life), in favour of a thought of the conjunctive becomings of the *assemblage*. Assemblages ensnare all of life in a web of relations, linking living beings with one another and with the nonhuman entities that populate the territorial "milieus" of this life (Deleuze and Guattari 1987: 313). Affects, relations and events ensure the "openness" of the assemblage to the irruption of new associations that "qualitatively" transform that assemblage's "dynamic nature" (Massumi 2002: 224). Assemblages like life, an individual, a subject, an idea, a concept, are composed in and of relations, and the events, affects and sensations that relations draw together.

It is for these reasons, moreover, that the intensive "intersections" (Jensen and Rödje 2010) that describe the conceptualisation of relations, affects and events within Deleuze's empiricism must be emphasised in any attempt to use or apply his methods. Transcendental empiricism is itself an intensive multiplicity inasmuch as it is the *force of the convergence of concepts within this multiplicity* that accounts for its pragmatic, ontological and epistemological impact. Isolating and removing concepts from this multiplicity greatly reduces their impact, limiting the creative force of individual concepts while eliminating the synergistic insights that follow from the interaction of concepts like relation, affect and event. This is why I have criticised the practice of selectively abstracting concepts from Deleuze's thought, and then redeploying them in the service of novel empirical inquiry. While this approach has no doubt provided a palatable entrée to Deleuze's philosophy among scholars otherwise wary of his appeal, much of the force of Deleuze's concepts is lost in this way. The concepts that comprise transcendental empiricism are bound one to the other in a system of intensive, differential relations (Deleuze 1994: 129–138). Each concept affects, and is affected by, other concepts immanent to this system in the production of thought. Concepts emerge on a plane of immanence (the 'image of thought'); they act together in dissonance and in sympathy, producing the effects of thought, the movement of thinking/living/affecting enacted in the *encounter* with thought (de Beistegui 2010: 5–18). The adoption of Deleuze's concepts thus requires "relating each concept to variables that explain its mutations" (Deleuze 1995: 31), rather than rigid adherence to a definitional logic or the simple application of a rule or theorem. Deleuze's concepts cannot be treated as 'ready-made' tools for empirical inquiry. Each must be assessed in relation to other concepts in Deleuze's system, both to grasp their heterogenetic character (their 'continuous variations') and to extract the maximum ontological and methodological force of their 'acting together'.

The application of Deleuze's empiricism to problems in the health and social sciences must acknowledge this relational quality if the full measure of Deleuze's innovation is to be realised. To this end, it is critical that the assemblage be regarded as both the *proper object and the preferred method* of a minor science of health. It is important that I briefly clarify this methodological point before considering how Deleuze's empiricism may be applied in the renovation of health science research. Deleuze's empiricism necessarily "proceeds to a direct exposition of concepts" (Rajchman 2000: 21) in order to develop a series of openings into (or engagements with) the "conditions of real experience" (Alliez 2004: 112). The methods and concepts necessary to explore these conditions must invariably shift and evolve as the contours of 'real experience' shift and evolve (Rajchman 2000: 21–23). This is another of the reasons why Deleuze's concepts are routinely characterised in terms of their 'heterogenesis' given that the constituent parts that make up concepts are necessarily assembled with the problem/contexts to which they are drawn. Hence, concepts are defined by the work they do in particular contexts, in relation to particular problems, rather than by their logical consistency (Massumi 2010: 10–12). It follows that transcendental empiricism ought to be understood as an intensive multiplicity *that emerges in the event of thought's encounter with the sensible*, with real experience. What's more, each concept immanent to this encounter inevitably affects each other concept within a "method assemblage" as their relations proliferate (Law 2004: 83–85). Deleuze's empiricism is fashioned after the assemblage because the 'real experience' it is concerned to explicate can only be understood in terms of the assemblage. Just as the objects of empirical inquiry are assembled, so too must methods equal to this assemblage be pieced together from varied sources.

As such, the 'thinking together' of relations, affects and events attempted in this chapter provides both a methodological model for investigating assemblages of health, as well as an empirical explanation for how such assemblages are composed, constructed and maintained. Deleuze's empiricism thus establishes both *explanans* and *explanandum* in its treatment of the conditions of real experience. This suggests, more directly, that assemblages of health are composed in distinctive events, affects and relations, whereby diverse elements converge and resonate in the experience of health. It follows that health may reasonably be construed as the product of qualitative relations of force, affect and becoming, "actualised" in events and 'states of affairs' and composed on planes or territories. It is worth briefly noting the manner of this 'actualisation' before examining how assemblages produce qualities or identities like health. Buchanan (2000: 120) argues that assemblages are created in two distinct operations "that logically succeed one another but in actual fact take place simultaneously". The first operation entails an "autonomous process of selection", a "grouping together" of heterogeneous elements. The second involves the "consolidation" of this selection and the "actualization of the potential" effected in the connections and flows created between these consolidated elements (Buchanan 2000: 120–121). The actualization of potential – understood as the release of affect, energy/matter or force in the grouping together of flows/elements – explains the active and autonomous character of assemblages. It also explains why assemblages of health should not be understood as a composite of forces that may somehow be disassembled to reveal each constituent element. On the contrary, assemblages are "intensive multiplicities" insofar as each assembled element is transformed in its relations with other elements such that it no longer makes sense to speak of constituent parts (Deleuze and Parnet 1987: 132). The key is to grasp how each element connects with others in a "constellation of singularities and traits, deducted from the flow" of interactions and processes in life (Deleuze and Guattari 1987: 406).

It is for this reason somewhat misleading to distinguish the constitutive properties of assemblages of health in terms of individual relations, affects and events, for each assemblage is composed in intensive conjunctions that are only intelligible in terms of their assembling or "putting together" (Wise 2005: 77). The active power of assemblages lies, moreover, in the *force* of these events, relations and affects. To understand this power one must consider how events necessarily entail encounters between heterogeneous elements, which combine in intensive relations that generate divergent affects marked by a transition in the perfection or power of acting of each of the elements so assembled. Caroline Williams (2010: 249) provides a useful summary of the relationality that sustains all assemblages of health when she notes that the "relation is literally a 'taking in hand', a production of something that did not exist before and which, through the process of relation, becomes an aspect of that thing's existence". Elements are not folded into some pre-existent entity, in other words, but rather contribute their affective and relational force to the ongoing modification of an assemblage of health in the event of their encounters with it. I want to close this chapter with an assessment of how this logic may be applied in ways that do justice to the "heterogenetic" character of the assemblage. This should also provide a better sense of the methodological promise of Deleuze's empiricism in preparation for the analyses to follow in the two case studies. Anticipating the content of these case studies, I will focus on the character and experience of (human) life and the manner of its expression in an assemblage of health (or illness).

2.4 Towards a 'Minor Science' of Health

Despite widespread engagement with poststructuralist critiques of a naturalised *a priori* subject, most empirical studies in the health and social sciences still endorse traditional ontological assumptions about human life (see Fox 2002; Moore and Fraser 2006; Lupton 1999). As a result, these sciences appear caught between a nostalgic affection for positivism with its assurances of a stable 'objective' reality, and various iterations of constructivism with their bewilderingly "messy" accounts of scientific discourses acting on (or modifying) the realities they supposedly merely describe (see Law 2004: 2–10). This leaves the 'subject' of health caught between its traditional ontological securities and the 'decentrings' of discourse, power and knowledge common to all poststructuralisms (Foucault 1983). Charting a course between these familiar antinomies, Deleuze's empiricism provides a compelling methodological template for the reorientation of studies of health and illness, and the more specific investigation of the production of healthy and ill subjects. In particular, transcendental empiricism provides a means of interrogating the nonhuman, social and structural dimensions of health, and the ways social and structural forces mediate the production of assemblages of health and illness in discrete settings (Fox 2012). Deleuze's empiricism satisfies this goal by indicating how relations, affects and events may serve as the *focus* of empirical research (see also Brown 2010).

Taken together, the analysis of relations, affects and events establishes a pragmatic ontology of subjects, bodies and worlds, of the assemblages that compose them and the diverse becomings by which they are transformed. This logic arguably presents something of a breakthrough in recent attempts to *operationalize* the 'posthuman' subject in empirical research. Hence, to conceive of transcendental empiricism as a methodology that might be applied to diverse problems in the study of health and illness, is to logically prioritise the analysis of the relations, affects and events that express (human) life, however provisionally. The task calls for analysis of the varied extensive parts or simple bodies that make up an assemblage of health. This should, in turn, present some basis for determining the mechanisms (the events, affects and relations) of a body's becoming well or ill, bearing in mind that this body is always, already an assemblage of diverse simple bodies, human and nonhuman. Such an approach suggests the importance of investigating the *ethological composition* of bodies and subjects in order to identify the specific relations, affects and events that enable joyous (or healthy) encounters between bodies, and those that precipitate sad (or unhealthy) relations. Ethology proposes a means of distinguishing between elements, forces or relations that promote the power of acting of a given assemblage of health, and those which decompose or frustrate this power. Extending Deleuze's ethology to include that particular set of relations, affects and events that support a body's health and wellbeing suggests grounds for a *novel empirical study* of health and development that in the next chapter will be called a 'developmental ethology'.

Developmental ethology treats the lived experience of health and illness as a complex of affective and relational transitions within the various assemblages which express human life. This logic can be applied to the study of any event, or set of encounters, by which the health and wellbeing of a particular assemblage is mediated. Following Bruno Latour's (2005) lead, it is arguable that no specific *a priori* criteria are needed to delimit specific 'health-related' events; rather one should 'follow the actors' in assessing the specific relations, affects and events that actors themselves nominate (or reveal) in the process of becoming healthy. Such ambition gestures towards a renewed *empiricism of the body* and its milieus such that the character of health may be refined along with the affects and relations that express it. Health should, in this sense, be understood as a particular modulation of (human) life, produced in an assemblage of relations, affects and events. Deleuze's empiricism provides a means of interrogating this assemblage, rejecting any *a priori* notion of a naturally healthy body. In proposing an "expanded empirical field" (Massumi 2002: 235) for the study of health and illness, Deleuze's work affords a basis for eliciting *positive accounts* of health, highlighting the specific affects, events and relations by which health may be sustained or promoted in 'real experience'.

This expanded empirical field should also enable novel explorations of the (nonhuman) social and structural determinants of health and health inequalities. I noted in the previous chapter that the social and structural dimensions of health were first described in research conducted in the 1970s indicating sharp differences in health outcomes between poorer groups and those with higher social and economic status (Marmot 2005). Subsequent studies have revealed the role of various social, structural and political factors in the production of these health inequalities. As a result of this research, it is now routinely accepted that health is a function not merely of individual biology, or the expression of genetic variance, but of diverse social and political contexts, comprising divergent structural forces, as well (Green and Labonte 2008). Among the most significant structural factors identified thus far are poverty and income inequality; differentials in educational attainment and/or employment security; access to essential services like health care, transport and income support; as well as 'cultural' factors associated with help seeking behaviour, health literacy, and health related beliefs, attitudes and practices (Gorin and Arnold 2006). These factors have each been shown to mediate (or act on) health outcomes, leading to calls for comprehensive public health interventions targeting the social determinants in an effort to improve health outcomes among disadvantaged groups.

Less clear however, are the specific mechanisms by which structures (or contexts) actually mediate health outcomes. In promoting the figure of the assemblage, and by describing the means of the assemblage's composition or emergence, transcendental empiricism provides a means of exploring these mechanisms in the articulation of a novel causal analytics. Yet the first task in any reassessment of the social determinants of health ought to entail the replacement of the notion of context with that of the assemblage. I should think that the notion of 'determinants' will have to go too if the problem of causality is to be properly interrogated. As Deleuze would have it, nothing is *determined* in life, for the events, affects and relations which define it are never closed and rarely linear. It follows that there are no distal factors in the experience of health and contexts are never structural or remote. Entities, bodies, structures or forces participate in health by entering into an assemblage; if they are not involved in this assemblage they cannot be said to affect the health that it expressed or performed in it. There is, as such, no sense distinguishing health problems from their social contexts, for surely the goal of analysis is to properly characterise these problems in terms of the bodies or forces which produce them.

Starting with the relations, affects and events which comprise the assemblage, Deleuze's empiricism establishes a means of tracing the connections by which social processes (bodies and actors) shape the experience of health and illness. Relation by relation, affect by affect, event by event, transcendental empiricism should allow for the documentation of processes that materially impact the health status of individuals and groups, including that bundle of relations, affects and events that constitute 'the social', as well as the more immediate relations typical of 'local' interactions. Each domain is critical to the production and maintenance of assemblages of health and illness, indicating the array of human and nonhuman entities active in the expression of health. The properly empirical task is to investigate a given assemblage to demonstrate how it is composed, and the specific causal mechanisms by which social and/or structural processes enter into it. Social and structural actors must by definition leave a relational and affective trail by which their ingress within the assemblage may be documented. Following this trail will, however, require switching focus from subjects, bodies, structures and contexts to the assemblage proper. Such a move may also yield novel strategies for transforming the range of social and structural factors at work in these assemblages in the interests of promoting health conceived as a property of the entire assemblage. Such at least is the promise of a Deleuzian health science.

Realising this promise will require the articulation of new problems, new challenges and new directions for thought. I would conclude that the most compelling of these directions is Deleuze's exhortation to expose human life to more of its *nonhuman* becomings (Grosz 2011: 26–39). Such a task suggests grounds for significant innovation in the health and social sciences, yet it is also profoundly disruptive of the basic epistemological and methodological assumptions that govern most contemporary research in these fields (Brown 2010). The most important of these disruptions involves the displacement of the subject and meaning-making from the centre of empirical inquiry (Fox 2011: 435–438). In making this point I am not suggesting dispensing altogether with the study of subjectivity and/or hermeneutics in the human sciences. Rather, I wish to propose an alternative set of methodological techniques for the analysis of health and human life. As Deleuze (1994) has so powerfully shown, the subject cannot stand as an ontological and epistemological foundation for empirical inquiry. The subject must itself be explained.

As it stands, the health and social sciences rely far too heavily on a static, obdurate account of subjectivity, even though the 'subject' of health is increasingly regarded as a function of deeper, more elusive social, discursive and relational processes (Mansfield 2000). This settlement introduces great confusion to the study of health and illness, for it is rarely clear what the most appropriate unit of empirical analysis should be (Latour 2005: 27–30). Should one focus on individuals and groups, their experiences, practices and beliefs, or should one explore the mechanisms by which individuals and groups are 'formed', such as discourse, power and socialisation? Is the subject the foundation of theoretical and empirical understanding, or the very abstraction that the human sciences must explain? Even those approaches which ostensibly tackle each side of this dyadic puzzle almost inevitably emphasise one side at the expense of the other (Law 2004: 68–69). Deleuze's empiricism provides a way out of this bind, emphasising the analysis of relations, affects and events in the work of explaining human life and the assemblages in which it is expressed. The task now, to anticipate the work of the next three chapters, is to mobilise Deleuze's conceptual inventions in the design of novel empirical studies of health and illness.

Much remains to be done in the development of this inquiry, yet the discussion here provides some indication of the rudiments of a Deleuzian approach to the study of health and illness. In what may be regarded as a provisional research program for a minor science of health and illness, I should like to recall the various research goals identified earlier in this chapter following the review of existing Deleuzian inspired research in the health and social sciences. First, I stressed the importance of eschewing the subject/object, human/nonhuman and body/society dyads. In their place should stand the figure of the assemblage and the analysis of relations, affects and events required to describe it. Studies of the assemblage's formation, and the actors, entities, bodies, affects, forces and signs active therein, ought to serve as the second research priority for a minor science of health and illness. Determining how health may itself be conceptualised in terms of the assemblage, and the spaces, forces, affects, signs, relations and events by which it is expressed, should stand as the third principal research priority for such a science. Methodologies alert to these three challenges are beginning to emerge in science and technology studies (Latour 2005), psychology (Brown and Stenner 2009), anthropology (Jensen and Rödje 2010), geography (Anderson and Harrison 2010) and sociology (Fox 2012). While the prospect of a Deleuzian health science may seem remote, 'lines of flight' are everywhere apparent in contemporary health and social science research. The next three chapters pursue the most significant of these lines in an attempt to lead the health sciences back to the 'real experience' of (human) life in all its plenitude.

References

Albertsen, N., and B. Diken. 2006. Society with/out organs. In *Deleuze and the social*, ed. M. Fuglsang and B. Sørensen, 231–249. Edinburgh: Edinburgh University Press.

Alliez, E. 2004. *The signature of the world: What is Deleuze and Guattari's philosophy?* London: Continuum.

Anderson, B. 2009. Affective atmospheres. *Emotion, Space & Society* 2(2): 77–81.

Anderson, B., and P. Harrison (eds.). 2010. *Taking place: Non-representational theories and geography*. London: Ashgate.

Anderson, B., M. Kearnes, C. McFarlane, and D. Swanton. 2012. On assemblages and geography. *Dialogues in Human Geography* 2(2): 171–189.

Armstrong, A. 1997. Some reflections on Deleuze's Spinoza: Composition and agency. In *Deleuze and philosophy: The difference engineer*, ed. K. Ansell-Pearson, 44–57. London: Routledge.

Arnold, J., and L. Breen. 2006. Images of health. In *Health promotion in practice*, ed. S. Gorin and J. Arnold, 3–20. London: Wiley.

Audi, R. (ed.) 1995. *The Cambridge Dictionary of Philosophy*. Cambridge: Cambridge University Press.

Avgerou, C., C. Ciborra, and F. Land (eds.). 2004. *The social study of information and communication technology: Innovation, actors and contexts*. Oxford: Oxford University Press.

Bains, P. 2002. Subjectless subjectivities. In *A shock to thought: Expressionism in philosophy and Deleuze and Guattari*, ed. B. Massumi. New York: Routledge.

Barad, K. 2007. *Meeting the universe halfway: Quantum physics and the entanglement of matter and meaning*. Durham: Duke University Press.

Baugh, B. 1992. Transcendental empiricism: Deleuze's response to Hegel. *Man and World* 25(2): 133–148.

Bell, J. 2009. *Deleuze's Hume: Philosophy, culture and the Scottish enlightenment*. Edinburgh: Edinburgh University Press.

Bennett, J. 2010. *Vibrant matter: A political ecology of things*. Durham: Duke University Press.

Blackman, L., and M. Featherstone. 2010. Re-visioning body & society. *Body and Society* 16(1): 1–5.
Bogard, W. 1998. Sense and segmentarity: Some makers of a Deleuzian – Guattarian sociology. *Sociological Theory* 16(1): 52–74.
Bogue, R. 2004. Search, swim and see: Deleuze's apprenticeship in signs and pedagogy of images. *Educational Philosophy and Theory* 36(3): 327–342.
Bonta, M. 2009. Taking Deleuze into the field: Machinic ethnography for the social sciences. *Deleuze Studies* 3(1): 135–142.
Bouchard, D. (ed.). 1980. *Language, counter-memory, practice: Selected essays and interviews by Michel Foucault*. Cornell: Cornell University Press.
Boundas, C. 1991. Translator's introduction. In *Empiricism and Subjectivity: An Essay on Hume's Theory of Human Nature*, ed. G. Deleuze. Trans. C. Boundas. New York: Columbia University Press.
Boundas, C. 1994. Deleuze: Serialization and subject-formation. In *Gilles Deleuze and the theatre of philosophy*, ed. C. Boundas and D. Olkowski. London: Routledge.
Braidotti, R. 1994. *Nomadic subjects: Embodiment and sexual difference in contemporary feminist theory*. New York: Columbia University Press.
Brown, S. 2010. Between the planes: Deleuze and social science. In *Deleuzian intersections: Science, technology and anthropology*, ed. C. Jensen and K. Rödje. Oxford: Berghahn.
Brown, S., and P. Stenner. 2009. *Psychology without foundations: History, philosophy and psychosocial theory*. London: Sage.
Bryant, L. 2008. *Difference and givenness: Deleuze's transcendental empiricism and the ontology of immanence*. Evanston: Northwestern University Press.
Buchanan, I. 1997a. The problem of the body in Deleuze and Guattari, or, what can a body do? *Body and Society* 3(3): 73–91.
Buchanan, I. 1997b. Deleuze and cultural studies. *South Atlantic Quarterly* 96(3): 483–497.
Buchanan, I. 2000. *Deleuzism: A metacommentary*. Durham: Duke University Press.
Colebrook, C. 2002. *Gilles Deleuze*. London: Routledge.
Colebrook, C., and I. Buchanan (eds.). 2000. *Deleuze and feminist theory*. Edinburgh: Edinburgh University Press.
Colwell, C. 1997. Deleuze and the prepersonal. *Philosophy Today* 41(1): 18–23.
Cresswell, T. 2010. Towards a politics of mobility. *Environment and Planning. D, Society and Space* 28(1): 17–29.
De Beistegui, M. 2010. *Immanence: Deleuze and philosophy*. Edinburgh: Edinburgh University Press.
De Landa, M. 2002. *Intensive science and virtual philosophy*. London: Continuum.
De Landa, M. 2006. *A new philosophy of society: Assemblage theory and social complexity*. London: Continuum.
Deleuze, G. 1978. Lecture transcripts on Spinoza's concept of affect (Cours Vincennes 24th January 1978). Published online at http://www.webdeleuze.com/php/sommaire.html. Accessed 15 Mar 2011.
Deleuze, G. 1988a. *Spinoza: Practical philosophy*. San Francisco: City Lights.
Deleuze, G. 1988b. *Bergsonism*. New York: Zone Books.
Deleuze, G. 1990. *The Logic of Sense*. Trans. Mark Lester with C. Stivale. New York: Columbia University Press.
Deleuze, G. 1991. *Empiricism and Subjectivity: An Essay on Hume's Theory of Human Nature*. Trans. C. Boundas. New York: Columbia University Press.
Deleuze, G. 1992. *Expressionism in Philosophy: Spinoza*. Trans. Martin Joughin. New York: Zone Books.
Deleuze, G. 1993. *The fold: Leibniz and the Baroque*. London: Athlone Press.
Deleuze, G. 1994. *Difference and repetition*. London: The Athlone Press.
Deleuze, G. 1995. *Negotiations: 1972–1990*. Trans. Martin Joughin. New York: Columbia University Press.

Deleuze, G. 2001. *Pure Immanence: Essays on a Life*. Trans. Anne Boyman. New York: Zone Books.

Deleuze, G. 2004. *Desert Islands and Other Texts (1953–1974)*. Trans. Mike Taormina. New York: Semiotext(e).

Deleuze, G., and F. Guattari. 1987. *A Thousand Plateaus: Capitalism and Schizophrenia*. Trans. Brian Massumi. Minnesota: University of Minnesota Press.

Deleuze, G., and C. Parnet. 1987. *Dialogues*. London: Athlone Press.

Dewsbury, J. 2011. The Deleuze-Guattarian assemblage: Plastic habits. *Area* 43(2): 148–153.

Duff, C. 2007. Towards a theory of drug use contexts: Space, embodiment and practice. *Addiction Research and Theory* 15(5): 503–519.

Duff, C. 2011. Networks, resources and agencies: On the character and production of enabling places. *Health and Place* 17(1): 149–156.

Fitzgerald, J. 1997. An assemblage of desire, drugs and techno. *Angelaki: Journal of the Theoretical Humanities* 3(2): 41–57.

Foucault, M. 1983. Afterword: The subject and power. In *Michel Foucault: Beyond structuralism and hermeneutics*, 2nd ed, ed. H. Dreyfus and P. Rabinow. Chicago: University of Chicago Press.

Fox, N. 1993. *Postmodernism, sociology and health*. London: Open University Press.

Fox, N. 2002. Refracting 'health': Deleuze, Guattari and body-self. *Health* 6(3): 347–363.

Fox, N. 2011. The ill-health assemblage: Beyond the body-with-organs. *Health Sociology Review* 20(4): 434–446.

Fox, N. 2012. *The body*. Cambridge: Polity Press.

Fraser, M. 2006. Event. *Theory, Culture & Society* 23(2–3): 129–132.

Friedman, J. 1978. An overview of Spinoza's ethics. *Synthese* 37(1): 67–106.

Fuglsang, M., and B. Sørensen (eds.). 2006. *Deleuze and the social*. Edinburgh: Edinburgh University Press.

Gatens, M. 2000. Feminism as 'Password': Re-thinking the 'Possible' with Spinoza and Deleuze. *Hypatia* 15(2): 59–75.

Goodchild, P. 1996. *Deleuze and Guattari: An introduction to the politics of desire*. London: Sage.

Gorin, S., and J. Arnold (eds.). 2006. *Health promotion in practice*. London: Wiley.

Green, J., and R. Labonte (eds.). 2008. *Critical perspectives in public health*. London: Routledge.

Grosz, E. 1994. *Volatile bodies: Towards a corporeal feminism*. Bloomington: Indiana University Press.

Grosz, E. 2005. *Time travels: Feminism, nature, power*. Durham: Duke University Press.

Grosz, E. 2008. *Chaos, territory, art: Deleuze and the framing of the earth*. New York: Columbia University Press.

Grosz, E. 2011. *Becoming undone: Darwinian reflections on life, politics and art*. Durham: Duke University Press.

Haraway, D. 1997. *Modest–Witness@ Second Millennium. FemaleMan meets OncoMouse: Feminism and technoscience*. New York: Psychology Press.

Hardt, M. 1993. *Gilles Deleuze: An apprenticeship in philosophy*. Minneapolis: University of Minnesota Press.

Harrison, P. 2000. Making sense: Embodiment and the sensibilities of the everyday. *Environment and Planning D: Society and Space* 18(4): 497–517.

Hayden, P. 1995. From relations to practice in the empiricism of Gilles Deleuze. *Man and World* 28(3): 283–302.

Hickey-Moody, A. 2007. Little war machines: Posthuman pedagogy and its media. *Journal of Literary & Cultural Disability Studies* 3(3): 273–280.

Hickey-Moody, A. 2009. *Unimaginable bodies: Intellectual disability, performance and becomings*. Rotterdam: Sense Publishers.

Hughes, J. 2011. Pity the meat? Deleuze and the body. In *Deleuze and the body*, ed. I. Buchanan and J. Hughes, 1–6. Edinburgh: Edinburgh University Press.

Jensen, C., and K. Rödje (eds.). 2010. *Deleuzian intersections: Science, technology and anthropology*. Oxford: Berghahn.

Jones, M. 2009. Phase space: Geography, relational thinking, and beyond. *Progress in Human Geography* 33(4): 487–506.

Kuppers, P., and J. Overboe. 2009. Deleuze, disability and difference. *Journal of Literary & Cultural Disability Studies* 3(3): 217–220.

Lash, S. 1984. Genealogy and the body: Foucault/Deleuze/Nietzsche. *Theory, Culture & Society* 2(2): 1–17.

Latour, B. 2005. *Reassembling the social: An introduction to actor-network theory*. Oxford: Oxford University Press.

Law, J. 2004. *After method: Mess in social science research*. London: Routledge.

Law, J. 2009. Actor network theory and material semiotics. In *The New Blackwell companion to social theory*, ed. B. Turner, 141–158. London: Blackwell.

Lee, N., and J. Hassard. 1999. Organization unbound: Actor-network theory, research strategy and institutional flexibility. *Organization* 6(3): 391–404.

Lloyd, G. 2001. *Spinoza: The reception and influence of Spinoza's philosophy*. London: Routledge.

Lupton, D. (ed.). 1999. *Risk and sociocultural theory: New directions and perspectives*. Cambridge: Cambridge University Press.

Malins, P. 2004. Body-space assemblages and folds: Theorizing the relationship between injecting drug user bodies and urban space. *Continuum: Journal of Media and Cultural Studies*. 18(4): 483–495.

Manning, E. 2009. *Relationscapes: Movement, art, philosophy*. Cambridge: MIT Press.

Mansfield, N. 2000. *Subjectivity: Theories of the self from Freud to Haraway*. Sydney: Allen and Unwin.

Marcus, G., and E. Saka. 2006. Assemblage. *Theory, Culture & Society* 23(2–3): 101–106.

Marks, J. 1998. *Gilles Deleuze: Vitalism and multiplicity*. London: Pluto Press.

Marmot, M. 2005. *The status syndrome: How social standing affects our health and longevity*. London: Holt Paperbacks.

Marrati, P. 2006. Time and affects: Deleuze on gender and sexual difference. *Australian Feminist Studies* 21(51): 313–325.

Marston, S., J.P. Jones III, and K. Woodward. 2005. Human geography without scale. *Transactions of the Institute of British Geographers* 30: 416–432.

Massumi, B. 2002. *Parables for the virtual: Movement, affect, sensation*. Durham: Duke University Press.

Massumi, B. 2010. What concepts do: Preface to the Chinese translation of a thousand plateaus. *Deleuze Studies* 4(1): 1–15.

Mitchell, D. 1996. Postmodernism, health and illness. *Journal of Advanced Nursing* 23(1): 201–205.

Mol, A. 2002. *The body multiple: Ontology in medical practice*. Durham: Duke University Press.

Moore, D., and S. Fraser. 2006. Putting at risk what we know: Reflecting on the drug-using subject in harm reduction and its political implications. *Social Science & Medicine* 62(12): 3035–3047

Patton, P. 2000. *Deleuze and the political*. London: Routledge.

Patton, P. 2006. The event of colonisation. In *Deleuze and the contemporary world*, ed. I. Buchanan and A. Parr, 108–124. Edinburgh: Edinburgh University Press.

Pile, S. 2010. Emotions and affect in recent human geography. *Transactions of the Institute of British Geography* 35(1): 5–20.

Probyn, E. 2004. Teaching bodies: Affects in the classroom. *Body and Society* 10(4): 21–43.

Rajchman, J. 2000. *The Deleuze connections*. Cambridge: MIT Press.

Roberts, M. 2005. Time, human being and mental health care: An introduction to Gilles Deleuze. *Nursing Philosophy* 6(3): 161–173.

Robinson, K. (ed.). 2009. *Deleuze, Whitehead, Bergson: Rhizomatic connections*. New York: Palgrave MacMillan.

Rolli, M. 2009. Deleuze on intensity differentials and the being of the sensible. *Deleuze Studies* 3(1): 26–53.

Semetsky, I. 2004. Experiencing Deleuze. *Educational Philosophy and Theory* 36(3): 227–231.

Semetsky, I. 2010. The folds of experience, or: Constructing the pedagogy of values. *Educational Philosophy and Theory* 42(4): 476–488.

Shaviro, S. 2009. *Without criteria: Kant, Whitehead, Deleuze and Aesthetics*. Cambridge: MIT Press.

Sismondo, S. 2010. *An introduction to science and technology studies*, 2nd ed. Oxford: Wiley/Blackwell.

Smith, D. 2010. Deleuze: Concepts as continuous variation. *Journal of Philosophy: A Cross-Disciplinary Inquiry* 5(11): 57–60.

Smith, D. 2012. *Essays on Deleuze*. Edinburgh: Edinburgh University Press.

Stengers, I. 2011. *Thinking with whitehead: A free and wild creation of concepts*. Harvard: Harvard University Press.

Thrift, N. 1999. Steps to an ecology of place. In *Human geography today*, ed. D. Massey, J. Allen, and P. Sarre, 295–323. Cambridge: Polity Press.

Thrift, N. 2007. *Non-representational theory: Space, politics, affect*. London: Routledge.

Tucker, I. 2010. Mental health service user territories: Enacting 'safe spaces' in the community. *Health* 14(4): 434–448.

Turner, B. 2008. *The body & society: Explorations in social theory*, 3rd ed. London: Sage.

Vitellone, N. 2010. Just another night in the shooting gallery? The syringe, space and affect. *Environment and Planning D: Society and Space* 28: 867–880.

Viveiros de Castro, E. 2010. Intensive filiation and demonic alliance. In *Deleuzian intersections: Science, technology and anthropology*, ed. C. Jensen and K. Rödje. Oxford: Berghahn.

Williams, J. 2005. *Understanding poststructuralism*. London: Acumen.

Williams, J. 2008. *Gilles Deleuze's logic of sense: A critical introduction and guide*. Edinburgh: Edinburgh University Press.

Williams, C. 2010. Affective processes without a subject: Rethinking the relation between subjectivity and affect with Spinoza. *Subjectivity* 3(3): 245–262.

Williams, J. ND. *Deleuze, Whitehead, Stengers: The Fold, the Leibniz lectures and the free and wild creation of concepts*. Unpublished Manuscript. Available at: http://www.dundee.ac.uk/media/dundeewebsite/philosophy/documents/williams/Deleuze_Whitehead_Stengers.pdf. Accessed 22 Mar 2012.

Wise, J. 2005. Assemblage. In *Gilles Deleuze: Key concepts*, ed. C. Stivale, 77–87. Toronto: Queens University Press.

Zembylas, M. 2007. The specters of bodies and affects in the classroom: A rhizo-ethological approach. *Pedagogy, Culture & Society* 15(1): 19–35.

Chapter 3
Health, Ethology, Life

Slowly, the ideas and concepts conveyed in Deleuze's mature philosophy are being absorbed in contemporary health debates (Fox 2011). The faltering dynamics of this engagement are striking given the extensive treatment of Deleuze's oeuvre in most social science disciplines, including those studies reviewed in the previous chapter. Despite the centrality of affect, desire and embodiment to Deleuze's thinking, and the salience of these concerns in much contemporary analysis of health and human development (Tucker 2012: 772–775; Fox 2011: 435–437), the emergence of a distinctly Deleuzian health science remains uncertain. The ambivalence of this reception is likely a reflection of the diversity of Deleuze's thought and the strange complexion of so many of his ideas. Yet as I have argued in each of the previous chapters, Deleuze's empiricism affords a host of intellectual resources for the study of health and illness. Rejoining this argument, the present chapter offers a minor science of health and human development modelled on Deleuze's 'biophilosophy' (Ansell Pearson 1999). This will first entail a *pragmatic reconceptualisation of health,* and a discussion of how it may be used to guide research innovation across the health and social sciences. To this end, I will focus on assessing how Deleuze's empiricism may inspire novel accounts of the processes, events, affects and relations by which bodies, signs and technologies converge in the formation of assemblages of health and illness. Conceiving of health in these terms will require greater acknowledgment of the force of organic and non-organic life, the human and the nonhuman, and the role each plays in the becomings that transform embodied experience (Grosz 2011).

Building on the review of Deleuze's empiricism offered in the previous chapter, the present chapter is concerned to elucidate the characteristic features of assemblages of health and illness; the varied processes by which such assemblages are formed; and the ways health itself should be construed, maintained and promoted. Analysis of each of these issues will further indicate how Deleuze's unique refiguring of (human) life may inspire novel lines of inquiry in the health sciences. In the first chapter I noted that Deleuze effectively distributes (or spatialises) human life in and among diverse assemblages of matter, force, affect and technology. This suggests that the embodied subject is more like a network, or a collocation of

C. Duff, *Assemblages of Health: Deleuze's Empiricism and the Ethology of Life*,
DOI 10.1007/978-94-017-8893-9_3,

interacting associations, than a discrete ontological 'fact' (Latour 2004: 206–214). However, it is not yet clear how this distributed body/subject may be regarded as either healthy or ill; or how the assemblages which effect this distribution may be manipulated in an effort to promote health. What in other words is the proper object of a 'minor science' of health and illness? The primary conjecture underpinning the analysis offered below – and in each of the case studies to follow – is that the subject of contemporary biomedical research is a cultural and ideological artifact; a product of scientific reflection rather than a discrete feature of the 'real' (see also De Landa 2002; Grosz 2011; Law 2004). The philosophers of science Bruno Latour (2004), Annemarie Mol (2002) and Nikolas Rose (2007), among others, insist that biomedicine necessarily *creates a stable body* in the course of ontologically and epistemologically securing the objects of its analysis. This is not to deny that such processes are scientifically important. It is rather to insist that the conceptualisations of embodiment advanced in contemporary biomedicine do not exhaust the range of ontological suppositions that might profitably explain the character of human life, or embodied experience, however defined.

So how else may the subject of health and illness be construed? And what advantages might follow from the work of expanding our ontological command of the body and its ailments and capacities? This chapter offers a necessarily speculative account of the ways empirical inquiry in the health sciences may orient itself to a *posthuman, distributed and relational body/subject* (Law 2007: 597–600). As traditional ontological distinctions separating body and world, human and nonhuman, subject and object recede, the benefit of a Deleuzian account of health and embodiment arguably lies in the development of rival ontological and epistemological suppositions to guide research innovation in the health and social sciences (see also Fox 2011). Such is the posthuman challenge that Deleuze's biophilosophy, and the empiricism which supports it, may assist the health sciences to negotiate. I would add that the most interesting aspect of this challenge concerns the need to rethink the relationship between 'body' and 'society', 'agency' and 'structure', 'nature' and 'culture'. Efforts to overturn these epistemological pairings are a feature of research innovation across the health and social sciences, although each such science still subsists on the epistemic distinction of biology and culture; on the idea that bodies in their discrete facticity both act and are acted upon by an equally discrete cast of social or cultural 'actors' (Mol and Law 2004: 54–59). Despite the apparent self-evidence of the ontological distinction of humans and nonhumans (subjects and objects), scholars in various disciplines are beginning to question this distinction for its failure to accommodate the imbrications of biology, culture, media and technology that characterise 'technoscience' in the twenty-first century (Grosz 2011; Rose 2007). While I am not suggesting that Deleuze's empiricism may finally resolve the antinomy of subjects and objects, I would argue nonetheless that Deleuze provides a fresh conceptual vocabulary for rethinking the relationship between the human and the nonhuman, body and society, biology and culture in explicitly posthuman terms.

These should not be primarily theoretical or speculative reflections either, for Deleuze's biophilosophical account of (human) life should help inspire novel empirical studies of enduring health problems like mental illness and addiction, as the next two chapters will demonstrate (see also Fitzgerald 2009; Tucker 2010). The source of this innovation lies in Deleuze's articulation of a relational methodology capable of explaining the physical, social, political and experiential dimensions of health and illness. Calls for the establishment of novel relational methodologies have been a feature of epistemological debates in the health and social sciences for many years (Dewsbury 2011; Cummins et al. 2007). In each instance, scholars have called for methodologies capable of isolating and explaining the ramifying causal pathways that underpin complex health problems (Hollway 2008: 14–45). Despite the ongoing appeal of Foucault's genealogical technique, a number of scholars have recently turned to Deleuze's work in the search for a properly relational method (Dewsbury 2011: 149–151). Deleuze's account of the relationality of (human) life, and its composition in assemblages of affect, desire, practice and habit, highlights the mutually reinforcing associations that enmesh bodies in diverse physical, psychical, social and political milieus (Fox and Ward 2008: 1008). This account yields important insights into the experience of the 'person in context' and the varied associations that materially and affectively conjoin person and place, body and society. Steven Cummins and colleagues (2007: 1825) have recently argued for the "expansion of theoretical and empirical work investigating the role of contextual factors in the production and maintenance of health variation". Deleuze's treatment of the assemblages by which place, culture and politics are organised offers a far richer model of social context than is typically available in contemporary public health research. Similarly, Deleuze's account of territorialisation and deterritorialisation ought to afford a radical rethinking of the links between health and place. This chapter explores each of these themes, further indicating how the methods canvassed in Chap. 2 may be applied to the study of health and illness.

In developing this analysis, I will draw heavily from Deleuze's reading of the early Modern philosopher Baruch Spinoza. Deleuze's exegesis of Spinoza's central works provides a new way of conceptualising embodiment and the manner of the body's organisation in the "singular, partial or 'molecular' experiences" that give form to immanent life (Colebrook 2002: 82; see also Buchanan 1997: 79–83). As I noted in the previous chapter, Spinoza argues that a body's manifold encounters transform its affects and capacities, understood as expressions of that body's "power of acting" (Deleuze 1992: 225). Capacities (or powers) are not innate properties of (human) life but rather emerge in the body's disjunctive "enfolding" of diverse human and nonhuman milieus (Deleuze and Guattari 1987). This analysis highlights the emplacement or "embeddedness" of health and human development, and the importance of an *ethology* of affects, events and relations in the course of this development (Protevi 2010: 170–179). Keith Ansell-Pearson (1999: 2) adds that Deleuze's ethology advances empiricism "'beyond' the human condition", incorporating organic and "inorganic life" and thereby "opening up the human experience to a field of alterity". And yet Deleuze's ethology, like his empiricism, does not abandon 'human life', but rather seeks to expose it to more of the "inhuman", "nonhuman" and/or "superhuman" forces, affects and events that compose the 'human'. Deleuze (1994) argues that such a shift is essential for the work of founding a posthuman ethical practice capable of "expanding the horizons" of the human condition, "intensifying experience" and exposing human life to the force of its nonhuman ("more than human") becomings (see also Ansell Pearson 1999: 64–75).

The present chapter introduces the notion of a *developmental ethology* in the course of elaborating Deleuze's contributions to the study of health and human development. Taken from a Deleuzean perspective, health and development will be characterised as discontinuous processes of affective and relational change, whereby health is advanced in the provision of new affective sensitivities and new relational capacities. This analysis is broadly consistent with existing models of health and human development – particularly those associated with Amartya Sen's capabilities model (Alkire 2005: 115–116) – with the advantage of offering a more viable working theory of the ways developmental competencies are acquired, cultivated and maintained. Consistent with Deleuze's ethological account of bodies, spaces and territories, I will argue that *events, affects and relations* constitute the basic mechanisms by which developmental capacities are acquired or exchanged in encounters between bodies, and between bodies, worlds and contexts. This contention gives rise to a series of novel research problems, some of which will be reviewed below by way of conclusion. I will start, however with a brief review of more traditional definitions of health and human development, identifying various ontological and epistemological problems in these models and indicating how the application of Deleuze's ethology may help to resolve them. My goal is to generate a Deleuzian account of health and human development to guide the analysis offered in the two case studies to follow.

3.1 What Is Health and (Human) Development?

Attempts to define health – and its positive and substantive expression in the lived experience of the human animal – are as old as medicine itself (Blaxter 2004). The question has inspired philosophers, theologians, ethicists and scientists in every age, while the duty to attend to the "proper functioning" of the body, its ailments and dysfunctions, endures as a distinctive "practice of the self" observable in almost all cultures and historical contexts (Foucault 1985; Greco 2009). Still, it is arguable that the problem of defining health has latterly become even more difficult, as the very idea of health has evolved to include a litany of biological, genetic, physiological, psychical, social, cultural, political and economic phenomena (Metzl 2010; Lupton 1995). No longer can health be regarded as the sole province of the biological organism; as a measure of the fitness or due functioning of the 'body proper' (Metzl and Herzig 2007). Instead, health today is 'over-coded' with ever more redoubtable moral, ethical, ideological and philosophical connotations. As I argued in the first chapter, health is both a normalising index of the body's adherence to (or departure from) the norms of a scientifically hypostasized biology, as well as a normative injunction; a moral imperative to be well, to live in certain ways, and to comport the body in a manner befitting its genetic, cultural and physical inheritance. For many of these reasons, Monica Greco (2009) has recently described health as a kind of 'meta-value' central to the project of civil, cultural and economic governance in the West. Governmentality in the "health-society" relies upon a sometimes explicit, sometimes tacit "right to health" that functions as a revised social contract binding the governed and the governing (Greco 2009: 18–21). As such, health has become alternatively a verifiable 'fact' of the organismal body; a political value; a cultural norm; a set of desirable aesthetic qualities; and/or a suite of corporeal properties or characteristics. Health is, indeed, "indeterminate" in this diversity (Greco 2004: 6–9).

Perhaps it has always been this way. More commonly however, health has been defined simply enough as the absence of disease, illness, malady or dysfunction (Blaxter 2004). The idea that health may be defined in the negative – primarily in terms of the *failure to observe* a discrete set of ailments or conditions (Foucault 1973: ix–xi) – neatly dispenses, of course, with the challenge of identifying the ends to which health itself may aspire. Illness and dysfunction are readily discernible according to the deviations they describe from what might be regarded as 'normal functioning', even though efforts to determine the precise biological character of 'normal functioning' have mainly been in vain (Greco 2009). In other words, the study of illness seems only incidentally to elucidate the nature of health. Enduring focus on the etiology of illness is significant in that it serves to establish health as a normative moral category – something to which all bodies ought to strive – at the same time as it relentlessly dictates the criteria by which designated bodies may be regarded as failing this normative test. Almost by definition, illness is regarded as a diminution or failure of the body proper, such that the 'ill' are commonly regarded as somehow deficient (or 'incomplete') compared to the 'well' (Manderson 2011: 93–96). And so being 'healthy' is conflated with being 'normal'; the 'norm' with the 'normative' (Greco 2009: 27–29). In the absence of substantive definitions, and in the preponderance of the negative, health becomes a kind of 'empty signifier' into which all manner of normative judgements may be invested. If this analysis seems overly cynical – or worse, dismissive of the wealth of technological and creative industry manifest in contemporary biomedicine, and the significant alleviation of suffering that such industry enables – the point is merely to observe the shortcomings associated with the propensity to define health in the negative (see also Arnold and Breen 2006: 5–6). This negativity has directed medicine towards the pragmatic investigation of illness and disease, and the invention of a panoply of technological, clinical and palliative interventions designed to arrest this 'disorder', even though each course has transformed the body into a kind of biological automaton; a discrete "physico-chemical system" (Arnold and Breen 2006: 5). It follows that health must logically be defined according to the functional or adaptive efficiency of this biological system, and not in ways that presume to divine the ends towards which such a system may tend (Blaxter 2004: 16–19). Biomedicine, in this sense, has little to say about the teleology of health, or the art of living, and so cannot meaningfully contribute to discussions about the *value* of health (see Greco 2009; Metzl 2010).

Of course, vibrant denunciations of the reductionist habits of biomedicine are a feature of contemporary debates across the health and social sciences, often leading to the search for more productive grounds for the study of health and illness. Recent interest in 'resiliency', 'thriving', 'strengths' and 'self-efficacy', amid a broader concern for the *quality of life*, are each indications of this effort to derive positive definitions to guide research and practice (see Dawson 2009). A number of scholars have been particularly drawn to the study of wellbeing – and its characteristic qualities, properties and effects – as a way of accounting for the positivities of health (Sen 2006). This task has typically involved the analytical privileging of 'balance', 'capacitation', 'empowerment', 'functionality', 'growth', 'development' and 'fitness' in assessments of the sources and features of wellbeing (see Arnold and Breen 2006; Blaxter 2004). A common goal has been to clarify the ways wellbeing is experienced as a *resource or capacity* by which individuals may determine the purpose of life. Much of this research has been informed by Amartya Sen's (1999) increasingly seminal treatment of freedom and human development. In reframing wellbeing as potentially "anything a person may value doing or being" (Sen 1999: 75), Sen shifts the focus of analysis from the quantifiable and/or objective status of the organism to the qualitative and/or subjective value of life as it is progressively lived (see also Alkire 2002). A number of scholars have recently drawn from this approach to argue that empowerment, development and wellbeing ought to be regarded as critical determinants of health, serving also as proxies by which health may be measured or assessed (see Blaxter 2004 for a review). According to this view, health must be understood as an always unfinished "project" or "work" which requires for its ongoing satisfaction varied resources, abilities, skills and relationships (Tengland 2007: 206).

The consequences of this reconceptualisation of health are at least twofold. First, the attempt to yield more positive definitions exposes health to a range of social, cultural, economic and political contexts. No longer confined to the epidemiology of bodies, populations, vectors and hosts, health must be reconceived as *a social and political artifact* insofar as the resources, capacities and opportunities necessary to maintain health are understood to be unevenly distributed throughout society (see Baum 2008; Scriven and Garman 2007). Health is politicised in other words. Secondly, in the search for more positive conceptualisations, health is converted into a subjective, rather than primarily normalising, value or quality. Individuals are encouraged or "empowered" to "realize their own health aims" with less interest in clarifying what these aims should or ought to be (Arnold and Breen 2006: 3). Perhaps the most obvious and far-reaching manifestation of this concern for empowerment is the concomitant valorisation of wellbeing noted above. Often simply eliding health and wellness, scholars in public health in particular have taken to regarding the purpose of health care to be the ongoing promotion of wellbeing, however poorly defined. Indeed, this position is enshrined in the World Health Organisation's (1986: 1) celebrated Ottawa Charter, and its characterisation of health as a "resource for everyday life, not the objective of living".

Notable here is the characterisation of health as an instrumental resource, divorced from any consideration of the "objective" purpose to which this resource investment ought to be oriented. Health is something to be used (or enjoyed) in the subjective pursuit of life goals, which themselves need not necessarily concern health professionals (see also Sen 1999). Whatever may result from the pursuit of life goals objectively or practically injurious to the maintenance of health and wellbeing is, of course, routinely neglected. My point is that the conflation of health and wellbeing, while extending the analysis of health beyond the objective verifications of biomedical science, commonly serves to forestall discussion by substituting the notion of health with more or less cognate synonyms such as functionality, fitness or freedom. Suggesting that health in its substantive expression ought to be reconceived in terms of wellbeing, resiliency, empowerment, freedom or growth is a kind of artful prestidigitation that leaves open the problem of determining how empowerment is lived as a quantum improvement in one's health; the kinds of 'personal growth' that are health-related; how freedom is related to wellbeing or how one's relationship to particular settings or contexts promotes health.

If much of the substantive character of health remains obscured in recent discussions of wellbeing, empowerment and/or functionality, a very different picture emerges in the narrower study of human development. This study offers important insights into the characteristic features of health and wellbeing, insofar as the study of human development is concerned to reveal the ecological advantages of "adaptive fit" (Arnold and Breen 2006: 10–12). Most contemporary models position human development as an always unfinished process of communication and exchange between bodies and environments (Sigelman and Rider 2011: 30–35). Human development is said to proceed in a series of *functional adaptations* that extend the organism's "scope of activity" (Sen 1999: 39–51), serving in turn as an index of the organism's responsiveness to adaptive pressures within its environment (Lerner 2002). This kind of approach lends itself to the more discrete study of "human flourishing", and the particular environmental, genetic and/or ecological conditions that support the acquisition of novel developmental capacities (Deneulin and Shahani 2009). Endorsed, for example, in Sen's (1999) aforementioned "capabilities approach" it follows that health may be understood as the sum effect of the adaptive advantages enacted in the acquisition of new capacities (Alkire 2002: 184–193). Health, in this sense, is what capacities enable individuals and groups to 'do' or 'be' (Sen 1999: 74–76). It is notable that the ideas of health and development become almost interchangeable in this account, with health serving as the putative function of positive development conceived as the acquisition of new capacities which extend an individual's scope of activity. Taken together, then, the study of health and human development advances beyond traditional understandings of the physical or biological maturation of the organism to include a range of contextual factors that are said to be essential for that organism's 'normal functioning' (Rogoff 2003). Human development must not, therefore, be regarded as the mere unfolding of some innate biological code, but rather entails the dynamic convergence of various "cultural, historical, biological and ideological processes"

(Colby 1996: 327). All of which suggests that human development should be understood to involve the *ontogenetic interaction* of biology and environment, and the effects of this interaction on health and wellbeing across the life-course (Keller et al. 2002: 384–388).

Such conclusions are a central feature of Sen's capabilities model, and his conviction that human development involves the ongoing acquisition (and/or divestment) of social, cognitive, emotional, physical and moral capacities within a web of social, cultural and biological interactions (Sen 1999; see also Cattell et al. 2008; Rogoff 2003). Indeed, almost all contemporary understandings of human development now include various social and moral phenomena – such as the maintenance of social networks, the creative role of self-expression, and the development of practical reason – in addition to more traditional objects of inquiry such as physical and/or biological development (Alkire 2002: 187–189). Encompassing therefore the genetic and the epigenetic, the biological and the cultural, human development is increasingly regarded as a complex process involving the acquisition and ongoing cultivation of *a mix of capabilities*, and the social, cultural, environmental and biological processes or conditions that support this functional capacitation. More specifically, the process by which individuals cultivate specific capabilities may be described as developmental insofar as it entails "organised or systematic" transformations in that individual's "characteristic functioning" (Lerner 2002: 16).

Human development entails a "qualitative change in organization rather than a quantitative increment" such that development must be distinguished from the mere fact of ageing, or organismal "growth" (Colby 1996: 333). Qualitative changes are developmental to the extent that they entail a distinctive chronological trajectory in which "changes seen at a later time are at least in part influenced by changes that occurred at an earlier time" (Lerner 2002: 16). Development is recursive in this sense but that does not mean that it is linear or uni-directional, or that development always entails movement from simpler to more complex forms of organisation. Development involves a continuous modification of one's capacities and relationships, sometimes in ways that involve an increase in such capacities, sometimes in ways that involve a decrease, and sometimes in both senses at once. Whereas earlier models of human development posited neat, sequential stages of development, always from simpler to more complex forms, contemporary accounts emphasise the dynamic and contingent character of human development in specific contexts (see Keller et al. 2002: 392–396). As noted, a feature of this shift away from sequential models of development has been the identification of various developmental domains in excess of strictly biological or physiological aspects (see Nussbaum and Sen 1993). Alkire (2002: 182–183) observes that most contemporary models of human development share this logic, despite considerable divergence of emphasis and terminology. As such, human development is increasingly regarded as a nonlinear process that transpires in *social, emotional, cognitive, physical* and *moral* domains or contexts at the same time. Alkire (2002: 186) adds that these overlapping or concurrent domains are "non-hierarchical, irreducible, incommensurable and hence (constitute) basic kinds of human ends".

Turning briefly to consider the character of these developmental domains, recent accounts of social development emphasise the acquisition of diverse interpersonal skills necessary for the maintenance of 'pro-social' personal and peer relationships; for solving interpersonal conflict; for planning for the future; for setting goals, and for modulating one's behaviour to achieve these goals (Linley and Joseph 2004). Social development may also refer to the cultivation of "prosocial and health-enhancing values and beliefs" (Catalano et al. 2004: 103). Emotional development refers to the capacity for self-reflection and empathy that underpins the capacity to "form attachments to things and persons outside ourselves" (Nussbaum cited in Alkire 2002: 188). It entails the capacity to accurately identify and respond to feelings and emotional reactions in oneself and others, and to manage these feelings and reactions in reducing stress and maximising contentment. Social and emotional competencies are, in turn, vital for the maintenance of peer relationships and the broader organisation of human communities (Payton et al. 2000). Hence, the acquisition of social and emotional competencies is regarded as essential to both health and human development in that each ultimately determines the extent to which individuals are able to avail themselves of the varied developmental resources available in their community (Jessor et al. 1996). The acquisition of social competencies is both a "basic kind of human end", as Alkire (2002: 186) insists, and a mechanism or resource by which other kinds of developmental competencies may be realised (see also Payton et al. 2000).

Cognitive development includes the range of analytical skills necessary for effective problem solving, as well as the planning and decision-making involved in formal intellectual development and/or academic achievement. It also refers to the more subtle processes of self-awareness, reflection and contemplation central to the maintenance of positive personal identity and self-respect (Nussbaum and Sen 1993). Cognitive competencies also describe the kinds of practical reasoning that underpin everyday habits, practices and social interactions (Alkire 2002). This includes the mastery of both verbal and non-verbal communication, and the physical and/or action oriented competencies required to execute personal action decisions. In what is still perhaps the most familiar aspect of human development, the notion of physical development refers primarily to observable changes in the functional structure and physiological character of the human organism as it ages (Lerner 2002). More broadly, the idea of physical competencies concerns the acquisition of those skills deemed by any given community to be central to the basic character of everyday life including mobility and comportment, the maintenance of health and safety, security, sustenance and nutrition, hygiene and the maintenance of "bodily integrity" (Nussbaum cited in Alkire 2002: 188). An interest in physical competence is also a hallmark of epigenetic accounts of human development, which tend to highlight the role of material conditions in physical developmental, insofar as the material environment mediates or "regulates" gene expression (Francis 2011: 1–9). The notion of material development is, in this way, strongly linked to the kinds of physical and/or biological maturation common to more traditional conceptions of human development. Yet material development should also be taken to include the acquisition of skills and competencies necessary to transform or modify one's material circumstances (Sen 1999: 3–12). This includes the capacity to participate in political processes concerning the production and distribution of material resources, and the various ways resources are differentially allocated or utilised (Lerner 2002).

Finally, moral development involves the "ability to assess and respond to the ethical, affective or social-justice dimensions of a situation" (Catalano et al. 2004: 105). It concerns the development of normative judgements about the world and the capacity to distinguish between divergent normative claims. Moral development has sometimes been described as the highest accomplishment of human endeavour, permitting individuals to transcend the dictates of biology and circumstance in the generation of a moral philosophy to guide industry, expression and contemplation (Nussbaum and Sen 1993). Wary of the temptation to rank the relative significance of the various domains of human development noted above, it may be safer to observe that where individuals and groups report high levels of self-efficacy in relation to either social, emotional, cognitive, physical and/or moral development, they also tend to report high levels of subjective wellbeing, or 'healthy' development.

The question of how these varied social, emotional, cognitive, physical and moral competencies are *acquired* is the subject of considerable inquiry and debate (Bronfenbrenner 2005). Most scholars agree that developmental competencies are acquired or cultivated through the individual's active engagement with their social, political and/or cultural environment (Sen 1999; Thiers and Travers 2005). Richard Lerner (2002: 45) for example, stresses that the relationship between the individual and their social context "constitutes the basic process of human development". This relationship determines the array of developmental opportunities that are available to individuals and groups, with greater levels of engagement associated with greater human development. Practical links between social context and development may be observed in the varied social, emotional and behavioural interactions individuals experience as part of everyday life, as well as discrete environmental factors which serve as the effective context for these interactions (Linley and Joseph 2004). They are equally discernible in the ecological relationships that support (or fail to support) the organism's physiological development, such as diet and caloric availability, physical activity, immunological development, the presence and absence of pathogens in the environment and the organism's antigenic responses to them, and so on (see Francis 2011; Polan and Taylor 2007). In this respect, all developmental competencies are a function of specific processes of *socialisation, enculturation and biological interaction* with different cultural and ecological contexts providing different kinds of developmental support (Jessor et al. 1996). Beyond the basic biology of the organism's exposure to its environment, cultural contexts known to impact human development range from formal settings such as the family, education, training and the workplace, through to more private contexts and the rich array of interactions that support social and emotional development (Payton et al. 2000; Rogoff 2003). This is not to deny the political and economic *structuration* of developmental opportunities and their unequal distribution; it is rather to highlight the contention that all developmental processes are a function of an individual's engagement in and with their social and physical environment (Francis 2011).

Yet the *nature of this engagement* – and its specific character in specific settings – is much less clearly delineated in the existing literature. The development of physiological capacities, for example, is almost always treated as a kind of autonomic *fait accompli* (Sigelman and Rider 2011). While physical development may potentially be disrupted or retarded in the face of environmental obstacles, in otherwise "normal" circumstances physical development is regarded as a "natural" response to extant "internal" and "external" stimuli (Polan and Taylor 2007: 55–57). Meanwhile, most accounts of the acquisition of cultural competencies rely on a simple model of socialisation, or social learning theory, in which individuals adopt with varying degrees of success the capabilities modelled for them in their social milieus (Rogoff 2003: 3–24). The acquisition of social, moral and/or emotional competencies is, in this sense, presented as a kind of mimetic achievement, which remains dependent on the stock of developmental resources available in any given setting. Yet, it is arguable that much of the literature in which these kinds of claims appear presents the acquisition of developmental competencies as a taken for granted function of social life; as an inevitable product of "positive" social interaction and "positive" community engagement (see Catalano et al. 2004: 98–105; Modell 1996: 493–501; Rogoff 2003: 3–5). While the specific developmental competencies derived from this engagement may differ from one context to another, the *mechanism of developmental capacitation* is either ignored, or held to remain constant across all settings. There is no doubt some value in existing accounts of the acquisition of developmental competencies, and the role of socialisation in particular. However, I would argue that a much fuller treatment of the *specific mechanisms* of this acquisition promises fresh insights into the broad dynamics of human development.

Deleuze's transcendental empiricism provides considerable methodological support for the development of this inquiry. Deleuze's elaboration of the work of Baruch Spinoza suggests that human development proceeds according to the individual's idiosyncratic encounters, and the affects and relations that these encounters afford. Furthermore, the realisation of developmental capacities is akin to Spinoza's account of the body's acquisition of 'external parts' (described in the previous chapter), and the ways these parts transform the body's affective and relational capacities, or its power of acting. Deleuze's work is also consonant with research regarding the contextualisation of human development, and the ways development advances and stalls in response to particular features of place or context (see Jessor et al. 1996). In each of these respects, Deleuze's reading of Spinoza draws attention to the *relational composition* of health and human development in diverse social, political, biological and material processes, while also indicating grounds for the development of more theoretically refined methodologies for the analysis of this development (on the need for such methodologies see Cummins et al. 2007: 1826–1828). At the same time however, and as I have noted in previous chapters, Deleuze's mature philosophy disrupts most conventional understandings of the 'human', as well as associated notions of the 'individual', the 'body' and 'subjectivity', which remain central to the study of health and development. Applying Deleuze's methods to the study of health and human development will therefore require a kind of 'erasure' of the 'human', the 'body' and the 'individual' in order to achieve a more *molecular understanding* of the activity of life in its becoming (Grosz 2011: 28–39). Indeed, one must suspend the notion of the 'human' in human development in order to reveal more of the molecular movement (or 'becomings') by which life exceeds itself in the transformation of being. Such a suspension recalls Derrida's (1997: xiv) deconstructive erasures, whereby terms regarded as inaccurate or misleading, though without adequate substitution, are crossed through, or "placed under erasure". And so "since the word is inaccurate, it is crossed out. Since the word is necessary, it remains legible" (Derrida 1997: xiv). Without conceiving of the gesture in quite these terms, Deleuze's thought too elicits a suspension of the human with far reaching implications for the analysis of health and human development. By way of *denoting this suspension* in subsequent analyses, I will bracket, rather than erase, the 'human' [hence (human) development hereafter].

3.2 A Deleuzian 'Life' Science

Throughout his life, Deleuze vehemently rejected 'organic' conceptions of 'individual' human life for their insistence on the temporal and spatial coherence of the body/organism. In his later collaborations with Felix Guattari (1987: 158), Deleuze went so far as to declare that "the organism is the enemy" in presenting a highly idiosyncratic account of the events, affects and relations by which bodies are assembled or expressed. Yet as Ansell-Pearson (1999: 96–99) notes, Deleuze's opposition to the 'organism' does not amount to an ontological dismissal of 'the human', or a kind of rabid anti-humanism. While Deleuze rejects the idea of a *fixed human entity* somehow distinct from the nonhuman, animal and material becomings that surround it, he offers in its place a "more than human" conception of life, and an ethics by which these nonhuman becomings may be harnessed in the cultivation of a "superior human nature" (Ansell Pearson 1999: 59). Grosz (2011: 16) adds that such a gesture inaugurates the search for a "humanities in which the human is no longer the norm, rule or object, but instead life itself, in its open multiplicity, comes to provide the object of analysis". It follows, therefore, that the ideas of health and development are not somehow inconsistent with Deleuze's project, alone or in his collaborations with Felix Guattari. It is nonetheless true that the deployment of Deleuze's concepts in the analysis of health and (human) development will remain highly disruptive of most existing conceptions of health and wellbeing. The dividend to be gleaned from this disruption involves the development of novel responses to some of the outstanding challenges confronting scholars in the health and social sciences. I have already described the first of these challenges in noting the support Deleuze offers for the identification of the means by which developmental capacities are acquired, cultivated, transmitted and divested in particular contexts or milieus. Another problem, cited in each of the previous chapters, is the promise of a substantive account of health, more inclusive of the various organic and nonorganic (human and nonhuman) forces active in the assemblages by which health and illness are composed. Moving beyond an 'anthropocentric' understanding of health should enable greater elucidation of the nonhuman actors at work in the modulations of health, including the various social and structural actors long catalogued in established accounts of the social determinants of health. Giving force to this 'minor science' of health and (human) development is Deleuze's inventive account of 'life'.

In an interview conducted close to the end of his career, Deleuze (1995: 143) observed that "everything I've written is vitalistic, at least I hope it is, and amounts to a theory of signs and events". Deleuze's work teems with this vitalism, with the affects, percepts, signs and forces pursuant to life, and the boundless becomings that transform it. Deleuze (1994) is committed in the first instance to *immanent* life; to a philosophy that conceives of life as an autopoietic process that draws matter and force together in the differentiation of organic and inorganic life. Life is the vitalist impulse – the *elan vital* for Bergson (1998) and for Spinoza (2005) the *conatus* – that forces matter to differentiate in the continuous variations by which all becomings are enacted (Grosz 2011). Life is self-organising in this regard insofar as it *effects a plane of composition* ("a block of space-time") on which the material, affective, social, expressive and territorial elements necessary for the continuation of life are assembled (Deleuze and Guattari 1987: 313). There is, as such, "no form or correct structure imposed from without or above but rather an articulation from within" (Deleuze and Guattari 1987: 328). Life must not, in other words, be construed as the complex manifestation of some primal set of codes, laws or axioms; life prefigured in a grand transcendental injunction. Life evolves, differing from itself according to forces, selective pressures and territorial opportunities immanent to life itself. There is no 'correct structure' only 'articulation from within'; only the force of life in its assembling. Life is always composed in this way; in assemblages of matter, force, affect, territory, communication, metabolism, energy, expression and duration (Deleuze and Guattari 1987: 323–326). As such, "the living thing has an exterior milieu of materials, an interior milieu of composing elements and composed substances, an intermediary milieu of membranes and limits, and an annexed milieu of energy sources and actions-perceptions" (Deleuze and Guattari 1987: 313). Each of these milieus constitutes the *life* of the living thing; all continually "pass into one another" as life differentiates in its becomings (Deleuze and Guattari 1987: 313). It follows that life cannot be reduced to the material or organic forms by which it is 'actualised' (Grosz 2011). Life is always distributed in and among a series of territories or milieus; a multiplicity or assemblage of forces rather than a singular, stable organismal form.

Life, vitalism, force, affect, territorialisation, difference, becoming, matter, signs and event; Deleuze's biophilosophy is replete with the conceptual innovation necessary to think life in the *force of its living*, its striving to persevere (Ansell Pearson 1999). Such interest in the force of life ultimately informs Deleuze's discrimination of the 'actual' and the 'virtual', a distinction which remains central to the basic ontological structure of his entire philosophy. What is 'given' to observation are the 'actual', extensive properties, qualities, traits and orientations of life in its variegated plenum. This 'actual' form provides the basis for the great taxonomical systems by which life is observed and catalogued in the organisation of species, genera, orders, classes, phylum and so on. While the 'order of things' that emerges in observation may account for the diversity of life, it fails to explain its generative, differentiating impulse. Concealed among its extensive properties are a series of virtual, *intensive*, processes that give force to life, causing it to evolve, to differentiate in becomings that take life beyond itself. This intensive domain comprises myriad singular forces, including the affects, percepts, desires, qualities, sensations, durations and events that constitute, or give form to, "extended life" (Rolli 2009: 36–44). Each of these forces provides the "resources" necessary for becoming; for the "individuations and self-actualisations" life "requires to continue and develop itself" (Grosz 2011: 38) In this way, intensive processes add a virtual dimension to life: each is "real without being actual"; all are immanent to life (Deleuze 1988c: 96). More directly, the intensive processes that impel life are actualised as they "ascribe themselves to some persistent object" (Rolli 2009: 29). Intensive life is actualised, therefore, in the familiar extended forms matter adopts, and yet these same intensive forces continually disturb matter, such that life must be understood as a *process* by which matter exceeds itself in its differentiations. By the same token, life cannot be conceived as some superordinate spark or catalyst that gives force to inert matter. Matter, rather, provides a *medium* for the actualisation of the virtual, whereby life "draws from matter the forces it requires to ... persist, to grow ... to extend, to prolong, to differ from itself" (Grosz 2011: 33–35). Life, indeed, is nothing but the "ever more complex elaboration of difference" (Grosz 2011: 3).

The work of elaborating difference, of *explicating difference,* lies at the heart of Deleuze's biophilosophy, providing the basis for distinguishing the actual from the virtual, the extensive from the intensive processes that compose life. Grosz (2011: 45) adds that for Deleuze, "difference is the methodology of life"; it is in the very order of living. It is also true that the work of elaborating difference calls for a superior empiricism equal to the intensive and extensive modulations of this life. It calls for "new ways of thinking and conceptualising the real as dynamic, temporally sensitive forms of becoming" (Grosz 2011: 41). The question is how to think becoming; how to fashion a mode of thought capable of tracing its rhizomatic lines such that one may expose oneself to more of the force of becoming. *Such is the properly philosophical and ethical achievement of a transcendental empiricism.* In the last chapter I argued that Deleuze's empiricism establishes a method for the interrogation of the actual and the virtual dimensions of "real experience". Reframing this argument somewhat in the language of the present chapter, it is equally plausible to suggest that 'life' is the *persistent medium* of this experience. As Eric Alliez (2004: 21) notes, transcendental empiricism provides a means of "diagnosing" the "real experience of becoming" in all its particularities. Alert to the intensive becomings that transform life – the inorganic/nonhuman/'more than human' affects, forces and relations that "fracture" subjective life (Deleuze 1994: 169) – transcendental empiricism establishes a means of extending or intensifying the "immediate present" of real experience; what Keith Ansell-Pearson (1999:

8–15) calls "germinal life". Germinal life is intensive. It encompasses the virtual elements that comprise life; the singularities, affects, desires, events, territories, signs and relations that constitute "the preindividual, the real or matter" (Grosz 2011: 38). Indeed, life is not distinct from matter; it is always coincident with it (Deleuze 1994). Life, therefore, establishes the conditions for real experience and in so doing furnishes the proper object of transcendental empiricism.

Or perhaps it is more accurate to say that *life in its becomings* ought to remain the proper object of transcendental empiricism. Such a conversion establishes, finally, an analytical link between the study of life, becoming, development and health insofar as the becomings that most interest Deleuze are precisely those becomings which involve "the ongoing exploration of and experimentation with the forms of bodily activity that living things are capable of undertaking" (Grosz 2011: 22). Grosz (2011: 22) adds that "this is perhaps the only ethics internal to life itself: to maximise action, *to enable the proliferation of actions, movements*" (emphasis added). The idea of an ethics which entails as its primary objective the 'proliferation' of 'forms of bodily activity' that extend a body's range of movement arguably provides the clearest exposition yet of a Deleuzian life science. It also provides further indications of a Deleuzian account of health. Health, like development, may be understood to involve those forms of bodily activity that extend a body's range of action – construed as the array of bodies, entities, things and processes that such a body may affect and/or be affected by – along with the variety of human and nonhuman, organic and material relations that subtend this activity. To the extent that a body is able to establish novel relations that extend the array of actions it may participate in (and so extend the array of things it may affect and be affected by), that body may be said to have acquired a novel developmental competency. To the extent that these relations affect a body with an increase in its power of acting, that body may also be said to have become healthy (or maintained its health). This suggests, in turn, the merits of retaining an analytical distinction between health and (human) development. As such, development may be construed as the *expressed quality or manifestation* of health, while health may be understood as a quantum of a body's power of acting. Health, in other words, is the affective and relational force that impels a body's developmental trajectory, giving rise to the acquisition of novel competencies and thereby extending a body's scope of activity. What remains to be established are the specific mechanisms of the body's becoming healthy, along with the actual mechanisms of its development. Following Deleuze's empiricism once more, these mechanisms may be said to concern the events, affects and relations that constitute real experience; or life in all its manifold diversity. Health and (human) development proceed in those specific events, relations and affects which extend a body's manifest activity. Events are always primary after all.

In the previous chapter I noted Deleuze's eschewal of an ontology of substance or identity, and his subsequent valorisation of a processual ontology emphasising change, becoming and differenc/tiation. Deleuze (1994) is primarily concerned to found a relational ontology, more sensitive to the change that all things undergo, notwithstanding the challenges associated with the attempt to ground an ontology in a process that is forever differing from itself (see Ansell Pearson 1999: 90–96).

Applied to the analysis of (human) development, Deleuze's ontology calls attention to the *becoming of development*, rather than the human subject who notionally experiences (or enjoys) this development. Most traditional models of human development rely on a seemingly 'preformationist' logic in which 'life' serves as a ready-made homunculus awaiting its realisation in the dynamic of human experience (see Lerner 2002). In this view, development is merely the preordained manifestation of an existing biological imperative. While the phenotypic expressions of development may differ from one individual to another, the fundamental structures of development remain unalterable. Events, in other words, are in the order of the phenotype, leaving the genotype subject to other, more primal forces. Deleuze utterly rejects this view for its failure to explain the diversity (or differentiation) of development, and the more specific failure to address the causes of the modifications or mutations common to all genetic 'codes' (see Ansell Pearson 1999: 2–14). The genotype, like the phenotype, must be explained in ways that avoid the common habit of regarding substance (genotype) as primary and change (phenotypic expression) as secondary. Deleuze's creative solution is to position the intensive, virtual or 'pure' event as the primary force of becoming, whereby events effect divergent or disjunctive individuations that carry the individual beyond itself.

The event, in this sense, expresses the force of individuation by which bodies are transformed. Such individuating differences are the very motor of becoming. The idea of individuation, taken from Gilbert Simondon (see Deleuze 2004: 86–90), attends to the processes of formation and/or subjectivation that transpire in the event. The individual is never prior to the event, figuring as the subject for whom (or to whom) 'things happen'. Rather, the event happens, or more accurately "is happening" (Deleuze 1990: 16–19), drawing together myriad intensive elements – expressions, affects, desires, relations, signs, behaviours, movements – which are each individuated in discrete "packets of relations" (Ansell Pearson 1999: 175). These packets may be understood as *fragments of subjectivity* which circulate in and through the event attaching themselves to bodies in intensive, affective associations. Bodies are affected by the event in a series of combinatorial expressions of subjectivity (affects, desires, memories, postures, gestures, behaviours). Such are the individuations by which bodies become subject. It follows that bodies are continually transformed in the events they experience, or through which experience unfolds for them. Events unleash the intensive forces central to becoming, and so provide the key to understanding a more Deleuzian model of (human) development. The principal advantage of such a model is the emphasis it places on the *mechanisms of development*; the actual/virtual processes by which development proceeds. In an earlier Section I noted that almost all contemporary models of human development endorse an ontogenetic logic whereby individual development is said to advance via a process of social and/or contextual engagement (Rogoff 2003). Yet it is never quite clear what engagement actually consists of and how, moreover, developmental competencies are actually acquired. Deleuze's account of the event of individuation provides the conceptual heft necessary to address these shortcomings.

Deleuze's notion of the event suggests very strongly that (human) development advances in a series of individuations 'actualised' in events of human and nonhuman interaction or engagement. Events avail the various affective and material resources necessary for the progress of (human) development. Events of parental bonding for example, draw bodies together in a commingling of forces and relations (affection, trust, reciprocity, anxiety, relief, sustenance and satisfaction), which affect infant and parent alike with *a force of attraction*. The nursing infant is primarily affected by the event of material, maternal interaction. Yet the force of this interaction is for the most part intensive. The infant body is affected by the presence of the maternal body in an exchange of forces. The nature of these forces will differ from event to event, ensuring that the fragments of subjectivity available in these events will differ also. The infant is, in fact, individuated anew in each event of parental interaction, sometimes subtly, and sometimes more profoundly. The extent to which particular events provide the resources necessary to impel development depends on the character of the relations established in the event, and the affective valence of these relations (Grosz 2011). If (human) development is to be construed as the ongoing establishment of diverse relational capacities (understood as the *capacity to be affected* by an ever wider cast of bodies or subjects), then the developmental utility of individual bodies or relations must be assessed in and through this affective force.

Drawing on the review of Deleuze's reading of Spinoza's ethics offered in the previous chapter, it may be argued further that affects establish both the particular emotional valence of individual developmental events or relations, as well as the specific transition in the respective powers of acting of those bodies so subjected. Any given event may be regarded as developmental to the extent that it entails the acquisition of novel skills or capacities. Such capacitation must, in turn, be primarily regarded as an affective process; capacities have to stick to the body after all. Acquiring a novel developmental competency from language acquisition and the capacity to form legible words using pencil and paper, to the capacity to drive a car or swing a tennis racquet, must henceforth be regarded as *affective processes* by which bodies establish novel means of affecting the world around them. Capacities are developed in a slow process whereby bodies acquire novel extensive parts and establish novel affective relations between these parts. And so, the pencil slowly becomes part of the extensive capacities of the prehensile hand; the phonemes by which languages are expressed slowly affect the material architecture of the mouth, tongue, larynx and lips; the racquet is differentially gripped by the hand and the shoulders begin to affect the hips and legs in novel ways as the body 'learns' to essay a forehand drive; the mind is affected by love and acquires a moral sensitivity.

(Human) development is primarily affective in other words, advancing and retreating in a series of intensive transitions, exposing the force of the varied assemblages in which the human body is composed. Still, this formulation leaves unresolved the issue of explaining how the assemblages which figure as the effective expression of (human) development are themselves composed. How, in other words, do affective sensitivities and developmental competencies settle into the human assemblage and so obtain the *consistency* that remains perhaps the most striking feature of 'actual' human experience? How, moreover, does the assemblage hold together, and how are developmental and affective competencies once acquired, subsequently retained? The first part of Deleuze's response to these problems concerns the notion of the 'fold' borrowed from Michel Foucault, and his second, more sustained response, involves the elaboration of Spinoza's ethology. To start with, Deleuze (2006) takes up Foucault's eschewal of the separation of the inside and the outside; the idea of a human consciousness or "interiority" that remains separate and distinct from the exteriority of life, which serves also as the primary object of interiority. In overturning this dualism, Deleuze (2006: 96–97) follows Foucault's lead in arguing that "the outside is not a fixed limit but a moving matter animated by peristaltic movements, folds and folding that together make up an inside; they are not something other than the outside, but precisely the inside *of* the outside". The human assemblage may, on this basis, be regarded as a function of this folding of the outside, whereby an interiority like subjectivity is established. What's more, the notion of the fold provides a compelling basis for determining how developmental competencies (understood as novel affective and relational capacities) are subsumed within the assemblage. The idea of the fold may also serve to distinguish the affective intensity of different events in terms of the relative developmental trajectories they unleash. Each of these related courses should help distinguish events which merely involve bodies (the human assemblage), from those events which affect a more *enduring developmental transition* by facilitating the acquisition of new competencies.

Development is, in this respect, "conditioned by the fold" as forces are folded back on themselves in their subsumption within the (human) assemblage (Deleuze 2006: 106). The *force* of the fold is the force of difference and repetition. It is the affective and intensive force of a body exposed to novel capacities as it takes on novel extensive parts in the acquisition of novel developmental competencies. The acquisition of the capacity to read and write, for example, involves the repetitive folding within the body of the force of language and communication; into the hand as it is affected by the technology of pen and paper, or keyboard and screen, and so begins to affect each tool differently; and within the spaces of the body itself as it is ergonomically oriented to the chair/keyboard/desk/screen assemblage. Each involves the force, or folding, of habit, repetition and memory (Deleuze 2006: 106–108). The fold is in this sense, always, already *a folding*. It involves the ongoing habitual, corporeal, affective and durational repetition of intensive and extensive movements and force-relations. And so, the hand slowly acquires the capacity to fold the force of inscription within itself, thus acquiring the capacity to write, along with the force of communication and the capacity to emit signs. Or, the body orients itself to the musical instrument, folding the scales, notations and timbres of musical theory, affecting sound, repeating exercises, establishing a capacity to affect the instrument and so produce sound and rhythm; the lyricism of the musical assemblage, the joys of the refrain (Deleuze and Guattari 1987: 313–315). The more repetitive the folding, the more intensively the differences of germinal life are lived within the assembled, developmental body. *Folding is the repetition of difference habituated within the body.* It is how bodies acquire developmental competencies. As Deleuze (2006: 114) observes "as a force among forces, man does not fold the forces that compose him without the outside folding itself, and creating a self within man". This finally provides a basis for distinguishing between events, affects and relations which impel, reposition or otherwise involve bodies, and those which effect a more significant developmental change. The fold – among the related notions of habit, difference and repetition – is the proper index by which this distinction may be drawn. Indeed, the more repetitive the folding, the more enduring the developmental becoming will be.

Deleuze (1994) adds, of course, that this logic holds for both the biological development of the body, as well as its social, cultural and material becomings. Just as the forces of language and culture are folded into a body made of habits, so too are the body's biological codes folded and repeated, albeit according to different spatial and temporal rhythms (Ansell Pearson 1999: 145–152). And so, the ovum's fertilisation initiates an ongoing sequence of cell division by which the gestating foetus folds within itself the genomic inheritance of its biological parents. The foldings or 'invaginations' of embryonic, foetal and neonatal development express a body's morphogenesis, understood as a process of differentiation and specialisation by which complex organism's develop and evolve (Deleuze and Guattari 1987; Ansell Pearson 1999). In each instance, the folding of code, matter, energy and affect is repeated in a ceaseless process of individuation, which holds no less for the body's biological inheritance than its cultural endowment. Indeed, if development may be said to advance in the rigors of the individual's engagement with a 'nature', 'territory' 'space' or 'context', then the fold provides the effective measure of this engagement (Protevi 2012: 213–226). The fold is not in this sense, simply change; it serves as the primary mechanism of a body's becoming; its development in the language of this chapter. The concept of the fold introduces, in turn, a series of properly ethical and developmental questions: "what can I do, what power can I claim and what resistances may I counter? What can I be, with what folds can I surround myself or how can I produce myself as a subject?" (Deleuze 2006: 114). Such questions receive their most sustained treatment in Deleuze's reading of Spinoza's ethology. This ethology also provides the strongest empirical support for the job of describing health and development in context. As such, further application of Deleuze's account of Spinoza's ethology should provide fresh insights into the mechanisms of (human) development and the specific ways particular competencies are folded into the body.

3.3 A Developmental Ethology (Events, Affects, Relations)

I suggested in the last chapter that Spinoza's ethics establish a new model for philosophy: a philosophy of the body, of encounters and relations, ideas and affects (Deleuze 1988b: 17). Spinoza grounds this philosophy by inquiring into what a body can (or might) do. I have argued further that such inquiry holds the key to the articulation of a more Deleuzian account of health and (human) development, proffering new ways of conceiving of the processes and characteristic features of this development (Fox 2012). The task now is to indicate how Deleuze's specific adoption of Spinoza's ethology may help to clarify how bodies acquire novel developmental competencies, amid the more general dynamics of (human) development and the assemblage's becomings. To briefly recap, Spinoza regarded the body as a mobile, ever modulating ensemble of simple parts, human and nonhuman, material and affective, connected in distinctive relational encounters. In describing a body, whether human or nonhuman, Spinoza was ever alert to this relational and affective congeries, a commitment Deleuze (1988b) himself embraced in his characterization of the body as an assemblage. Deleuze's account includes material bodies, as well as bodies of ideas, thoughts, processes and practices. The body as such, is not a singular ontological essence deserving of some *a priori* regard. Instead, the body *emerges* in a series of affective and relational becomings, each of which shapes a body's distinctive capacities or powers. This position yields an avowedly *ethological* understanding of bodies, their affects and relations in life.

Such an ethology requires, of course, that one consider individual bodies in terms of their "power of acting", where this power stands as *an index* of the body's capacity to enter into diverse relations and experience diverse affects (Deleuze 1992: 256). A body's power grows as it becomes more capable of entering into novel relations with other bodies, and thus more capable of affecting and being affected by these bodies. In drawing such conclusions, Deleuze, like Spinoza before him, highlights the role of affects and encounters in transforming a body's characteristic composition, or the relations between its extensive parts. As such, the ethology that emerges in Deleuze's reading of Spinoza provides a basis for identifying the mechanisms of the body's capacitation; or the specific means by which bodies acquire new capacities or powers in certain encounters, just as capacities are lost in other contexts. *Affects and the encounters which generate them are the means by which bodies acquire novel capacities.* Indeed, Spinoza's characterization of ethics as the sum total of practices or techniques by which individuals strive to organise their encounters in an attempt to maximise the experience of joyful affects, may itself stand as a fitting characterization of (human) development. Deleuze (1992: 212) goes onto argue that Spinoza's ethics requires an "*empirical study of bodies* in order to know their relations and how they are combined" (emphasis added) such that they might be recombined otherwise. One might add that this kind of 'empirical' study of bodies, relations and affects ought to advance the study of (human) development in equal measure. The problem of how this study may be applied in the analysis of (human) development, and its characteristic features, is the object of what I would call a developmental ethology.

Such innovation draws on the paradigmatic insight of Deleuze's ethology – the contention that bodies can only be known on the basis of their idiosyncratic affects and relations – and applies it to the problem of (human) development. This is a development of *continuous variation* as the body is transformed in its myriad encounters, both with other bodies and with the objects and processes that constitute place and social context. Developmental ethology does away with the idea of phenotypic maturation in favour of the empirical study of *bodies and their milieus*

(Ansell Pearson 1999). Milieus themselves 'enfold' diverse material elements within a particular environment, in addition to a host of immaterial (or inorganic) elements such as ideas, affects, habits, forces, energy and action-perceptions (Deleuze and Guattari 1987: 313). It follows that milieus are inherently unstable or dynamic, incorporating diverse affective, material, biological, geographical, cultural, economic and symbolic components (Ballantyne 2007: 84–87). What's more, the *relational imbrication* of bodies and milieus admits of no ontological distinction between the two, and instead conjures an immanent plane of coextensive becomings. Bodies, territories and milieus are composed together in manifold assemblages, comprised of an indefinite number of parts, forms and processes (Patton 2000: 44). Indeed, the affects generated in encounters with milieus are, for Deleuze, just as significant as the affects generated between bodies (see Bogue 2003: 55–58). As such, milieus are important vectors of affective transmission in the body's power of acting, and hence, important sources of developmental capabilities in their own right. Foregrounding the relations that bodies establish between milieus – and the ways milieus shape a body's capacities in their territorial and affective specificity – provides the properly empirical basis for the generation of a developmental ethology. Such an ethology is founded in the open "communication" established between bodies and milieus, as milieus "pass into one another" and bodies "pass from one milieu to another" (Deleuze and Guattari 1987: 313). More directly, communication describes the body's *territorialisation* of place, or the distinctive processes of movement and affective engagement that define the body's 'emplacements' (Patton 2000; Grosz 2011). Territorialisations are effected in the unique array of affects and relations that bodies establish with the external and internal milieus, membranes and limits, energy sources and actions-perceptions that constitute place (or social context). This position is consistent, I would argue, with established views in human development regarding the role of contextual engagement, even if the terms are unfamiliar.

More precisely, processes of de/territorialisation involve the relational transference of "codes", such as energy, affect, matter, percepts, capacities and action-potential, from milieus to bodies, and from bodies to milieus (Deleuze and Guattari 1987: 313–316). This transference is the *medium of communication* that links all bodies with their constitutive contexts or milieus. An ethology of bodies, relations and territories contends, moreover, that (human) development arises as a result of this communication, this territorial engagement, and the differential developmental opportunities that attend the communicative and relational exploration of diverse milieus. And so, the character of developmental opportunities in any particular setting remains a function of the affective and relational intensity of communication in and between milieus (see Bogue 2003: 55–58). The more intensive a body's territorialisations, and the greater the array of milieus that this territorialisation occurs in, the greater that body's developmental becomings will be. Given the relational and affective nature of territorialisation, it follows that the body's territorial engagements involve a transition in that body's power of action, understood as the subsumption (or divestment) of social, affective and material resources within the human assemblage, which are then availed in the course of extending that body's range of activity (Ansell Pearson 1999: 170–189). Put another way, transitions in a body's power of action are a product of that body's communicative (or territorial) encounters in and with diverse milieus, and the distinctive transferences, or additions and reductions in that body's extensive parts, that attend these encounters. Indeed, such variation in the body's capacities is the primary feature of all (human) development (see also Grosz 2011).

(Human) development should therefore be regarded as a processual function of a body's diverse territorialisations. The empirical study of (human) development necessarily entails the examination of such territorialisations and the transferences that accompany them. It requires the more specific study of the distinctive affects, percepts, capacities and action-potential that are "communicated" in the event of a body's territorialisations. It was noted earlier that contemporary accounts of human development emphasise two related processes: the acquisition and maintenance of select developmental competencies and the engagements with place and context that enable this acquisition. A developmental ethology satisfies each condition of this study in foregrounding the role of *territorialisation.* This notion implies an alternative theoretical impetus for the study of contextual engagement and the terms and processes of (human) development. Developmental ethology contends that territorialisation (deterritorialisation and reterritorialisation) is the mechanism by which bodies acquire additional developmental competencies (or affective capacities) in specific milieus, just as these competencies are lost or retarded in others. Territorialisation, or developmental capacitation, is the dynamic process that links bodies and milieus in the *affective and relational transmission of capacities.* Milieus are themselves dynamically "encoded" assemblages that are forever evolving with the body's territorialisations, along with the modulations of the imbricative "molecular" forces that compose them (Deleuze and Guattari 1987: 315). Developmental ethology further suggests that affects and relations constitute the basic forces or processes by which capacities are exchanged or transmitted in encounters between bodies and between bodies and milieus. *The acquisition of new developmental capabilities is in this sense a thoroughly affective and relational phenomenon.* Capacitation always involves a transition in a body's affective sensitivities and relational repertoires.

This arguably holds for any of the developmental competencies described above in relation to the five key developmental domains of social, cognitive, emotional, physical and moral development (see also Alkire 2002). In each instance, capabilities are slowly acquired in affective and relational engagement, such that capabilities must themselves be regarded as affective and relational in nature. Social development, including sociality and group dynamics, exemplifies this affective and relational engagement. The encounters that subtend social engagement involve the transmission of affects and relations in ways that *compose sociality as a particular way of being in the world* (see also Thrift 2004). Sociality slowly accretes in the embodied subject as it is modified in turn by the affective transitions of social interaction, with its obligations and reciprocities. Facial expressions, habits of speaking and listening, comportment and social spaces, for example, are folded into the body as affective orientations or dispositions. In each instance, the affects and relations that comprise this embodied sociality add to the body's extensive parts (Massumi 2002: 1–21). Sociality entails the *expression of these extensive parts* in that each part extends the array of social interactions a body may be capable of. The more diverse a body's social interactions, the more diverse its affective and relational transitions are likely to be, and the greater its social or developmental capacitation.

Bruno Latour's (1999) notion of "relative existence" and the related ideas of association and substitution, further clarify the nature of these processes, and the broader contours of a developmental ethology. In keeping with Deleuze's account of the ethological flux of the body's affects and relations, Latour is concerned to identify the means by which bodies acquire (or lose) associational "elements". Latour argues that relational processes like (human) development are advanced in the provision of new associations and novel collaborations. Latour (1999: 158) notes that "an entity gains in reality if it is associated with many others that are viewed as collaborating with it. It loses in reality if, on the contrary, it has to shed associates or collaborators (human and nonhuman)". Despite differences of nomenclature, the conceptual consonance between this position and Deleuze's ethology is striking. Each helps to elucidate the manner of a body's composition and decomposition; or the means by which the body acquires and/or loses external parts, or "collaborating entities" (see Bell 2009: 4–5). This process determines a body's relative existence at any one time, subject to modifications in that body's associations or substitutions. 'Association' describes the array of elements that "cohere" with an entity over time, including the various human and nonhuman actors that such an entity "collaborates" with and the ways these relations affect that entity (Latour 1999: 158–159). 'Substitution' in turn, describes the processes of modification or accommodation that transpire as entities enter into relations with new actors, and the impacts these actors have on that entity's existing collaborations. Given the considerable variability in these two processes, an entity's relative existence "waxes and wanes relative to the number of human and nonhuman associations it has established within a network" (Bell 2009: 71). It is arguably just as plausible to contend that health and development involve an *intensification* of an individual's relative existence (Latour 2004: 206–214).

This is close to the original conception of Spinoza's ethics and the argument that joy is associated with the acquisition of novel extensive parts and an increase in the body's force of existence, or power of acting. From an ethological perspective, this power is a function of the territorialisations and deterritorialisations that accompany the acquisition of extensive parts. (Human) development is advanced in the diversification of the body's territorialisations, and the intensification of the affective transitions that attend these territorialisations. It follows that positive (human) development is a product of those territorialisations that involve the communication or expression of the specific affects, percepts, capacities, energies and/or action-potential that affect a body with joy and an increase in that body's force of existing. *Joy is the primary index of positive (human) development in this sense*. Given that the particular affects that may affect a body with joy can't be known in advance but must rather be discovered through active engagement with the world, (human) development itself demands the empirical study of ethology, of affects and relations, in specific milieus, such that the force of development in life may be determined (see Bell 2009). This may also entail analysis of the force or process of territorialisation and deterritorialisation, such that the actual conduct of development in context may be better appreciated. This, finally, is the course by which Deleuze's ethology may be taken up in contemporary health debates, particularly those concerning the ecological dimensions of (human) development. A provisional research agenda consistent with this ethology is offered below by way of introduction to the case studies to follow.

3.4 Ethology, Health and Becoming

Contemporary assessments of health and human development emphasise the ontogenetic significance of the relationship between individuals and their social context. Various theoretical models of this contextual engagement exist, yet few surpass the ontological and empirical rigour provided in Deleuze's mature philosophy. The ethological account of (human) life furnished in Deleuze's transcendental empiricism sets out a novel methodological frame for the study of (human) development, furnishing new methods for analysis and suggesting new objects of inquiry (Fox and Ward 2008). Deleuze's work highlights the relationality of all developmental processes, including the affective and material engagement that grounds the person in context (the body in its territories). Taken from an ethological perspective, (human) development may be regarded as a discontinuous process of becoming, rather than a linear record of the organism's ontogenetic complexification. What's more, Deleuze's empiricism establishes a means of studying these discontinuous becomings, and the developmental transitions they entail, *in vivo*. It emphasises the progress and retreats of the developmental trajectory; the asynchronous acquisition and loss of developmental capacities, and the dynamic character of epigenetic engagement. Ethology suggests that development does not terminate in some final 'mature' state but rather persists across the life-course as bodies encounter one another, establishing new relations and affective sensitivities.

The consonance between Deleuze's idiosyncratic ethology and the capabilities approach to human development, introduced in an earlier section, should by now be apparent. Amartya Sen (1999) defines human development in terms of the *expansion of capabilities*, where these capabilities are not established *a priori*, but rather follow from the specific and contingent activities of individuals and groups (see also Alkire 2002). Sen (1999: 75) describes capabilities as any "thing a person may value doing or being" and so avoids establishing an exhaustive list of the kinds of capabilities or functionings that might advance human development in some universal way. Valuable functionings are determined in dynamic social contexts and their value is subject to recurrent negotiation and experimentation. This is consistent with Spinoza's views regarding the character of joyful affects, and their role in facilitating one's ethical engagement with the world. Like Sen, Deleuze and

Spinoza insist that it is not possible to determine in advance some core set of affects and encounters that may guarantee health and/or (human) development in every instance. There can, after all, be no reliable blueprint for development (or health), and so positive development must rely instead on an experimental ethos; even a lust for life. In any case, various commonalities are clearly discernible between Sen and Deleuze's rival understandings of health and development – each for example emphasises the significance of functionings, capabilities, activities or powers in the course of (human) development – suggesting that Deleuze's intervention is less an unprecedented, or unrecognisable, departure for scholars interested in health and development, and more a kind of conceptual reinvention designed to call attention to the dynamics of development in context. Deleuze's ethology, and the superior empiricism which supports it, helps to clarify the affective and relational character of (human) functioning, and the ways capabilities may promote development in specific contexts.

However, I would stress that Deleuze's ethology offers the considerable advantage of fostering a more viable working theory of the *specific mechanisms* by which capabilities and competencies are acquired, cultivated, maintained and lost. Sen and others have certainly attended to this problem, though it is arguably among the weakest elements of the capabilities approach (see Crocker 1992; Alkire 2005). Deleuze's ethology furnishes various concepts useful for identifying the means of a body's capacitation, including the fold, de/territorialisation, affect, event, communication, relationality and the assemblage. Each of these concepts provides fresh ways of conceiving of (human) development, building on the insights of Sen's capabilities approach rather than undermining or displacing them (Buchanan 1997).

The pursuit of a more Deleuzian approach to the study of health and (human) development offers further insights by acknowledging a cast of nonhuman, material and/or inorganic entities active in the advances and retreats of development; a cast which has hitherto been largely relegated to the nominal status of 'social context' (Keller et al. 2002; Latour 2004). Rather than regard these nonhuman or material factors as mere 'props' in support of an otherwise *naturalised* human development, Deleuze emphasises the relational entwinement of the human and the nonhuman, and the inseparability of organic and inorganic life in the course of development. There can be no account of (human) development in the absence of the nonhuman, just as there can be no account of the embodied subject in the absence of the material or inorganic. Organic and inorganic life are forever folded within the (human) assemblage, drawing from the territorial milieus that serve as the proper context of (human) development, extending the range of movement or activity that such an assemblage may express or participate in. Following Foucault, this suggests that the differentiation of the inside and the outside, the human and the nonhuman, the subject and the object, the biological and the cultural, obscures rather than elucidates the everyday course of (human) development. Retaining such ontological distinctions almost inevitably reifies the hierarchisation of nature and culture, reproducing what are often unhelpful conventions regarding the primacy of the human and its mastery over the cultural, material or natural world. If the differentiation of the human and the nonhuman ever made sense in the study of human development, it is surely untenable now given the relentless imbrication of the body and technology, biology and culture in the age of 'biopolitics' (Protevi 2009). It is simply impossible to imagine the contours of (human) development in the absence of technology, and culture more generally. While this fact is openly acknowledged in contemporary studies of human development (Bronfenbrenner 2005), the stubborn adherence to the ontological distinction of the human and nonhuman (subjects and objects) seems ultimately to defy the logical corollary of any attempt to devise a cultural model of development.

Better, like Deleuze, to abandon the separation of the human and the nonhuman in the articulation of a truly relational ontology of the imbrications of (human) life. As I noted in the introduction to this chapter, such a conclusion does not 'do away' with the idea of the human, much less does it abandon the notion or merits of (human) development. The point, as Ansell-Pearson (1999: 2–3) observes, is not to dismiss the human condition, but rather to "go beyond" it in the search for those "animal", "inhuman" or "more than human" becomings whereby a body might be carried away from itself *into life* in all its manifold, vital, abundance. Such ambitions conjure the allure of a "superior human nature beyond the human condition" (Ansell Pearson 1999: 59), alive to the developmental opportunities of the diverse territorial milieus life inhabits or passes through (or, more accurately, that pass through it). This finally is the proper objective of a developmental ethology, and the major intellectual achievement of the effort to derive a Deleuzian account of health and development.

Indeed, in describing the means by which bodies acquire extensive parts, Deleuze and Spinoza establish grounds for a novel empirical study of (human) development; what I have here called a developmental ethology. Developmental ethology treats the lived experience of (human) development as a complex of affective and relational transitions, each effectuated in diverse encounters. This logic can be applied to the study of any moment, or set of moments, in the developmental trajectory, and any specific developmental milieu. On offer is a deeper understanding of the body and its milieus such that the character of (human) development might be refined, along with the affects and relations that support the acquisition of discrete capabilities (see also Thrift 2008). Such analysis suggests an expanded empirical field for the study of (human) development, and an empirical study of affects and relations in particular (Massumi 2002: 235). Each will require a specific kind of empirical study, consistent with the methods of a transcendental empiricism described in the previous chapter. This is an empiricism concerned both with the contingent formation of life, knowledge and experience, as well as the *contingency of the subject of this life, knowledge and experience*. It calls attention, in particular, to the array of intensive affects, relations, events, durations, signs, habits and memories by which all developmental processes advance. The challenge now is to apply this logic in the design of novel empirical accounts of the affective and relational dimensions of (human) development. The following might stand as provisional research priorities in the pursuit of this work.

Traditionally, studies of human development have privileged the investigation of child and adolescent development, often in carefully controlled environments (see Keller et al. 2002). A developmental ethology demands a broader remit. Development does not terminate in some final mature state but rather persists across the life-course, as individuals encounter new relations and establish new affective sensitivities. This is to argue for an empirical study of (human) development across the life-course, taking in the key developmental thresholds associated with early childhood and adolescence, in addition to the developmental vicissitudes of adulthood and middle age. Applied to the study of adolescence, for example, a developmental ethology ought to concern itself with the manner in which specific developmental competencies are acquired in relational and affective engagement within diverse milieus, including schools, the family, peer settings and so on. Such an ethology suggests that the acquisition of developmental competencies involves the slow modification of the body's affects and relations in ways that leave it more *sensitive or receptive* to the expression or realisation of diverse developmental skills or capabilities. What has recently been labelled social and emotional learning offers an obvious example of the centrality of affects and relations in the acquisition of developmental competencies (see Payton et al. 2000). Social and emotional learning involves the acquisition of competencies such as empathy, reflection, prosocial engagement and emotional expressiveness, which together assist with the development of "self-control, social awareness and responsible decision making" (Payton et al. 2000: 184). The techniques and strategies associated with this pedagogy each entail the modification of a body's characteristic relations in order to affect that body with enhanced reflexive and allocentric sensitivities. In applying a developmental ethology to the study of social and emotional learning, the goal once more must be to specify how such sensitivities or capacities are acquired; the kinds of territorial assemblages they call forth; and the ways they are communicated between bodies in the exchange of 'simple' parts.

Developmental ethology thus proposes to treat a phenomenon like social and emotional learning as a problem of affective engagement, and to study this engagement primarily through the analysis of (human and nonhuman) bodies and the affective and relational transitions that attend social learning. It is perhaps more interesting however, to apply such a logic to the study of instances where (human) development is less commonly anticipated. To study development during later phases of life requires the consideration of different kinds of developmental processes and different kinds of developmental outcomes. What does it mean, in other words, to consider (human) development in relation to the middle aged father of three, gainfully employed and socially engaged? Or the young graduate student about to complete her doctorate? (Human) development in such contexts may be rather more subtle and convoluted than the functionally adaptive advances observable in earlier stages of life. Yet development indubitably persists in these circumstances, just as its contours may be the subject of observation and analysis. What's more, the logic of a developmental ethology is ideally suited to this kind of empirical inquiry. To study (human) development in early and middle adulthood, according to the methodological imperatives of a developmental ethology, will likely highlight the ways bodies slowly evolve in their affective and relational capacities. Examples include the way specific skills acquired in adolescence or early adulthood, such as playing a musical instrument or learning to cook, slowly change according to a body's diverse experiences and engagements. Similarly, emotional expressivity, sociality and self-awareness are forever evolving with the body's affective and relational modulations (or becomings). Each of a body's varied practical, social and emotional, cognitive and physical capabilities evolve in this way. Moreover, the study of such becomings promises an important contribution to contemporary debates regarding the ecological dimensions of (human) development. While the environmental mediation of human development is well established, *the distinctive mechanisms* of this interaction are not (see Keller et al. 2002; Jessor et al. 1996).

Deleuze's philosophy addresses this problem in a highly original way, emphasising the affective and relational investments that attend a body's explorations of diverse milieus, and the ways these investments facilitate the acquisition of novel developmental competencies (see also Fox 2011). By concentrating on those encounters that facilitate (human) development in the maximisation of a body's manifold joys, Deleuze's methods should open up new approaches to the promotion of (human) development in diverse settings. This is to more formally distinguish between those elements, forces or relations which promote the power of acting of a given assemblage of health, and those which decompose or frustrate this power. I would further insist that these insights should elucidate any event, or set of encounters, by which the health and wellbeing of a particular assemblage is mediated. The extent to which such a project succeeds is one important measure of the utility of Deleuze's work in the analysis of discrete health problems. This, at least, is the wager cashed out in the next two chapters as I apply Deleuze's empiricism, along with his ethology, to the analysis of problems associated with mental illness and addiction. The goal throughout is to indicate how Deleuze's method may contribute to a careful reassessment of these problems in the interests of promoting life, health and development. The promotion of health and (human) development, in the ways these processes have been conceived in this chapter, entails a bending of the force of the outside, *the force of life*, within those assemblages by which health is sustained. Here in an assemblage of health "among the folds...in a zone of subjectivation" one may become "master of one's speed...master of one's molecules and particular features" (Deleuze 1988a: 123). Strong, reasonable and free.

References

Alkire, S. 2002. Dimensions of human development. *World Development* 30(2): 181–205.

Alkire, S. 2005. Why the capability approach? *Journal of Human Development* 6(1): 115–135.

Alliez, E. 2004. *The signature of the world: What is Deleuze and Guattari's philosophy?* London: Continuum.

Ansell Pearson, K. 1999. *Germinal life: The difference and repetition of Gilles Deleuze*. London: Routledge.

Arnold, J., and L. Breen. 2006. Images of health. In *Health promotion in practice*, ed. S. Gorin and J. Arnold, 3–20. London: Wiley.
Ballantyne, A. 2007. *Deleuze & Guattari for architects*. London: Routledge.
Baum, F. 2008. *The new public health*, 3rd ed. Melbourne: Oxford University Press.
Bell, J. 2009. *Deleuze's Hume: Philosophy, culture and the Scottish enlightenment*. Edinburgh: Edinburgh University Press.
Bergson, H. 1998 [1911]. *Creative Evolution*. Trans. Arthur Mitchell. New York: Dover.
Blaxter, M. 2004. *Health: Key concepts*. London: Wiley.
Bogue, R. 2003. *Deleuze on music, painting and the arts*. London: Routledge.
Bronfenbrenner, U. (ed.). 2005. *Making human beings human: Bioecological perspectives on human development*. Thousand Oaks: Sage.
Buchanan, I. 1997. The problem of the body in Deleuze and Guattari, or, what can a body do? *Body and Society* 3(3): 73–91.
Catalano, R., M.L. Berglund, J. Ryan, H. Lonczak, and J.D. Hawkins. 2004. Positive youth development in the United States: Research findings on evaluations of positive youth development programs. *Annals of the American Academy of Political and Social Science* 98: 98–124.
Cattell, V., N. Dines, W. Gesler, and S. Curtis. 2008. Mingling, observing, and lingering: Everyday public spaces and their implications for wellbeing and social relations. *Health and Place* 14(3): 544–556.
Colby, A. 1996. The multiple contexts of human development. In *Ethnography and human development: Context and meaning in social inquiry*, ed. R. Jessor, A. Colby, and R. Shweder. Chicago: University of Chicago Press.
Colebrook, C. 2002. *Gilles Deleuze*. London: Routledge.
Crocker, D. 1992. Functioning and capability: The foundations of Sen's and Nussbaum's development ethic. *Political Theory* 20(4): 584–612.
Cummins, S., S. Curtis, A. Diez-Roux, and S. Macintyre. 2007. Understanding and representing place in health research: A relational approach. *Social Science and Medicine* 65(10): 1825–1838.
Dawson, A. (ed.). 2009. *The philosophy of public health*. London: Ashgate.
De Landa, M. 2002. *Intensive science and virtual philosophy*. London: Continuum.
Deleuze, G. 1988a. *Bergsonism*. New York: Zone Books.
Deleuze, G. 1988b. *Spinoza: Practical philosophy*. San Francisco: City Lights.
Deleuze, G. 1988c. *Foucault*. London: The Athlone Press.
Deleuze, G. 1990. *The Logic of Sense*. Trans. Mark Lester with C. Stivale. New York: Columbia University Press.
Deleuze, G. 1992. *Expressionism in Philosophy: Spinoza*. Trans. Martin Joughin. New York: Zone Books.
Deleuze, G. 1994. *Difference and repetition*. London: The Athlone Press.
Deleuze, G. 1995. *Negotiations: 1972–1990*. Trans. Martin Joughin. New York: Columbia University Press.
Deleuze, G. 2004. *Desert Islands and Other Texts (1953–1974)*. Trans. Mike Taormina. New York: Semiotext(e).
Deleuze, G. 2006. *Two regimes of madness. Texts and interviews 1975 – 1995*. New York: Semiotext(e).
Deleuze, G., and F. Guattari. 1987. *A Thousand Plateaus: Capitalism and Schizophrenia*. Trans. Brian Massumi. Minnesota: University of Minnesota Press.
Deneulin, S., and L. Shahani (eds.). 2009. *An introduction to the human development and capability approach: Freedom and agency*. London: Earthscan.
Derrida, J. 1997. *Of Grammatology*. Trans. G. Spivak. Baltimore: Johns Hopkins University Press.
Dewsbury, J. 2011. The Deleuze-Guattarian assemblage: Plastic habits. *Area* 43(2): 148–153.
Fitzgerald, J. 2009. Mapping the experience of drug dealing risk environments: An ethnographic case study. *International Journal of Drug Policy* 20(3): 261–269.

Foucault, M. 1973. *The birth of the clinic*. London: Routledge.
Foucault, M. 1985. *The history of sexuality*, The use of pleasure, vol. 2. London: Penguin.
Fox, N. 2011. The ill-health assemblage: Beyond the body-with-organs. *Health Sociology Review* 20(4): 434–446.
Fox, N. 2012. *The body*. Cambridge: Polity Press.
Fox, N., and K. Ward. 2008. What are health identities and how may we study them? *Sociology of Health and Illness* 30(7): 1007–1021.
Francis, R. 2011. *Epigenetics: The ultimate mystery of inheritance*. New York: W. W. Norton and Company.
Greco, M. 2004. The politics of indeterminacy and the right to health. *Theory, Culture and Society* 21(6): 1–22.
Greco, M. 2009. Thinking beyond polemics: Approaching the health society through Foucault. *Oesterreichische Zeitschrift fuer Soziologie* 34(2): 13–27.
Grosz, E. 2011. *Becoming undone: Darwinian reflections on life, politics and art*. Durham: Duke University Press.
Hollway, W. 2008. The importance of relational thinking in the practice of psycho-social research: Ontology, epistemology, methodology and ethics. In *Object relations and social relations: The implications of the relational turn in psychoanalysis*, ed. S. Clarke, P. Hoggett, and H. Hahn, 137–162. London: Karnac.
Jessor, R., A. Colby, and R. Shweder (eds.). 1996. *Ethnography and human development: Context and meaning in social inquiry*. Chicago: University of Chicago Press.
Keller, H., Y. Poortinga, and A. Schölmerich (eds.). 2002. *Between culture and biology: Perspectives on ontogenetic development*. Cambridge: Cambridge University Press.
Latour, B. 1999. *Pandora's hope: Essays on the reality of science studies*. Harvard: Harvard University Press.
Latour, B. 2004. How to talk about the body? The normative dimension of science studies. *Body and Society* 10(2–3): 205–229.
Law, J. 2004. *After method: Mess in social science research*. London: Routledge.
Law, J. 2007. Making a mess with method. In *The SAGE handbook of social science methodology*, ed. W. Outhwaite and S. Turner. London: Sage.
Lerner, M. 2002. *Concepts and theories of human development*, 3rd ed. New York: Lawrence Erlbaum Associates.
Linley, P., and S. Joseph (eds.). 2004. *Positive psychology in practice*. Hoboken: Wiley.
Lupton, D. 1995. *The imperative of health: Public health and the regulated body*. London: Sage.
Manderson, L. 2011. *Surface tensions: Surgery, bodily boundaries and the social self*. San Francisco: Left Coast Press.
Massumi, B. 2002. *Parables for the virtual: Movement, affect, sensation*. Durham: Duke University Press.
Metzl, J. 2010. Introduction: Why against health? In *Against health: How health became the new morality*, ed. J. Metzl and A. Kirkland. New York: New York University Press.
Metzl, J., and R. Herzig. 2007. Medicalisation in the 21st century: Introduction. *The Lancet* 369 (9562): 697–698.
Modell, J. 1996. The uneasy engagement of human development and ethnography. In *Ethnography and human development: Context and meaning in social inquiry*, ed. R. Jessor, A. Colby, and R. Shweder. Chicago: University of Chicago Press.
Mol, A. 2002. *The body multiple: Ontology in medical practice*. Durham: Duke University Press.
Mol, A., and J. Law. 2004. Embodied action, enacted bodies: The example of hypoglycaemia. *Body and Society* 10(2–3): 43–62.
Nussbaum, M., and A. Sen (eds.). 1993. *The quality of life*. Oxford: Oxford University Press.
Patton, P. 2000. *Deleuze and the political*. London: Routledge.
Payton, J., D. Wardlaw, P. Graczyk, M. Bloodworth, C. Tompsett, and R. Weissberg. 2000. Social and emotional learning: A framework for promoting mental health and reducing risk behaviours in children and youth. *Journal of School Health* 70(5): 179–185.

Polan, E., and D. Taylor. 2007. *Journey across the life span: Human development and health promotion*. Los Angeles: FA Davis.
Protevi, J. 2009. *Political affect: Connecting the social and the somatic*. Minneapolis: University of Minnesota Press.
Protevi, J. 2010. Deleuze and Wexler: Thinking brain, body and affect in social context. In *Cognitive architecture: From Bio-politics to Noo-politics. Architecture and mind in the age of communication and information*, ed. D. Hauptmann and W. Neidich. Rotterdam: 010 Publishers.
Protevi, J. 2012. Deleuze and life. In *The Cambridge companion to Deleuze*, ed. D. Smith and H. Somers-Hall, 239–264. Cambridge: Cambridge University Press.
Rogoff, B. 2003. *The cultural nature of human development*. New York: Oxford University Press.
Rolli, M. 2009. Deleuze on intensity differentials and the being of the sensible. *Deleuze Studies* 3(1): 26–53.
Rose, N. 2007. *The politics of life itself: Biomedicine, power, and subjectivity in the twenty-first century*. Princeton: Princeton University Press.
Scriven, A., and S. Garman (eds.). 2007. *Public health: Social context and action*. London: Open University Press.
Sen, A. 1999. *Development as freedom*. Oxford: Oxford University Press.
Sen, A. 2006. Why health equity? In *Public health, ethics and equity*, ed. S. Anand, F. Peter, and A. Sen. Oxford: Oxford University Press.
Sigelman, C., and E. Rider. 2011. *Life-span human development*, 7th ed. Belmont: Wadsworth Learning.
Spinoza, B. 2005. *Ethics*. Edited and Introduced by Edmund Curley. New York: Penguin Classics.
Tengland, P. 2007. Empowerment: A goal or a means for health promotion? *Medicine, Health Care and Philosophy* 10(2): 197–207.
Thiers, K., and J. Travers (eds.). 2005. *Handbook of human development for health care professionals*. New York: Jones and Bartlett Publishers.
Thrift, N. 2004. Intensities of feeling: Towards a spatial politics of affect. *Geografiska Annaler* 86B(1): 57–78.
Thrift, N. 2008. I just don't know what got into me: Where is the subject? *Subjectivity* 22(1): 82–89.
Tucker, I. 2010. Mental health service user territories: Enacting 'safe spaces' in the community. *Health* 14(4): 434–448.
Tucker, I. 2012. Deleuze, sense, and life: Marking the parameters of a psychology of individuation. *Theory and Psychology* 22(6): 771–785.
World Health Organisation. 1986. *The Ottawa charter for health promotion*. Geneva: WHO.

Chapter 4
The Assemblage in Recovery (Mental Health)

Hinting at the contours of a minor science of health and illness, Deleuze (1992: 212) once observed that Spinoza's ethics demand an "empirical study of bodies in order to know their relations, and how they are combined". This chapter offers the first of two case studies modelled on this empiricism and the biophilosophy that Deleuze derives from Spinoza and Bergson. Each case should help elucidate a unique *ethics of the event* whereby the becomings that Deleuze (1994) regards as central to all life may be accelerated or promoted (see also Grosz 2011: 50–56). Complementing recent efforts to 'think with' Deleuze in the design of novel methodologies for the health sciences (see Fox 2011; Malins 2004; Tucker 2010), I intend in this chapter to draw on the developmental ethology described in the last to explore the mechanisms by which bodies territorialise place, amid the processes by which places territorialise bodies. My conjecture is that such analysis should help to establish an 'ethico-ethology' of health capable of explaining the becomings that obtain in health and illness. I then apply this conjecture to the analysis of qualitative data recently collected in Melbourne, Australia among individuals recovering from a mental illness. On the basis of this analysis, I will argue that recovery may be construed as a process of learning to manipulate the affects, signs, territories and events of one's 'becoming well'. Recovery is a process, an open extended event, by which the recovering body becomes sensitive to an array of affects and relations emitted in diverse internal, intermediary and external milieus (Tucker 2010: 436–439). These are the affects and events by which bodies become well. The always unfinished event of recovery links diverse human and nonhuman signs, bodies, territories and relations in the joint expression of an enhanced capacity to affect (and be affected by) other bodies. One of the most important of these capacities in the promotion of recovery from mental illness is the means of reterritorialising place in the expression of belonging to, or feeling included in, the socius (Protevi 2009: 33–42). I will close with a discussion of how this insight may inspire novel ways of understanding the role of social inclusion, place and community in promoting recovery from mental illness.

C. Duff, *Assemblages of Health: Deleuze's Empiricism and the Ethology of Life*,

DOI 10.1007/978-94-017-8893-9_4,

This discussion will be characterised by an attempt to apply the logic presented in Deleuze's empiricism – and the developmental ethology I have derived from it – to the task of identifying and describing the array of human and nonhuman bodies, forces, affects and relations active in the *event* of recovery. My goal is to depart from most existing accounts of recovery, which tend to emphasise the near voluntarist capacities of individual clinicians, consumers and carers, to enable more variegated assessments of the particular assemblages of health and illness in which recovery is enacted. Rather than regard recovery as a process or phenomenon that *happens to* individuals living with mental health problems, I wish to reframe recovery in terms of the broad assemblages of health which sustain recovery in particular territories or milieus. This more ethological perspective suggests that recovery occurs in and among an assemblage of human and nonhuman forces, as that assemblage's capacity to affect the varied forces it encounters grows or expands. It is, properly speaking, the assemblage which recovers, rather than individual bodies or forces within it. I would stress that the advantage of such a formulation lies in the attention it draws to the variety of *nonhuman* entities, forces, affects and relations active in any event of recovery. Of course, the importance of pharmacotherapies in the travails of illness and recovery is well understood, yet medication should not be regarded as the only nonhuman entity active in recovery. Research in social and community psychology, anthropology, sociology, public health and cultural studies is slowly revealing an ever wider cast of nonhuman entities and their role in the everyday work of recovery. Examples include research confirming the role of place attachments in mediating recovery (Tucker 2010); the importance of everyday objects and effects in shaping recovery trajectories (Hodgetts et al. 2010); as well as the security that derives from enduring attachments to 'home' and housing (Duff et al. 2013). These studies hint at the prospect of manipulating or affecting select nonhuman entities in an effort to promote recovery in diverse settings. This is not to deny the significance of human subjects in the course of recovery. Instead, the goal is to resist the de facto privileging of 'the human' to the neglect of other nonhuman ('more-than-human') vectors of recovery. I would add that the application of tools derived from Deleuze's empiricism should provide a means of synthesising recent evidence indicating the significance of nonhuman forces in promoting recovery from mental illness. This should, in turn, support the articulation of an ethological understanding of recovery sensitive to the diversity of human and nonhuman bodies, affects and relations active in the diverse assemblages which give force to recovery in life. First, a brief introduction to debates regarding the nature and experience of recovery is required.

4.1 Mental Illness, Wellbeing and Recovery

For many decades, the vast majority of mental illnesses like schizophrenia, depression and bipolar disorder were regarded as incurable, chronic conditions, associated with significant disability and reduced quality of life (Ramon and Williams 2005).

Even with the emergence of dedicated pharmacotherapies and their progressive refinement, the goal of treatment was largely confined to the successful management of symptoms, and the longer term 'stabilization' of the disorder. This was typically true of treatment regimes for adults, for adolescents and for youth, even though the character of mental health problems was known to differ significantly across the life-course (see Cattan and Tilford 2006; Rickwood et al. 2005). Underpinning such prognoses was a largely biological and/or organic model of mental illness, which regarded such disorders as a function of pathological brain function. This 'biomedical' model of mental illness, and its discrete etiology, remains hugely influential in contemporary responses to mental illness, despite the recent appearance of more holistic paradigms which contest many of the key assumptions underpinning biomedical accounts of mental health (see Henderson and Walter 2009 for a review). Including 'psycho-social' models, along with various strengths and resiliency frameworks, a range of competing accounts of mental illness has emerged, featuring divergent etiological explanations and diverse treatment indications (see Leamy et al. 2011 for a review). Importantly, most contemporary models dispute earlier claims regarding the chronic nature of mental illness, while criticising biomedical accounts for ignoring the social and political contexts of mental illness (see Andresen et al. 2011: 15–24). All emphasise the significance of recovery in identifying appropriate treatment goals for individuals living with mental illness.

The emergence of holistic understandings of recovery has influenced the treatment of mental health problems in many parts of the world, as clinicians and service providers have become more aware of the stigmatising effects of mental illness diagnoses, and the vast differences in illness trajectories reported among those experiencing mental health problems (Cattan and Tilford 2006). This has led to calls for greater sensitivity in the assessment and diagnosis of mental illness, and greater attention to the diversity of lived experiences of mental health problems (Andreson et al. 2011). Of particular importance has been the development of the idea of 'functional recovery' to describe everyday improvements in quality of life despite the lingering experience of symptoms associated with mental illness (Harvey and Bellack 2009: 300–303). Ongoing refinement of the idea of 'functional recovery' has been part of a broader move to repudiate the characterisation of recovery as 'cure', understood as the complete remission of symptoms caused by mental illness (Rowling 2006: 101–106). For example, in sketching the first outlines of a 'biopsychosocial' approach to health care, including the treatment of mental illness, George Engel (1977) stressed that early understandings of recovery were overly narrow, and failed to capture the diversity of treatment outcomes experienced by people living with mental illness, particularly adolescents and young adults (see also Rowling 2006; Rudnick 2012). Engel's biopsychosocial model, which has influenced the design and delivery of mental health care internationally (Andresen et al. 2011), acknowledges the interplay between biological (symptoms, genetic influence), psychological (cognitions, emotions, behaviour), environmental (access to support networks) and socio-political factors (stigma, mental health care) in both the etiology and lived experience of mental illness.

It also acknowledges that individuals may lead healthy, productive and fulfilling lives despite the ongoing experience of symptoms associated with mental illness. Most contemporary understandings of recovery build on Engel's model in adding existential, social and political dimensions to established biomedical accounts of mental illness (see Ritter and Lampkin 2012).

The growing significance of the biopsychosocial paradigm has been further abetted in the last two decades by an international consumer advocacy movement led by individuals living with mental illness, their families and supporters (Beeble and Salem 2009; Bradshaw et al. 2007). This movement has contributed to the emergence of more dynamic understandings of recovery as consumers have provided testimony of their own experience of mental health. Subsequent shifts in the conceptualisation of recovery have also drawn on longitudinal studies demonstrating that recovery from mental illness is possible (Harrison et al. 2001; Jobe and Harrow 2005; Lysaker and Buck 2008). In a systematic review of this literature, Calabrese and Corrigan (2005) report that between 36 and 77 % of individuals recover from mental illnesses like schizophrenia, regardless of treatment modality. The authors conclude that recovery requires more than just passive compliance with pharmacological regimes, and that recovery is more of a process than a static outcome (see also Leamy et al. 2011). These conclusions are echoed in recent socio-cultural accounts of mental health, which stress that recovery is unique to each person, and that treatment ought to focus on improving quality of life rather than focusing solely on mitigating symptoms associated with mental illness (see Ritter and Lampkin 2012 for a review). Other researchers have emphasised the traumas experienced by individuals as a result of diagnosis, treatment and/or hospitalisation, adding that recovery should involve some palliation of these traumas in addition to the physical and psychological problems caused by mental illness (Deegan 2001; Hinshaw 2005). All of this suggests the need to treat the consequences of mental illness, not just the illness.

These kinds of arguments have inspired recent attempts to transform the very idea of recovery, away from an emphasis on the complete remission of symptoms in favour of the notion of managing mental illness across the life-course (see Rudnick 2012 for a review). While these moves have prompted some confusion regarding the diagnostic 'meaning' of recovery, and doubtless accelerated the proliferation of popular understandings of the term, they also reflect the diversity of lived experience of mental illness. Indeed, contemporary understandings of recovery are grounded in the observation that most consumers report some capacity to manage a mental illness while successfully pursuing their nominated life goals (Andresen et al. 2011; Hinshaw 2005; Hopper 2007; Rickwood et al. 2005; Rowling 2006; Sawyer et al. 2001). Such insights are reflected more formally in the range of recovery models in use in both adult and youth mental health services in many countries, including the 'Boston Model', the 'Collaborative Model', 'Strengths and Resiliency' frameworks and the 'Functional Recovery' model (see Ritter and Lampkin 2012). Despite differences of orientation and terminology, each of these models endorses a broad-based biopsychosocial approach in proposing mental health treatment modalities to support the recovery of individuals and groups affected by mental illness. While there is not the scope here to provide a full account of these models, and their application in the design of mental health services, each shares an underlying set of values, principles and orientations (see Leamy et al. 2011). It is worth briefly describing these common terms by way of further contextualising the empirical analysis to follow later in the chapter. Some accounting of these principles should also shed further light on the formal properties of the assemblages of health enacted in each event of recovery.

Briefly, almost all recovery models currently in use in the provision of mental health services in developed countries endorse holistic understandings of recovery that go well beyond the healthy or 'normal' bio-psychological functioning of the individual to include an array of social, familial, cultural, existential and economic aspects. The following six principles are common characteristics of recovery models informing the design of mental health care in Australia, Canada, the United States, the United Kingdom and beyond. The list has been derived from systematic reviews compiled by Andresen and colleagues (2011: 45–52), Leamy and colleagues (2011: 445–452), Boardman (2010: 37–41), Patel and colleagues (2007) and Ritter and Lampkin (2012). First, all existing recovery models stress that individuals living with mental illness can learn, change, grow and adapt to their illness experience. Recovery is thus said to occur through continued learning, experimentation, collaboration, hope and support. Second, recovery models work from a 'strengths' and/or 'resiliency' framework to identify and promote the strengths, capabilities and aspirations of individuals in recovery. This contrasts with traditional biomedical models which focus on alleviating symptoms and remediating 'deficits'. By acting to enhance or promote strengths and resiliency, individuals and groups living with mental illness are affirmed in their capacity to contribute to their own recovery, to combat the specific effects of their illness, and to develop a more positive self-identity. Third, recovery models endorse an equal, open and collaborative relationship between consumers, family, carers and health-care providers. All are regarded as having important contributions to make to the everyday experience of recovery for individuals and groups living with mental illness. Four, all recovery models emphasise a person's right to self-determination in the development of specific recovery goals, including the right to make choices that may lead to mistakes, what is sometimes called the "dignity of risk" (see Anthony 2000). Five, recovery models typically identify the wider community as the most important source of the resources needed to facilitate growth and recovery for people living with mental illness, as opposed to emphasising the 'helping' resources available in formal, clinical services. Finally, recovery models commonly assert that the most effective 'recovery work' occurs in the 'natural context' of an individual consumer's private, family and community life (Parr 2008).

4.2 The Role of Social Inclusion in Promoting Recovery

One of the key features of the emergence and ongoing development of the recovery paradigm in the provision of mental health services has been recognition of the importance of community participation and/or social inclusion for individuals and groups living with a mental illness (Boardman et al. 2010). Indeed, most of the principles nominated in the list of 'recovery values' identified above explicitly endorse the importance of community participation in promoting recovery from mental illness. Arguments regarding the therapeutic utility of community participation typically assert the importance of various assets or resources that may be available locally to facilitate the 'work' of recovery. Moreover, emerging interest in the importance of social inclusion reflects decades of research indicating that individuals experiencing mental illness are at greater risk than other groups of being excluded from full participation in community life (Repper and Perkins 2003: 29–40). This includes the risk of exclusion from post-secondary education, meaningful employment, the development of peer and intimate relationships, and participation in civil associations (Boardman 2010: 22–25). In seeking to combat these risks, policy makers and service providers have supported initiatives designed to mitigate the effects of social exclusion and promote increased community participation for individuals living with mental illness. As such, social inclusion and community participation are each regarded as crucial factors in promoting the health and wellbeing of people living with mental illness. Indeed, it is arguable that social inclusion has become something of a synonym for recovery, given the movement noted above beyond conventional biomedical accounts of recovery in service delivery and policy development.

The apparent conflation of recovery and social inclusion nonetheless opens up the question of how local communities – and the wider social, symbolic, political and economic networks which sustain community life – actually promote or facilitate recovery from mental illness. Interestingly, endorsements of the links between social inclusion, community participation and recovery are a feature of formal mental health policy development in many countries, including Australia, New Zealand, Canada, the United States and the United Kingdom (Boardman et al. 2010; Repper and Perkins 2003; Ritter and Lampkin 2012). Typically, such policies emphasise the importance of delivering high quality mental health care in the community, in contrast to more traditional institutional settings like the clinic or the asylum (Pinfold 2000). In describing such aims, most policy statements seem to endorse the notionally therapeutic role of the *community itself* in supporting and promoting recovery. A common feature of policy development has been the recognition of everyday community settings in the promotion of mental health and/or wellbeing (Curtis 2010). Equally common is the call for action to address social exclusion among individuals living with a mental illness, primarily through partnerships with sporting, recreational and arts bodies to encourage greater participation in community life (see Parr 2008).

However, most recent national mental health strategies avoid explicit statements regarding the *means by which* community participation and increased social inclusion actually facilitate recovery from mental illness. Perhaps it is more charitable to observe that policy makers seem to regard these links as 'given' in light of research conducted over many years indicating the role of social inclusion and community participation in promoting recovery (see Curtis 2010: 35–40). Much of this research started in a more exploratory fashion with an interest in clarifying the role of community participation in facilitating health, wellbeing and recovery broadly defined (see Cummins et al. 2007; Macintyre et al. 2002). This work led to a series of insights regarding the links between place, social inclusion and health promotion, along with diverse theoretical models purporting to explain these links. Important examples include research and theory concerning the idea of 'therapeutic landscapes' (Williams, A. 2007), 'restorative settings' (Milligan and Bingley 2007) and 'enabling environments' (Steinfeld and Danford 1999). Taken together, the study of what might collectively be referred to as "enabling places" (Duff 2011), has consistently demonstrated a relationship between social inclusion and recovery from primary health problems. This research has largely focussed on the significance of individual aspects of community life – such as places and settings, community services, the provision of resources and supports, and the importance of family and peer relationships – in generating therapeutic benefits (Cummins et al. 2007). Such studies indicate that select community settings incorporate unique therapeutic qualities or "stress-buffering mechanisms", which facilitate wellbeing and mitigate health inequalities (Stockdale et al. 2007: 1870).

While it is important to stress that the bulk of existing studies have explored health in broad, generic terms, a small but rapidly growing literature indicates that these therapeutic qualities are also effective in facilitating recovery from mental illness (Cohen 2004; De Silva et al. 2005; Kawachi and Berkman 2001). Community integration, social inclusion and 'place-attachment' have been shown to be particularly important in promoting recovery, inasmuch as specific community places reportedly furnish an array of material, social and affective resources to facilitate health and recovery (Kawachi and Berkman 2001; Parr 2007; Stockdale et al. 2007). Available evidence indicates that these resources include opportunities for 'bridging' social networks and extending social ties (Kawachi and Berkman 2001); for personal reflection and the promotion of 'ontological security' (Hidalgo and Hernandez 2001); increased opportunities for leisure, aesthetic and/or recreational pursuits (Cattell et al. 2008); as well as relaxation, 'mental restoration' and the relief of stress and anxiety (Korpela et al. 2008). Other researchers have demonstrated the links between social inclusion and an increase in community 'belonging' and 'life purpose' (Boardman 2010); the development of 'social capital' (Boyd et al. 2008); as well as improvements in mood and wellbeing (Ritter and Lampkin 2012). Each of these processes has been shown to facilitate recovery from mental illness in specific instances, either through the promotion of physical health, enhanced psychological functioning, subjective wellbeing, or some combination thereof (Parr 2008). These kinds of findings also dovetail with recent studies of neighbourhood experience, concentrations of economic and social disadvantage, and the array of supports needed for successful community integration for individuals and groups recovering from mental illness (Boardman 2010; Curtis 2010; Kawachi and Berkman 2001). All of this again suggests the significance of social inclusion in facilitating recovery.

It must also be acknowledged however, that most of the existing research persists in identifying *associations* between social inclusion, community participation and recovery, without always clarifying the particular causal relations that generate these effects. To return, therefore, to the task of 'thinking with' Deleuze in an effort to explain the experience of recovery, it may be argued that existing research regarding social inclusion and recovery has largely failed to identify the 'conditions of real experience' involved in the *production of recovery* in specific territories or milieus. Subjecting the available literature to a more thoroughly Deleuzian interrogation then, one might say that social inclusion functions in support of recovery precisely to the extent that it affords expansion or reterritorialisation of the various assemblages of health active in each event of recovery. Hence, the 'actual experience' of social inclusion for people living with mental illness is one of ongoing enhancements in the array of bodies, affects, events, objects and processes they may affect and be affected by. To the extent that social inclusion actively promotes recovery, it succeeds by opening bodies (or assemblages) up to a more diverse range of affects, relations and events. Reflecting some of the most significant research findings drawn from the literature surveyed above, I would stress that the varied assemblages of health in which recovery is enacted or performed always contain *social, material and affective* forces, bodies and dimensions. I will briefly examine each domain before turning to consider the qualitative accounts of mental health and recovery collected in Melbourne, Australia. This analysis should also facilitate the articulation of a more ethological understanding of recovery to be completed in the chapter's final sections.

4.2.1 *The Social Assemblage*

It may be argued that social inclusion and community participation facilitate recovery from mental health problems to the extent that each promotes access to an array of *social, material and affective resources* which may then be utilised in the everyday work of recovery (see Duff 2010, 2012 for a review). Drawing on the 'empirico-ethological' account of health described in Chaps. 2 and 3, social resources may be understood to describe the varied processes and encounters – the relational, affective and embodied 'signs' and 'events' – which support the creation and maintenance of social networks in collocations of the human and the nonhuman. Social resources thus describe the means or processes by which social ties are cultivated and maintained. The real problem however, is to explain sociality itself in terms of the discrete resources that permit the realisation of *specifically social* relations. Such a concern speaks once more to the need to identify the 'conditions of real experience' immanent to the production of sociality, and its subsequent expression in the course of recovery from mental illness. In the absence of such analysis, sociality risks being 'naturalised' as innately healthy or therapeutic, leaving unresolved the question of how social interaction is mediated in a social field, and how sociality actually supports recovery. Suggestive indications of the links between sociality and recovery may be drawn from the literature on social capital, even though this literature rarely addresses the conditions of sociality itself (Duff 2011).

As it is conventionally understood, social capital comprises the myriad bonds of trust, reciprocity and cooperation that characterise social life (see Portes 1998). The model attempts to conceptualise the impact of social networks through the study of the social, affective and material resources on which they draw. Such resources have been shown to enable and extend the array of 'coordinated actions' realisable within particular networks (Hawe and Shiell 2000). While the specific resources individuals actually derive from their networks are always diverse, one's overall stock of social capital is fundamentally linked to the size, number and diversity of one's network connections, and the ways one can leverage these ties through the use of other forms of financial, intellectual, cultural and/or symbolic capital. Like these other forms, social capital 'flows' through networks in a series of formal and informal transactions. As such, social capital may be regarded as a fluid and potentially transferable resource useful for the realization of various goals or actions, including specific health related goals (Almedom 2005). Examples of social capital range from informational resources including job referrals, health care tips, and relationship counselling, through to the social transmission of material resources such as loans, 'gifts', bartering and other non-market based forms of exchange. What the extant literature on social capital largely lacks, however, is a compelling account of the character of sociality, and the mechanisms involved in the cultivation of social ties.

In other words, the notion of social capital may well describe the *varied benefits* that individuals and groups derive from their social networks – such as trust, solidarity, reciprocity and proximity to resources – yet these benefits do little themselves to explain how sociality unfolds in particular contexts (or territories). What is missing is an account of how 'the social' is generated, performed or enacted in relations between bodies (both human and nonhuman). Deleuze and Guattari's (1987) notion of the assemblage provides a unique way of thinking about social resources, and their distinctive modes of production and circulation. Such innovation relies on the idiosyncratic understanding of the 'social' conveyed in Deleuze and Guattari's (1987: 219–230) discussion of sociality and its modulation in "belief", "power" and "desire". According to their analysis, the 'social' does not comprise a discrete substance or domain. It should not be construed as a material infrastructure that guides or frames the myriad interactions that characterise everyday life (De Landa 2008b). Rather, the social ought to be understood in terms of a "field…animated by all kinds of movements of decoding and deterritorialization affecting 'masses' and operating at different speeds and paces" (Deleuze and Guattari 1987: 220). As such, the social is forever constituted or assembled in 'masses' comprising composite relations of desire, belief and force that each effect a kind of *sociality of the mass*. The social is, in this respect, a relation or connection by which associations between bodies, objects, ideas, beliefs, desires and events are created, maintained and contested in particular territories (see Dewsbury 2011: 149–151). The social is always relational and never the sum total of the elements so assembled. It follows that sociality is enacted in assemblages which collect or enfold bodies, forces, affects and relations in the creation of a 'social body'. What is commonly described as social must therefore be understood as a *flux of relational forces* that affect diverse bodies, objects, ideas and processes, temporarily folding these forces in the creation of a discrete mass. This flux is both the medium and the effect of the social.

Drawing on each of the last three chapters, the forces by which the social is enacted may be said to include the asubjective *desires* which conjoin bodies (human and nonhuman) in 'social interaction'; the *affects* generated in such interactions, along with the modulations in the power of acting of the bodies so assembled; the *beliefs* that galvanise practical action in 'social' contexts, such as the beliefs that lead bodies to assemble in pursuit of political, economic and/or 'social' goals; as well as the *power relations* involved in efforts to regulate the conduct of the varied bodies assembled in the social mass. Each of these forces combines in the composition or assembling of any social entity, encounter or context. They are at work, for example, in the forces assembled in crowds; in all social interaction and communication; and in every instance of intimacy or hostility enacted between bodies. Indeed, they are implicated in every encounter in which some kind of 'social' effect, relation or consideration may be said to be central (see also De Landa 2006: 47–67). Importantly, the desires, beliefs, affects, bodies and forces involved in the expression of sociality are each 'folded' into the assemblages that compose or enable human life, the embodied person. Sociality, as such, is expressed in "relations of exteriority established among the contents of experience" (De Landa 2006: 47). Social relations are 'exterior' inasmuch as beliefs, affects, signs and forces must be regarded as preindividual or "subpersonal" elements that are forever combining and recombining in the organisation of subjective life. There is no necessary (or internally determined) relation between these 'subpersonal' elements; rather they are combined in the various encounters by which social life is constituted. It is equally true that the subpersonal elements that combine in the expression of (human) sociality are not innate but must be acquired in concert with other bodies, other forces, other affects, other encounters. And so, as bodies (assemblages) assemble or enfold these 'social' competencies, they are able to establish more diverse relations with a greater array of bodies, and thus affect more diverse actions. It may be concluded therefore, that social resources inhere in the knot of associations that comprise assemblages, and in the individual territories that support these masses or 'social bodies' (De Landa 2008b: 255). As I will demonstrate in later sections, this logic provides grounds for identifying the varied social resources (beliefs, desires, affects and relations) involved in recovery from mental illness, insofar as recovery may be understood as a *qualitative transformation in the assemblages that express the recovering body*. Sociality (and the social resources which support it) remains, for this reason, one of the most important mechanisms through which assemblages of health are produced. Equally important is the selection and deployment of material resources in context.

4.2.2 The Material Assemblage

Deleuze and Guattari's (1987) account of the generation, composition and transformation of assemblages emphasises at every turn the coproduction of material spaces or territories. In addition to uniquely social, affective and/or semiotic elements, all assemblages have territorial components and so each assemblage must, at least in part, be regarded as a material achievement. More directly, assemblages draw together discrete material resources in the deterritorialisation and reterritorialisation of place. All assemblages create a territory in other words. Yet the material elements that comprise territories cannot be regarded as fixed – just as space should not itself be understood as a static, geometric array – in that each of the material elements available for the work of territorialisation circulates in relations of speed and slowness. All matter is in motion, even if this movement is sometimes imperceptible. As such, assemblages are created or expressed in a "double articulation" in which elements combine in "formed matters" subject to a variety of "relative movements" (Deleuze and Guattari 1987: 72). The first articulation involves the selection and combination of 'raw materials' out of which discrete territories are composed. Deleuze and Guattari (1987: 40) stress that the "first articulation chooses or deducts, from unstable particle-flows, metastable molecular or quasi-molecular units (substances) upon which it imposes a statistical order of connections and successions (forms)". As De Landa (2008a: 162) helpfully explains, this *process of selection* applies to the varied procedures by which "geological, biological and even social strata are formed". Each may be regarded as material processes insofar as each involves the combination or synthesis of material elements in the expression of discrete geological, biological or social territories. This includes, for example, the processes of selection and sedimentation which transpire over 'geological' time in the formation of physical structures; the combination of discrete material elements, forms and capacities in the evolution of biological life; and the convergence of material elements by which social entities are composed and/or recognised. In each case, the selection, attraction, synthesis and/or combination of material elements is 'articulated' in the creation of a territorial space unique to each geological, biological or social entity. And so, the sedimentation of materials settles in the space of the mountain; material elements are folded into the biological territory of the human body; just as the assemblage of crowd, bodies, communication, infrastructure and transportation expresses the social space of the modern city (see Thrift 2007).

The second articulation involves a "folding" that establishes "a stable functional structure" for the elements selected in the first articulation (Deleuze and Guattari 1987: 41). Put another way, the second articulation "establishes functional, compact, stable substances (forms), and constructs the molar compounds in which these structures are simultaneously actualized (substances)" (Deleuze and Guattari 1987: 41). The point is that each of the processes of selection and combination by which material elements are assembled in the expression of a territory (the first articulation), necessarily entails, in the second articulation, the expression of a series of explicit functions, capacities or forms. This second articulation establishes (or seeks to determine) the function, meaning, purpose or form of the territory effected in the first articulation. Moreover, the *molar* processes involved in the second articulation serve to limit the possible array of forms that may be attributed to a material territory. An interesting example may well be the human body itself and the way each of the material territories that make up the assembled body, such as the hand, is 'overcoded' in an attempt to delimit its function, form, capacity or purpose. Another example concerns the formation of crowds and the overcoding processes involved in the distinctions drawn between 'peaceable assemblies', insurrectionary mobs, incipient social movements and so on (see Thrift 2004). It is important to note however, as Deleuze and Guattari (1987) stress, that neither the first nor the second articulation is ever completed or fixed. Matter is continuously in motion, such that both the first and the second articulation need to be understood as a *movement towards stabilisation* rather than the final achievement of this state. Just as the 'raw materials' that combine in the creation of material entities are forever in motion, so too are the forms and functions that serve as the effective expressions of these processes. For De Landa (2008a: 164), this means that all material entities, forms, spaces and territories must be regarded as "objectively changeable: they may undergo destabilising processes affecting their materiality, their expressivity or both". This is why Deleuze and Guattari emphasise processes of territorialisation and deterritorialisation, in that all material forms, all assemblages, remain fluid and unstable ('objectively changeable') according to the historical, political, social and/or economic forces applied to, or expressed through, them. I should add that the means of this double articulation provide a range of insights into the formation of the varied assemblages of health central to the experience of recovery from mental illness.

Perhaps the most significant insight concerns the active role of material objects, assets or resources in the course of recovery. While the role of material resources is often highlighted in discussions of effective public health interventions (Baum 2008), these resources are usually regarded as means to other more substantive health-related goals, rather than active constituents of health and recovery in their own right. The therapeutic utility of material resources is especially salient in the case of financial benefits such as wages, welfare transfers and other allowances; material assistance associated with the delivery of essential services like health care and education; or in regards to goods and services accessed in relations of bartering or gifting (Portes 1998; Williams, A. 2007). These material resources are fundamental to the maintenance of health and wellbeing, shaping access to services and enabling all manner of health promoting activities (Baum 2008). Yet these resources are rarely regarded as constitutive of health and recovery in their own right. This, I would wager, is the primary contention of a more Deleuzian approach to the study of assemblages of health. Rather than regard material resources as tools or benefits of 'marginal utility' in the pursuit of health-related goals, material resources ought to be understood as functioning, active constituents of the various assemblages that accrue in the maintenance (or promotion) of health. While much recent work focuses on the links between the relative distribution of material resources and the creation of health inequalities between settings or regions (Cummins et al. 2007: 1830–1832), a more Deleuzian perspective calls attention to the *relational coproduction of health* in assemblages of organic, biological, social and material forces (see Fox 2011: 434–440). These forces are folded into the assemblage by way of a double articulation; first as materials made available for the work of health promotion; and then as they are enfolded into the body in the experience of health, in its becoming well.

Such arguments restore to material resources the full force of their activity (see also Latour 2005: 63–65). One of the most important features of Deleuze's empiricism is the symmetry it ascribes to humans, objects, technologies and events (Dewsbury 2011: 149–150). Deleuze does not regard agency as a unique function of human bodies, instead he spatialises and distributes agentic forces (or capacities) in and among an assemblage of human and nonhuman bodies, objects and entities. An activity like recovery is, in this respect, a function of the assemblages in which health is produced as an effect of relations established between an array of social, material, biological and physical forces, some of which are present at the moment of this action, while others are absent. This logic may be contrasted with much conventional thinking about health, where the individual human body is typically regarded as the sole agent involved in the activity of health promotion. One may well object that various biomedical technologies are central to this achievement, yet the activity (or health promoting utility) of these technologies is more commonly attributed to the manner of their selection and application at the discretion of (human) clinicians and/or bureaucrats. In insisting upon the activity of material forces, Deleuze provides a compelling basis for rethinking the therapeutic properties of matter itself. Indeed, his empiricism suggests that the production of assemblages in discrete territories generates a host of material resources useful for the maintenance of health or recovery. This includes material resources as they are conventionally understood, such as health care services, employment opportunities and welfare initiatives, as well as the objects, instruments and forces that comprise place in its very materiality. These latter forces potentially facilitate an array of therapeutic modifications in the assemblages which support or express health (and recovery). In each instance, the contours of the assemblage shift as novel forces are folded within it. This folding determines how the assemblage may affect (and be affected) by the material forces it encounters. Such affective modulations may themselves be regarded as therapeutic, to the extent that each potentially facilitates an array of health promoting activities. This finally speaks to the affective dimensions of assemblages of health.

4.2.3 The Affective Assemblage

All assemblages should be regarded as affective entities inasmuch as affective processes are at least partially responsible for the formations of the assemblage. This includes the modulations in the powers of acting of the bodies so assembled (see Massumi 2002: 32–39). Of course, Deleuze (1988) argues that affects are not the innate property of feeling, sensing bodies but rather obtain in *encounters between bodies*, both human and nonhuman. As I noted in Chap. 2, affect ought here to be understood in two distinctive ways. First, affect describes an array of feeling states such as anger, shame, fear, sorrow or happiness. Each of these states corresponds with a specific feeling such that envy, for example, is experienced as a qualitatively different condition than anger or sorrow. However, Deleuze (1988: 49–50) stresses that affects convey something more than a simple concatenation of feeling states. Affects also constitute the body's 'power of acting'; its unique capacity to affect (and be affected) by the world of bodies and things that it encounters. Deleuze (1992) insists that every encounter subtly transforms the body's affective orientations, either to enhance that body's power of acting or to diminish it. This affective modification involves a transfer of power, capacities or action-potential between bodies (Deleuze 1988: 48–50). The assembled body, itself a complex assemblage of simple elements both human and nonhuman, may in this way, be characterised by the ongoing modifications in its power of acting, occasioned by the encounters it experiences, or becomes capable of experiencing (Deleuze 1992).

The dynamic transmission of capacities or powers from one body to another should be understood as the primary feature of affective resources as they function in support of the ongoing modification of assemblages of health and illness. This process is defined by continuous variation as each encounter causes a relative shift in a body's capacities. Affects, in this sense, constitute the basic experiential mechanism by which capacities are acquired or lost to an assemblage. The affects associated with the experience of hope offer useful examples of this process, and its role in the 'real experience' of recovery from mental illness. Ben Anderson (2006: 733–735) argues that hope is always a belief in "something more", a belief in that which has "not yet become". This belief is generated in a range of affective encounters, insofar as hope is inspired in relation to diverse objects, places, bodies and events. However moving these encounters may be, hope is primarily experienced as a visceral enhancement of a body's capacity to act in response to these encounters. As a body becomes hopeful, a whole array of "capacities and capabilities are enabled" (Anderson 2006: 735). Hence, to feel hopeful is to feel more capable of the agency necessary to realise particular actions, to affect a more diverse array of bodies, or to compose relations with novel forces. The very generation of affective resources like hope, confidence or excitement facilitates the flow of capacities in and between bodies, sometimes in subtle ways, sometimes in more profound and transformative ways (Deleuze 1988). Indeed it is the question of how encounters generate novel capacities that is most relevant to my discussion of the lived experience of health and recovery, understood in terms of a qualitative increment in the assemblage's capacity to positively affect the bodies it encounters.

I would argue further that this question points the way to novel investigations of the role of affective resources like hope, optimism and confidence in the promotion and maintenance of mental health (see Leamy et al. 2011). Hope in particular, has been shown to shadow almost all aspects of mental illness, from the onset of symptoms to help seeking behaviour, compliance with treatment modalities and post intervention recovery (see Bernays et al. 2007; Eliott and Oliver 2007; Rickwood et al. 2005). Hope is, in this way, "linked to the capacity for behaviour change" (Bernays et al. 2007: S7) and the prospects for a return to good mental health. Confidence and optimism further confirm the relationship between affect and motivation (understood as a body's distinctive capacity for action), in that greater confidence and increased optimism are each associated with an increased predilection for health-related activity. Hope affects the entire assemblage in other words, investing it with greater scope in its power of acting, and so providing resources to support action consistent with the ongoing health (or recovery) of that assemblage. In characterising the ways affective forces like hope and confidence are folded into the assemblage (by way of the transfer of power between bodies), Deleuze provides an intriguing indication of the ways everyday affective encounters may be said to be productive of recovery. The point as always, is to uncover the 'conditions of real experience' immanent to the modulations of recovery in particular territories. Deleuze's ethology suggests that 'good' encounters facilitate the experience of recovery from mental illness to the extent that they involve a transfer of power between bodies. Recent accounts of the therapeutic aspects of social inclusion provide further illustrations of this process.

Studies investigating the relationship between place, belonging and "restorative experiences" (Korpela et al. 2008), provide concrete evidence of the affective modulations in a body's power of acting expressed in all healthy encounters. Early studies in environmental psychology, for example, examined the health-related benefits associated with "positive" encounters with place, particularly those which result in greater "place attachment" (Kaplan and Kaplan 1989). The critical idea is that place attachment is more than a simple emotional bond, for it also delivers discrete health related benefits. Research on 'restorative experiences' suggests that positive affective encounters in (or with) particular places do this by helping to reduce stress; by moderating mood and emotional balance; by restoring 'directed attention' and reducing fatigue; and by boosting 'positive' affects like joy, hope and wonder, while reducing 'negative' affects like anger, frustration and irritability (Korpela and Ylen 2009; Kuo and Sullivan 2001). Confirmed in studies all over the world, it has been shown that places that generate strong feelings of attachment, belonging and functional utility also generate a range of positive affects, while reducing fatigue and stress and restoring attentional and/or cognitive capacities (see Williams, A. 2007 for a review). Rendered in slightly more Deleuzian terms, it is arguable that these kinds of place attachments furnish affective resources useful for the everyday work of recovery, and the wider promotion of health and wellbeing. Certain places are, in effect, annexed to the recovering body and the particular assemblages of health which give form to this recovery. To the extent that bodies are able to enter into relations with specific places or territories, these places are folded into the assemblage, further accelerating the lines of 'becoming well' available to it.

In keeping with Deleuze's (2001) empirical method, the task is to patiently catalogue the kinds of affective resources generated in a given place – noting the characteristic features of the material setting, the activities of bodies and forces and the flux of events – in order to trace the modifications in affect and capacity experienced in that place. A place may be described as enabling of a body's recovery to the extent that it furnishes affective resources like hope, joy or confidence that extend that body's power of acting, even if only momentarily. Such is the 'real experience' of bodies recovering from mental illness in the context of an assemblage of health. Just as mental health may be understood in Deleuzian terms to exceed the individual body (ordinarily understood as the locus of mental illness), recovery too needs to be understood as a dynamic process that affects an assembled cast of human and nonhuman forces. As I have indicated in each of the last three sections, the assemblage incorporates select social, material and affective forces such that recovery ought to be understood as a relational achievement effected across the entire assemblage. Based on this assessment, it may be added that recovery involves an ever increasing capacity to enter into relations with these social, material and affective forces, within the milieus in which recovery 'takes place' (Tucker 2010). Understood in this way, it can be argued that a body recovers from mental illness as it incorporates and utilises select social, material and affective resources that enable or sustain its recovery. Picking up recent discussions of the importance of belonging and social inclusion in the course of recovery from mental illness (Boardman et al. 2010), it is likely that almost all 'social fields' provide access to the social, material and affective resources useful for the work of recovery, to a greater or lesser extent. What is yet to be established is the manner in which bodies identify, access, incorporate or utilise these resources in the ongoing expression of a discrete assemblages of health to support of their recovery. I will now explore this question in detail, taking up the tools provided in Deleuze's ethology in the analysis of qualitative reports of health, illness and recovery collected in Melbourne, Australia.

4.3 Assemblages of Recovery (Becoming Well)

The ideas assembled below are drawn from a series of qualitative studies completed in recent years in Melbourne among individuals and groups living with a mental illness (see Duff 2011, 2012; Duff et al. 2013 for details). Each study has sought to identify and explore the ways in which place, social inclusion and community participation may support the process of recovery from mental illness. Each moreover, has sought to document the 'real experience' of place, community and belonging in recovery, consistent with the theoretical resources described above. This necessarily required a high degree of methodological experimentation in an attempt to capture both the human and the nonhuman constituents of the varied assemblages of health in which recovery may be said to have accrued for participants. Each study utilised ethnographic and qualitative methods to generate rich descriptions of participant's experience of place and recovery. Yet I also sought to attend to the nonhuman constituents of recovery, adopting experimental visual and 'affective' methods in an attempt to capture more of the social, material and affective aspects of recovery. This included spatial and affective mapping exercises based on techniques described by Samuel Dennis and colleagues (Dennis et al. 2009); the 'go along' interview method introduced by Richard Carpiano (2009); visual methods including the film and photo-elicitation described by Wang and Burris (1997); as well as face-to-face interviews. Further detail regarding the methods, procedures, ethical approvals and analytical strategies deployed in these studies are available elsewhere (see Duff 2010, 2011, 2012).

The primary aim linking each study has been the effort to describe some of the conditions of recovery as they are experienced in the places, relations, encounters and affects that comprise the assemblages in which recovery from mental illness is enacted. For a long time now recovery from mental illness has been understood as an ongoing process of 'becoming well' in multiple 'life domains', including personal and family relationships, community participation, employment and education, housing security, physical and emotional health, identity and self esteem (see Leamy et al. 2011). It is further understood that recovery in each of these domains is a daily 'project' greatly facilitated by the kinds of assets or resources that individuals are able to access locally to support the 'work' of recovery. This incidentally is the primary rationale underpinning efforts to enhance the social inclusion of individuals living with mental health problems. In addition to combating the social exclusion many consumer's experience, it is argued that enhanced social inclusion is associated with increased access to varied social or community resources useful for the everyday work of recovery (see Boardman et al. 2010). Recovery is, in this sense, presented as a kind of instrumental calculus in which 'proximity to resources' figures as the primary variable determining an individual's likely progress towards, or retreat from, their nominated recovery goals (see Curtis 2010; Pinfold 2000). As applied in the mental health literature, this logic treats recovery as the outcome of the allocation, cultivation and deployment of local resources, inasmuch as greater access to these resources is associated with improved health (see Almedom 2005).

Yet this logic reveals very little about the 'real experience' of recovery in terms of the actual conditions in which the varying resources known to support recovery are identified, cultivated and deployed. This is where the concepts furnished in Deleuze's empiricism, and the developmental ethology I have derived from it, may prove most valuable. At issue is the task of explaining how recovery advances and retreats in the experience of bodies living with mental illness. The job is to explain the conditions of real experience immanent to recovery, and how these conditions articulate within the various assemblages of health in which recovery is expressed. I should add that such analysis ought to shed light on how social inclusion supports (or fails to support) the everyday work of recovery, and how social inclusion may be cultivated in support of recovery. The argument advanced above that social inclusion supports recovery to the extent that it facilitates access to select social, material and affective resources, suggests, in turn, that these resources ought to be amenable to empirical analysis. Recovery and social inclusion must be explained in other words. The various studies conducted in Melbourne confirm that social inclusion is one of the principal mechanisms by which bodies are transformed in the event of recovery. Each recovery event involves *social, material and affective* dimensions, as the assemblages which express recovery take on novel social, material and affective elements. Examples from the data should help to flesh these arguments out.

4.3.1 Recovery (The Role of the Social Assemblage)

Participants in the Melbourne studies endorsed the importance of social inclusion and community participation in support of their ongoing recovery. Most identified strong links between place and social inclusion, with most describing an array of local places vital to the everyday experience of recovery. This included sites long known to support sociality and/or social inclusion, like cafes, restaurants, parks, gardens, shopping malls and community centres (see Curtis 2010), as well as less familiar sites such as suburban street-scapes, cemeteries, train carriages and disused car-parks. Most often, 'place' was found to shape the character of social interaction, affording opportunities either for greater intimacy with friends or family, or for novel connections with peers and strangers (see also Clark and Uzzell 2002). At bottom however, sociality was found to involve a slow process of cultivating and developing social ties as the 'recovering body' becomes sensitive to the signs and events by which sociality accrues in real experience. As such, the recovering body establishes novel social relations, which both extend the array of actions that body is capable of enacting, while adding additional social bodies to the assemblages of health immanent to recovery. Participants described various social signs and events in the course of documenting their recovery. These signs and events ranged from sketchy indications of a willingness among others to engage in conversation; a sense of the appropriate time and place of sociality; greater sensitivity to the signs of social interaction and engagement (does that person want to talk to me? when has the conversation begun? when is it my turn to speak? what does silence 'mean'? how are bodies 'used' in the mechanics of social interaction?); as well as a sense of the affective depth of friendship and intimacy. A number of participants spoke of acquiring these sensitivities – *of learning how to be social* – by observing the signs and events of sociality in 'social' spaces like cafes, restaurants and shops, without actually engaging at that time in social interaction themselves. The point was to observe sociality from a seemingly 'safe distance', present within the social without necessarily being a part of it, acquiring a sense of the signs and events of interaction. Summing up this kind of experience, one participant (Robert)[1] noted that,

> I just like being around people not necessarily having to talk to people, just watching them you know, how they talk to each other, what they do when other people come along, trying to imagine what they're talking about. I spend hours doing this sometimes and it's amazing how no one seems to notice. I feel invisible sometimes I suppose but I just like watching everything.

---

[1] Note that participants in all studies were invited to nominate their own pseudonym or 'nickname' in the interest of preserving their anonymity in the presentation of research findings.

In the walking tours and other observational activities conducted with Robert it was noted that he frequently became interested in how people were interacting, particularly in cafes. Robert would observe how people engaged with one another, where they sat, whether they had any physical contact and so forth, using these observations as the basis for a series of speculations about the topic of the observed conversation and the nature of the relationship between the interlocutors. Quite unselfconsciously, Robert added that these experiences were all part of his recovery, helping him learn the norms of social etiquette, consistent with the ways "healthy people, you know the ones that aren't mad" socialise. Robert went on to say

> First coming here (café), it was really instrumental for me in restoring my ability to socialize with people, just watching people like I said. Then you start seeing people regularly who come every time the same time and you build up this non-threatening little community in a café, saying hello you know. One day you're sitting there and another regular comes along and you'll have a yarn and sometimes you can get into these really philosophical discussions.

When I asked Robert if this kind of experience might be a good example of social inclusion, he agreed, adding that

> most times, when people get sick (experience severe mental illness) you just lose all your friends. People don't want to know you so it's really important that you find ways to rebuild those connections. We all need friends right?!

Yet rebuilding social connections was found to be rarely straightforward, hence the importance of observing social interactions at a 'safe' distance, before risking a chance encounter, a brief conversation that might stimulate a more enduring connection. Again, the primary purpose of such observations seemed to be the opportunity to survey the varied signs and events of sociality such that one might become more sensitive to these signs in one's own subsequent interactions. Another participant, Cheryl, identified various social signs in describing the place of public transport in her recovery. Cheryl identified Melbourne's train network as one of the most important places or supports in her "recovery journey". Cheryl spoke of long trips on Melbourne's trains observing people coming and going, speculating about their purpose and their lives. Mostly however, Cheryl spoke of observing people's interactions; the ways school students gossiped, argued, flirted and misbehaved; how city bound office-workers protected themselves from apparently unwelcome social interactions by hiding behind sunglasses, headphones and a book; or how elderly commuters seemed intent on talking to strangers regardless of their enthusiasm (or lack thereof) for the conversation. She added that,

> The train is amazing really because it's like everyone from Melbourne is here in one place, normally I guess we try and avoid each other. But here on the train you have you know the unemployed next to office workers and city-types and kids and families and everyone is trying not to speak or something. So I just love watching people, how they try and avoid talking or how the oldies want to start talking to you about the footy or their grandkids or something.

The point once again is that the signs of sociality – or the rudiments of social interaction – may be learned in these quotidian events. Like Robert's observations,

Cheryl's experience appeared to function as an "apprenticeship" in the signs of sociality (Bogue 2004: 330–334). Each such sign affords further lessons in the art of the social; and so one learns if a stranger is receptive to conversation; what kinds of things friends talk about on the train; whether or not the train is a public or a private place for the purposes of sociality; or the proper etiquette of polite conversation should one happen upon a little known acquaintance. Each of these signs serves as a potential opening into a wider social network, furnishing opportunities (should one wish to take them) for the kinds of social networking by which social inclusion may be lived as a tangible feature of recovery. These are the actual conditions of recovery as they pertain to the roles of sociality and social inclusion in recovery.

Indeed, it was interesting to note just how often participants used the language of 'connection' or 'fitting in' to describe the benefits associated with social inclusion. It is no exaggeration to observe that participants mainly regarded social inclusion as a means of joining a wider 'social body'; entering an assemblage of health in the language of this chapter. As Melissa noted in describing a local hair salon:

> I might have holes in my shoes, but if my hair is looking good then I feel like I am getting better, looking better, fitting in I suppose. I am who I am supposed to be. It's also a great place to meet people and just talk, like lots of other women will be there with their kids or pets or whatever and you just have this time to talk to people, with no pressure, and it all just adds to my confidence.

The link Melissa observes here between 'social connection', wellbeing and recovery was explicitly endorsed by almost all participants, with many describing the onset of mental illness as a period of profound social disconnection. Social contact was subsequently regarded by most as an effective way of combating this disruption, of feeling connected to a community again. Noting the importance of enduring friendships, Mark added that;

> It's a very important thing in life to be connected with people who understand what you are going through. Being connected to friends is really important and now my friends know um, just where things are with my life. They are all really sensitive about it and that makes a huge difference, just like day to day.

Other participants emphasised the importance of supportive family networks, even though many acknowledged that such relations were often strained as a result of people's experience of mental illness and/or family member's individual responses to it. In an instructive remark Grant observed that "you can't underestimate how powerful it is for a person to be in touch with family." Gregory concurred, emphasising "how important families are in terms of just supporting each other through things, so many people with mental health issues end up disconnected from their family." Another informant, Al, noted of his family,

> They are all very supportive of me. I talk to them every week or two. I still lean on them as well at times you know like sometimes I borrow money from them. I'm a member of the family that does keep in touch with everyone, I support others and they support me.

Social and family connections were thus described as distinctive resources in their own right, useful both as a means of promoting recovery and sustaining a sense of wellbeing, but also for generating a more profound sense of hope and optimism for the future. Sociality ought to be regarded as a resource precisely because each connection reportedly provides support for the deepening of other connections. As Robert averred, each interaction makes the next one "that little bit easier", enhancing one's sense of wellbeing and recovery. Yet 'connection' was also reported to be dynamic in character in that the *conditions* of social connection – like self confidence, opportunity, patience, persistence and empathy – betray the complex links between social, affective and material resources in the place and promotion of recovery. Social connection may usefully be construed as a kind of relational union in this sense, in which the recovering body is augmented to include a wider array of forces. Each event of social connection adds to the body expressed or composed in this assemblage of health. In acquiring novel social 'parts', the body of recovery grows, 'becoming well' to the extent that each social interaction furnishes resources in support of recovery. It is not, as I have stressed, the individual body that recovers; recovery is always, already a social, relational, achievement. As the assemblage grows with each social connection, and as each social connection augments the bodies composed within this assemblage, health and recovery advance as a lived transition in the assemblage's power of acting. Robert, Cheryl, Melissa, Mark and Al observed as much in their accounts of recovery, even if they neglected to speak in the language of the assemblage. Robert's interactions in a local cafe; Cheryl's experience of public space on Melbourne's trains; Melissa's sense of 'fitting in' in a local hair salon; Mark's endorsement of the value of friendship; each in their own way speaks to the composition of an assemblage of health, drawing in diverse human and nonhuman bodies, objects and forces in the lived expression of recovery.

4.3.2 Recovery (The Role of the Material Assemblage)

The accounts of health and recovery provided by participants typically featured a range of material resources in addition to the social resources noted above. Often times, participant's efforts to explore their local communities were explicitly motivated by a desire to increase access to material resources useful for the work of recovery. For example, Mary's community map highlighted the significance of a charity store, which she went on to describe as one of her "favourite places". As Mary elaborated;

> I have my retail therapy here, it's therapy for me, absolute therapy. You can find the most amazing stuff here for 5 or 10 dollars, stuff I need for the house, or just stuff I might need one day. I love the unknown, you just never know what you're going to find there. I love it, if it closes down, I would be so depressed. It's like heaven really and it always boosts my mood, my endorphins go sky high here.

Mary's report further highlights the heterogeneity of the bodies and forces at work in the assemblages of health expressive of recovery. While the charity store might in the first instance increase Mary's access to a discrete material resource (the access to affordable material items), it also serves to promote her mood and general wellbeing ("my endorphins go sky high here"). Other participants spoke in a similar vein about the therapeutic significance of material objects themselves, and the ways such objects mediate the experience of recovery. Al, for example, spoke of the therapeutic character of his shed in terms of the materials, tools and objects contained therein, and the opportunities these tools presented for the ongoing work of recovery. Indeed, Al spoke very explicitly about the *work* of recovery in place:

> My shed holds my treasures. It's masculine too, like I build my life around the shed, it's part of my life. Like I work in my shed, I work on my recovery.

Another participant, Ric, spoke of the material significance of his home in terms of select objects and materials that he regarded as vital to his practice of recovery:

> Well it's my place, it's peaceful, secure, a really good feeling you know cos I have lived rough in the past. It's different here, where I have my DVD player and my radio and stuff, so I don't have to go anywhere. I'm better now that I have a place to call my own, it's an anchor for everything else in my life.

Intimate spaces like the home were identified by a number of participants. In every instance, the materiality of home was regarded as therapeutic to the extent that it afforded particular activities, practices and/or feeling states conducive to recovery. Sarah spoke in these sorts of terms when describing her garden;

> I just love to sit out here by myself, I have no idea what I think about when I'm out there, it's just that I feel safe and relaxed. The dogs often come and hop up each side of me, with the greenery around me, the breeze, it's lovely.

Jim spoke of the material benefits provided in a local community garden and the fresh produce it provided for his kitchen. He also talked about sharing this produce with friends and family as individual crops were harvested. Jim directly linked this practice of cultivation and sharing with a kind of 'self-care';

> I think we need to nurture ourselves regardless of whether we have a mental illness or not, but still with bipolar it's sometimes difficult to do that. And that's why I feel really grateful that I've actually got something (the garden) that is so solid. But also what it produces, besides being really good on an emotional level, the fact that I get beautiful food and the joy of being able to give away my produce, and that (giving it away) is part of nurturing as well I think.

A very different set of signs and events were identified by Marie, whose experience of social inclusion included local settings ideal for performing handstands. Marie regarded handstands as part of her recovery, likening the handstand to a contest or battle with her fears and anxieties:

> (m)ental illness is about feeling fearful or afraid a lot of the time and a handstand is like that, you are afraid of falling or hurting yourself. So the handstand has taught me how to live with fear, to do things anyway and then to prove that you can beat that fear.

Marie's "favourite" places included sites near her home that afforded the right material conditions for practising handstands. In describing these affordances (signs, affects, events, relations) Marie highlighted the importance of a space to move.

> The wall is very important when you are learning handstands. The wall takes away the fear of falling, so it kind of soaks up your anxiety. I've started seeing more walls now and going, just trying them out, looking for that feeling.

While Marie's handstands may seem incidental, her experience dramatises what is at stake in any ethological account of recovery and the assemblages of health which sustain it. As much as it solicits the expressive force of muscle, bone and desire, Marie's handstand also relies on the reassuring stability of the city's streetscapes; a wall, a locked door, a flat expanse of concrete. In learning how to do handstands, Marie has necessarily become alert to an array of signs and affects, and the ways these signs manifest in particular material spaces. All of a sudden, the right assemblage of wall, concrete, solitude, space and temperament is encountered as so many signs that the handstand is feasible. Each such sign is experienced as an affective and relational force; an opportunity to join a society of bodies (human and nonhuman) resonating together, acting together, affecting one another, insinuating themselves into place, into life. The wall, concrete, space, temperature, time and context are each folded into the assemblage; each is 'responsible' for the handstand. Like the tools in Al's shed, the books and DVDs in Ric's room or the produce in Jim's garden, a host of material objects are folded into the assemblage as it incorporates unique forces in the very expression of recovery. There is not a body 'in recovery' passively accessing and deploying equally passive material objects in the instrumental service of recovery. Recovery is a function of the entire assemblage, human and nonhuman. Remove one element and the assemblage morphs again, transforming the experience of recovery. Material forces thus provide the immanent conditions for recovery. They are not the 'tools' of recovery, *they embody recovery*.

4.3.3 Recovery (The Role of the Affective Assemblage)

Often explicitly, sometimes more tangentially, all participants spoke of the experience of place, social inclusion, community and recovery in a range of affective tones. Including both negative and positive affects, local places were said to provoke a range of affective responses, giving form to the actual experience of community. Most commonly, participants spoke of avoiding places that inspired negative affective responses, while seeking out places that generated more positive ones. Indeed, most participants traced the significance of what they regarded as their "favourite" places to the positive feelings states engendered therein. In describing these states, most participants explicitly canvassed the relationship between place, belonging and recovery from mental illness. Intriguingly, a number of participants spoke in terms that bore a striking consonance with Deleuze's understanding of affect, noted above. That is to say that in describing their 'favourite place' participants noted both an array of distinctive feeling states, as well as some sense of empowerment or motivation, an enhanced capacity to act (both *affectus* and *affectio* in the language of Chap. 2). A number of participant's favourite places attained this status because they inspired positive affective states, like improved mood, or a sense of "peace and quiet". Yet in almost every case, participant's spoke of valuing these states precisely because they were accompanied by an increased capacity to manage the "stress" or "problems" in one's life. While the places that were said to generate these kinds of affective responses included familiar sites including parks, beaches and gardens, other participants identified some rather unusual settings. Jed's favourite places included a local cemetery;

> I look at that cemetery and go, "It's great to be alive". I look at that river and go, "The river is still flowing Jed, you're still here". That river changes everyday, that's a reflection back on myself, like there's always something different about life. If I keep serving myself, it helps me maintain my recovery. So I always come away feeling more in control of my recovery or something.

Jed went on to describe the cemetery as a "peaceful, quiet place" that helped him to feel "more hopeful" about his own recovery, particularly on "down days". The significance of natural settings in inspiring greater optimism about the progress of one's recovery was noted by a number of participants. For many, contact with "nature" helped to combat feelings of isolation or loneliness. As Liz explained,

> I have always loved the Botanical Gardens, even as a child, but ever since I was diagnosed it has just been so important for me. It just makes me feel alive again, the greenery, all the plants, all that life all around. And the silence too, like I can just sit and watch things go by. It just makes me really happy.

For Melissa, parks and gardens in and around her local neighbourhood reminded her of the force of nature, the fact that "life just goes on". She added that these places provided a range of affective resources to support her recovery. Speaking specifically about the experience of one local park, Melissa added that,

> I drive about 5 minutes to get to the park almost every day. There's another park closer by but it doesn't give you the same feeling. The smell, water, trees, the birds, it's peaceful. I just always feel like I am getting better here, living better I suppose.

Like Jed, Liz and Melissa, many participants spoke about the impact of place in the management of "bad days". Summing up this view, Peter spoke alternatively of the importance of a local church and a bookshop;

> They are both important places for me when I am trying to cope with some of my negative emotions I guess you could call them. So I generally visit (the church or the bookstore) when I am feeling that way because I know they will help me. Just the feeling and the atmosphere of these places, it just helps me to relax, take my mind off things. I guess I feel like a different person there.

Other participants described experiencing these kinds of benefits in their own homes. In characterising these affective resources, most participants spoke in terms of solitude, safety and freedom. As James put it:

> At home I can be totally myself. I don't have to put on a facade or be worried about what other people think, or how they might react to me, and my moods, being sick I guess. I don't have to hide anything. I'm totally free to be myself.

April spoke in a similar fashion about her kitchen, describing it as the "most secure place" in her life. Asked to elaborate, April added that:

> It's become my sanctuary, a place just for me, for cooking, for trying out new things but also I guess just for the way it makes me feel. Like, pulling into the driveway, it's like entering another world for me. I know that when I get into the kitchen and make a cup of tea it will be me here, that's me and then the outside world. It (the kitchen) just makes me feel safe and in control of things.

In each of these reports, the *space* of the home ought to be regarded as critical in terms of the affective affordances it sustains to support recovery. Home is therapeutic or enabling for James and April to the extent that it furnishes affective resources like intimacy, solitude, safety and reflection to facilitate recovery and to sustain a more hopeful outlook. For Matt, this experience extended to the local streets around his home, although in contrast to most other participants, Matt was quick to emphasise the temporal significance of these places. These streets were only significant for Matt, only enabling, at particular times during particular activities:

> (g)oing for a walk at three o'clock in the morning, I feel quite safe on the street, cause its dark and there's no one around, everyone else is asleep. There's no energy floating around the air, you know people's manic energy, everybody's resting. So I find the streets around here quite calm and peaceful at night, even though it goes against what should be because you're not supposed to feel safe at night. I don't know but for me the darkness is safe. The world is at rest and it just makes be calmer.

Such is the body-becoming-street-becoming-night-becoming-calm of the recovering assemblage. Such is the affective rhythm of all assemblages of health. In each encounter, in each affective modulation, the recovering body takes on additional simple parts, both human and nonhuman, which enhance that body's power of acting. These simple parts – the bench in the cemetery overlooking the water; the "smell, water, trees, the birds" in the park; books lining shelves in a second hand bookshop; a kettle and cups resting on a kitchen counter – are each folded into the assemblage, adding to its capacities, furnishing an incremental improvement in the health and wellbeing of the recovering body. These are also examples of the affective resources available in communities, in the socius, to support social inclusion and to foster recovery for individuals and groups living with mental illness.

4.4 Becoming Well (Territories, Signs, Events)

Earlier I described recovery as an open, extended event, punctuated by the signs, affects and relations of a body's 'becoming well'. The advantage of such a characterisation lies in the attention it calls to the 'conditions of real experience' by which recovery advances (or stalls) in ordinary life. If recovery is now understood as a process without a determinate end-point (Andresen et al. 2011), then the problem for scholars, practitioners, clinicians and consumers alike is one of discerning the actual conditions in life, in social interaction, clinical intervention and support, which promote recovery understood as some incremental advance in the quality of life. Recovery, as such, ought to be construed as part of the affective, relational and intensive fabric of everyday life, expressed in moments of self-efficacy, connection and rapport; in the growing realisation of a body's power of acting. Recovery is an *affective and relational achievement* in this sense. The signs of this achievement were everywhere apparent in the research data introduced all too briefly above. The intimate conversation in a cafe that strengthens an emerging friendship; travelling aimlessly on the city's trains; the thrill of the handstand on a quiet street; browsing in a local charity store, each of these places and activities were described as therapeutic insofar as they manifest the signs and forces of recovery in life. Recovery traces a line of 'becoming well' in these forces, composing or assembling health from among the affects, signs, forces and events that inflect a body's power of acting. It is equally apparent that recovery involves a struggle to harness or cultivate these forces in an attempt to reterritorialise the fragments of subjectivity assembled in and for the 'ill' body. These fragments *overcode* the body, producing, in turns, the mental health 'patient'; the 'consumer'; the formerly well; the 'sick', 'mad' or 'insane' body (see also Foucault 1971). Each of these subjectivities is composed in an ethological assemblage, which must then be reterritorialised in an effort to produce the recovering body, the 'well' subject. This process of deterritorialisation and reterritorialisation ought to be regarded as the real work of recovery, expressed in the quotidian events, affects and relations of the assemblage's becoming well.

Recovery has to be invented, in other words, in each life so affected by the biological, cultural, social and existential experience of mental illness. *It demands an ethological transformation of the myriad assemblages by which the 'recovering subject' is expressed.* This includes the assemblage of 'home', family and identity; the peer and social assemblage; the citizen assemblage; the employment assemblage; and the affective and relational assemblages pursuant to love, intimacy and friendship. Each such assemblage must be transformed in the course of a body's becoming well, in a combinatorial reterritorialisation of the affects, percepts, gestures, forces, signs, utterances, expressions and events by which subjectivity is composed. I would stress that an 'ethico-ethology' of signs, affects and events is central to this praxis; an ethology that in every instance must be produced or effected in encounters before it can be expressed in life, and in health. Understood this way, recovery may be said to advance or retreat in the innumerable signs and events of everyday life; in interactions with the barista at the local cafe; in the comportment of passengers on the train; in the tactile feel of concrete pressing into palms in the moment before one launches into a handstand. What's more, each such sign or event presents a moment in which *social inclusion* may be expressed or enhanced in support of recovery. Each of these events reveals the forces by which social inclusion is lived as a virtual transformation in the assemblage expressing the recovering body. The data presented above confirm that social inclusion accelerates a body's becoming well, insofar as the process of inclusion affords opportunities for novel encounters; for the assembling of novel relations with bodies, objects, ideas and places which may extend a body's power of acting, and thus enhance its health or wellbeing. Social inclusion may be construed as a relational force between bodies, expressed in signs and events, which transform a body's power of acting, or its capacity to affect and be affected by the array of bodies it encounters in place, in life.

It is equally true that recovery may itself be reframed in these terms, as an *ethological practice* in which the recovering body is reterritorialised in the formation of novel affective and corporeal relations in and with the bodies both human and nonhuman that it encounters. Such a position highlights the array of forces that are active in all assemblages of recovery. Rather than heroicise the agentic capacity of individual clinicians, carers and consumers, recovery must be understood as an affective and relational effect of bodies (human and nonhuman) acting together. This includes the force or will of human bodies, in addition to the range of nonhuman bodies or objects at work in the assemblages of health and recovery described in the last section. The latter include the expanse of concrete that affords the handstand; the array of personal effects that constitute 'home'; the bench in the park, the wind in the trees; the tools arranged haphazardly in a much loved shed. Each of these nonhuman forces is active in the specific assemblages of health that express recovery in the life of the participants introduced above. In each life, in each assemblage, in each body, recovery advances in increments as that body establishes relations with the particular human and nonhuman forces that may promote some enhancement in its power of acting (see Fox 2012). This must stand as the principal conclusion of the empirical investigations of recovery and social inclusion canvassed above; just as it describes the primary lesson of Deleuze's ethology. Another way of approaching these findings is to regard them as indicative of the ethical dimensions of recovery and social inclusion. This introduces, at length, the problem of whether a formal ethico-ethology of recovery may ever be advanced in the treatment of mental health problems in the community (see Tucker 2010).

While the evidence assembled here provides little basis for a definitive response, I would like to close with a necessarily speculative assessment of the prospect of a creative ethics of recovery and social inclusion. I would argue that the ethology of affects and events outlined above (and its role in the lived practice of recovery and social inclusion more directly), suggests strong grounds for innovative community based mental health interventions. While it is tempting to suggest that the affects and events identified by research participants are inclusive or therapeutic precisely because participants have cultivated them themselves – that is to say that it is the *activity of working* on one's own recovery that is critical – it is nonetheless evident from the sketch presented above that participants who described some sensitivity to the signs and events of recovery also reported greater confidence in their recovery, and greater hope and optimism for the future. This suggests there may be an ethical role for community based mental health care services in promoting the *affective, relational and practical learning* essential to the everyday work of recovery. This will require a good deal of creative contemplation so that the signs, affects, relations and events central to recovery and social inclusion alike may be identified and assessed in ways that comprise an ethico-ethology of social inclusion, place and recovery.

Deleuze's idiosyncratic notion of learning suggests some basis for this creativity. Deleuze (1994) conceives of learning as the outcome of encounters that enable a body to increase the array of bodies, objects and entities it may affect and be affected by. Learning establishes a basis for assigning meaning to experience by furnishing grounds for explaining how and why bodies come to affect one another in their encounters. It follows that learning ought to be understood as an affective process in which bodies learn how to interact, relate to or 'compose themselves' with other bodies in the force of their encounter with them. Bodies learn in and through encounters which force them to think, to become and to change as they creatively adapt to novel circumstances. This is why Deleuze is so insistent that learning must be conceived as an intensive process, rather than a kind of technical training. Learning, as such, "is not a quality but a sign" (Deleuze 1994: 140). This suggests, in turn, that learning ought to be framed as an experiential and always experimental ethos, and not as some kind of felicitous dividend derived from the transfer and subsequent recognition of 'ideas'. The ethos proper to learning requires what Deleuze (2000: 4) memorably calls an "apprenticeship to signs". Just as the carpenter learns by "becoming sensitive to the signs of wood", and the physician acquires her skill by "becoming sensitive to the signs of disease" (Deleuze 2000: 4), learning no matter what the discipline, aim or objective entails a process of becoming sensitive to signs and events; learning how to identify, decipher and manipulate them; learning how to be affected by them, and to affect them in turn as one slowly acquires the capacity *to emit signs*. Recovery may itself be understood this way, inasmuch as the recovering body necessarily becomes sensitive to the specific signs and events by which its power of acting may be enhanced as it deterritorialises and reterritorialises the assemblages of health expressive of this recovery. The task ahead is to reframe such an ethological understanding of learning, social inclusion and recovery in ways that may support the articulation of novel assemblages of health in the ongoing promotion of recovery from mental illness in the community.

One obvious way of achieving this could be to involve mental health consumers in the creation of peer-support and mentoring programs to foster awareness of the myriad signs and events of recovery and social inclusion in various local milieus. Consumers are playing an increasingly important role in the provision of community based mental health care in many parts of the world, suggesting that a ready infrastructure is likely available in many places to support the kinds of innovations mooted here (see Andresen et al. 2011; Boardman et al. 2010). Indeed, many of the methods deployed in the empirical studies described earlier in this chapter – such as the spatial and affective mapping exercises and the various sensory and visual methods – could be used in a peer support setting to help consumers identify the signs and events of social inclusion and recovery in their own communities. It will no doubt be difficult to carry the notion of an ethico-ethology of affects, signs and events sufficient to promote the work of recovery, and yet the qualitative data presented above suggests that this kind of ethical praxis in an inescapable part of people's recovery, whether they are conscious of the effort or not. Such praxis draws one into the real conditions of mental health, recovery and social inclusion, forging meaning in the experience of recovery while cultivating an art of becoming well (Tucker 2010). This perhaps, is one more "apprenticeship to signs" occasioned by Deleuze's ethology. Another may be observed in the varied assemblages expressed in the event of drug use, including those affects, signs and relations that permit safe use.

References

Almedom, A. 2005. Social capital and mental health: An interdisciplinary review of primary evidence. *Social Science and Medicine* 61: 943–964.

Anderson, B. 2006. Becoming and being hopeful: Towards a theory of affect. *Environment and Planning D: Society and Space* 24(5): 733–752.

Andresen, R., L. Oades, and P. Caputi. 2011. *Psychological recovery: Beyond mental illness.* Sydney: Wiley Blackwell.

Anthony, W. 2000. A recovery oriented service system: Setting some system level standards. *Psychiatric Rehabilitation Journal* 24(2): 159–168.

Baum, F. 2008. *The new public health*, 3rd ed. Melbourne: Oxford University Press.

Beeble, M., and D. Salem. 2009. Understanding the phases of recovery from serious mental illness: The roles of referent and expert power in a mutual-help setting. *Journal of Community Psychology* 37(2): 249–267.

Bernays, S., T. Rhodes, and T. Barnett. 2007. Hope: A new way to look at the HIV epidemic. *AIDS* 21(5): S5–S11.

Boardman, J. 2010. Social exclusion of people with mental health problems and learning disabilities: Key aspects. In *Social inclusion and mental health*, ed. J. Boardman, A. Currie, H. Killaspy, and G. Mezey. London: RCPsych Publications.

Boardman, J., A. Currie, H. Killaspy, and G. Mezey (eds.). 2010. *Social inclusion and mental health.* London: RCPsych Publications.

Bogue, R. 2004. Search, swim and see: Deleuze's apprenticeship in signs and pedagogy of images. *Educational Philosophy and Theory* 36(3): 327–342.

Boyd, C., L. Hayes, R. Wilson, and C. Bearsley-Smith. 2008. Harnessing the social capital of rural communities for youth mental health: An asset-based community development framework. *Australian Journal of Rural Health* 16(4): 189–193.

Bradshaw, W., M. Armour, and D. Roseborough. 2007. Finding a place in the world: The experience of recovery from severe mental illness. *Qualitative Social Work* 6(27): 27–47.

Calabrese, J., and P. Corrigan. 2005. Beyond dementia praecox: Findings from long-term follow-up studies of schizophrenia. In *Recovery in mental illness: Broadening our understanding of wellness*, ed. R. Ralph and P. Corrigan, 63–84. Washington, DC: American Psychological Association.

Carpiano, R. 2009. Come take a walk with me: The "Go-Along" interview as a novel method for studying the implications of place for health and well-being. *Health and Place* 15(1): 263–272.

Cattan, M., and S. Tilford. 2006. *Mental health promotion: A lifespan approach.* London: Open University Press.

Cattell, V., N. Dines, W. Gesler, and S. Curtis. 2008. Mingling, observing, and lingering: Everyday public spaces and their implications for wellbeing and social relations. *Health and Place* 14(3): 544–556.

Clark, C., and D. Uzzell. 2002. The affordances of the home, neighbourhood, school and town centre for adolescents. *Journal of Environmental Psychology* 22(1–2): 95–108.

Cohen, S. 2004. Social relationships and health. *American Psychologist* 59(8): 676–684.

Cummins, S., S. Curtis, A. Diez-Roux, and S. Macintyre. 2007. Understanding and representing place in health research: A relational approach. *Social Science and Medicine* 65(10): 1825–1838.

Curtis, S. 2010. *Space, place and mental health*. London: Ashgate.

De Landa, M. 2006. *A new philosophy of society: Assemblage theory and social complexity*. London: Continuum.

De Landa, M. 2008a. Deleuze, materialism and politics. In *Deleuze and politics*, ed. I. Buchanan and N. Thoburn, 160–177. Edinburgh: Edinburgh University Press.

De Landa, M. 2008b. Deleuzian social ontology and assemblage theory. In *Deleuze and the social*, ed. M. Fuglsang and B. Sørensen, 250–266. Edinburgh: Edinburgh University Press.

De Silva, M., K. McKenzie, T. Harpham, and S. Huttly. 2005. Social capital and mental illness: A systematic review. *Journal of Epidemiology and Community Health* 59: 619–627.

Deegan, P. 2001. Recovery as a self-directed process of healing and transformation. In *Recovery and wellness: Models of hope and empowerment for people with mental illness*, ed. C. Brown, 5–21. New York: The Haworth Press.

Deleuze, G. 1988. *Spinoza: Practical philosophy*. San Francisco: City Lights.

Deleuze, G. 1992. *Expressionism in Philosophy: Spinoza*. Trans. Martin Joughin. New York: Zone Books.

Deleuze, G. 1994. *Difference and repetition*. London: The Athlone Press.

Deleuze, G. 2000. *Proust and signs*. Minneapolis: University of Minnesota Press.

Deleuze, G. 2001. *Pure Immanence: Essays on a Life*. Trans. Anne Boyman. New York: Zone Books.

Deleuze, G., and F. Guattari. 1987. *A Thousand Plateaus: Capitalism and Schizophrenia*. Trans. Brian Massumi. Minnesota: University of Minnesota Press.

Dennis, S., S. Gaulocher, R. Carpiano, and D. Brown. 2009. Participatory photo mapping (PPM): Exploring an integrated method for health and place research with young people. *Health and Place* 15(4): 466–473.

Dewsbury, J. 2011. The Deleuze – Guattarian assemblage: Plastic habits. *Area* 43(2): 148–153.

Duff, C. 2010. Towards a developmental ethology: Exploring Deleuze's contribution to the study of health and human development. *Health* 14(6): 619–634.

Duff, C. 2011. Networks, resources and agencies: On the character and production of enabling places. *Health and Place* 17(1): 149–156.

Duff, C. 2012. Exploring the role of 'Enabling Places' in promoting recovery from mental illness: A qualitative test of a relational model. *Health and Place* 18(6): 1388–1395.

Duff, C., S. Murray, S. Loo, and K. Jacobs. 2013. *The role of informal community resources in supporting independent housing for young people recovering from mental illness*. AHURI Final Report 199. Melbourne: AHURI Ltd.

Eliott, J., and I. Oliver. 2007. Hope and hoping in the talk of dying cancer patients. *Social Science and Medicine* 64(1): 138–149.

Engel, G. 1977. The need for a new medical model: A challenge for biomedicine. *Science* 196: 129–136.

Foucault, M. 1971. *Madness and civilisation: A history of insanity in the age of reason*. London: Routledge.

Fox, N. 2011. The ill-health assemblage: Beyond the body-with-organs. *Health Sociology Review* 20(4): 434–446.

Fox, N. 2012. *The body*. Cambridge: Polity Press.

Grosz, E. 2011. *Becoming undone: Darwinian reflections on life, politics and art*. Durham: Duke University Press.

Harrison, G., K. Kopper, T. Craig, E. Laska, C. Siegel, J. Wanderling, K.C. Dube, K. Ganev, R. Giel, W. An der Heiden, S.K. Holmberg, A. Janca, P.H. Lee, C.A. León, S. Malhotra,

A.J. Marsella, Y. Nakane, N. Sartorius, Y. Shen, C. Skoda, R. Thara, S.J. Tsirkin, V.K. Varma, D. Walsh, and D. Wiersma. 2001. Recovery from psychotic illness: A 15- and 25- year international follow-up study. *British Journal of Psychiatry* 178(6): 506–517.

Harvey, P., and A. Bellack. 2009. Toward a terminology for functional recovery in Schizophrenia: Is functional remission a viable concept? *Schizophrenia Bulletin* 35(2): 300–306.

Hawe, P., and A. Shiell. 2000. Social capital and health promotion: A review. *Social Science and Medicine* 51: 871–885.

Henderson, J., and B. Walter. 2009. Organising care for the mentally ill in Australia. In *Understanding the Australian health care system*, ed. E. Willis, L. Reynolds, and H. Keleher. Sydney: Elsevier.

Hidalgo, C., and B. Hernandez. 2001. Place attachment: Conceptual and empirical questions. *Journal of Environmental Psychology* 21(3): 273–281.

Hinshaw, S. 2005. The stigmatization of mental illness in children and parents: Developmental issues, family concerns, and research needs. *Journal of Child Psychology and Psychiatry* 46(7): 714–734.

Hodgetts, D., O. Stolte, K. Chamberlain, A. Radley, S. Groot, and L. Nikora. 2010. The mobile hermit and the city: Considering links between places, objects, and identities in social psychological research on homelessness. *British Journal of Social Psychology* 49(3): 285–303.

Hopper, K. 2007. Rethinking social recovery in Schizophrenia: What a capabilities approach might offer. *Social Science and Medicine* 65: 868–879.

Jobe, T., and M. Harrow. 2005. Long-term outcome of patients with schizophrenia: A review. *Canadian Journal of Psychiatry* 50(14): 892–900.

Kaplan, R., and S. Kaplan. 1989. *The experience of nature: A psychological perspective.* New York: Cambridge University Press.

Kawachi, I., and L. Berkman. 2001. Social ties and mental health. *Journal of Urban Health* 78(3): 458–467.

Korpela, K., and M. Ylen. 2009. Effectiveness of favourite place prescriptions. *American Journal of Preventive Medicine* 36(5): 435–438.

Korpela, K., M. Ylen, L. Tyrvainen, and H. Silvennoinen. 2008. Determinants of restorative experiences in everyday favourite places. *Health and Place* 14(4): 636–652.

Kuo, F. And, and W. Sullivan. 2001. Aggression and violence in the inner city: Effects of environment via mental fatigue. *Environment and Behaviour* 33: 543–571.

Latour, B. 2005. *Reassembling the social: An introduction to actor-network theory.* Oxford: Oxford University Press.

Leamy, M., V. Bird, C. Le Boutillier, J. Williams, and M. Slade. 2011. Conceptual framework for personal recovery in mental health: Systematic review and narrative synthesis. *British Journal of Psychiatry* 199: 445–452.

Lysaker, P., and K. Buck. 2008. Is recovery from schizophrenia possible? An overview of concepts, evidence, and clinical implications. *Primary Psychiatry* 15(6): 60–65.

MacIntyre, S., A. Ellaway, and S. Cummins. 2002. Place effects on health: How can we conceptualise, operationalise and measure them? *Social Science and Medicine* 55: 125–139.

Malins, P. 2004. Body-space assemblages and folds: Theorizing the relationship between injecting drug user bodies and urban space. *Continuum: Journal of Media and Cultural Studies* 18(4): 483–495.

Massumi, B. 2002. *Parables for the virtual: Movement, affect, sensation.* Durham: Duke University Press.

Milligan, C., and A. Bingley. 2007. Restorative places or scary places? The impact of woodland on the mental well-being of young adults. *Health and Place* 13: 799–811.

Parr, H. 2007. Mental health, nature work, and social inclusion. *Environment and Planning D: Space and Society* 25: 537–561.

Parr, H. 2008. *Mental health and social space: Towards inclusionary geographies?* London: Wiley Blackwell.

Patel, V., A. Flisher, S. Hetrick, and P. McGorry. 2007. Mental health of young people: A global public-health challenge. *The Lancet* 369(9569): 1302–1313.

Pinfold, V. 2000. Building up safe havens. . .all around the world: Users' experiences of living in the community with mental health problems. *Health and Place* 6(2): 201–212.

Portes, A. 1998. Social capital: Its origins and applications in modern sociology. *Annual Review of Sociology* 24: 1–24.

Protevi, J. 2009. *Political affect: Connecting the social and the somatic*. Minneapolis: University of Minnesota Press.

Ramon, S., and J. Williams (eds.). 2005. *Mental health at the crossroads: The promise of the psychosocial approach*. London: Ashgate.

Repper, J., and R. Perkins. 2003. *Social inclusion and recovery: A model for mental health practice*. London: Elsevier.

Rickwood, D., F. Deane, C. Wilson, and J. Ciarrochi. 2005. Young people's help-seeking for mental health problems. *Australian e-Journal for the Advancement of Mental Health* 4(3): 1–34, (Supplement).

Ritter, L., and S. Lampkin. 2012. *Community mental health*. Sudbury: Jones and Bartlett Learning.

Rowling, L. 2006. Adolescence and emerging adulthood. In *Mental health promotion: A lifespan approach*, ed. M. Cattan and S. Tilford. London: Open University Press.

Rudnick, A. (ed.). 2012. *Recovery of people with mental illness: Philosophical and related perspectives*. Oxford: Oxford University Press.

Sawyer, S., F. Arney, P. Baghurst, J. Clark, B. Graetz, R. Kosky, B. Nurcombe, G. Patton, M. Prior, B. Raphael, J. Rey, L. Whaites, and S. Zubrick. 2001. The mental health of young people in Australia: Key findings from the child and adolescent component of the national survey of mental health and well-being. *Australian and New Zealand Journal of Psychiatry* 35: 806–814.

Steinfeld, E., and G. Danford (eds.). 1999. *Enabling environments: Measuring the impact of environment on disability and rehabilitation*. New York: Springer.

Stockdale, S., K. Wells, L. Tang, T. Belin, L. Zhang, and C. Sherbourne. 2007. The importance of social context: Neighbourhood stressors, stress buffering supports and alcohol, drug and mental health disorders. *Social Science and Medicine* 65(10): 1867–1881.

Thrift, N. 2004. Intensities of feeling: Towards a spatial politics of affect. *Geografiska Annaler* 86B(1): 57–78.

Thrift, N. 2007. *Non-representational theory: Space, politics, affect*. London: Routledge.

Tucker, I. 2010. Mental health service user territories: Enacting 'safe spaces' in the community. *Health* 14(4): 434–448.

Wang, C., and M. Burris. 1997. Photovoice: Concept, methodology, and use for participatory needs assessment. *Health Education and Behaviour* 24(3): 369–387.

Williams, A. (ed.). 2007. *Therapeutic landscapes*. London: Ashgate.

Williams, C. 2007. Thinking the political in the wake of Spinoza: Power, affect and imagination in the Ethics. *Contemporary Political Theory* 6(3): 349–369.

Chapter 5
Assemblages of Drugs, Spaces and Bodies

The contention that alcohol and other drug (AOD) use is mediated in a social context is the inaugurating condition of a social science of drugs (Rhodes 2009: 193–195). It is equally implicit in all *social explanations* of the problems sometimes associated with this use. Indeed, the very promise of a 'science of drugs' sensitive to the force of social, political and cultural life is beholden to the conviction that such forces intervene somehow in the course of AOD use, changing it in ways that are amenable to empirical inquiry. What then, may be said to constitute a 'social explanation' of AOD use, including the problems associated with this consumption, and the most effective ways of reducing them? And what, more directly, does it mean to say that cultures and social contexts *mediate* AOD use? The present chapter addresses these questions in turn, adopting the conceptual resources furnished in earlier chapters to further test the methodological utility of transcendental empiricism. The study of AOD use provides fertile ground for this examination of Deleuze's methods, given enduring controversies regarding the social, biological, economic, neurological and political "causes" of problems like addiction, and the links between drug misuse and crime, violence and other social disorders (see Fraser and Moore 2011: 1–11). The health and social sciences alike have generated multiple, overlapping and often contradictory accounts of the etiology of problems like addiction and crime, tracing antecedents in neuropathology and psychological disorders (Carter et al. 2012); family dysfunction and deficits in education and employment opportunities (Durrant and Thakker 2003); shifts in consumption trends associated with the 'normalization' of illicit drug use (Aldridge et al. 2011); as well as global economic developments and the emergence of relatively stable international drug markets (Stortia and De Grauweb 2009). In their turn, proliferating causal explanations of drug misuse inform and endorse the vast apparatus devoted to solving problems associated with AOD use in diverse social and political contexts.

Despite decades of concerted political, economic and social endeavour, the effort to reduce the prevalence of AOD use, to mitigate the harms associated with consumption, even to delay the age at which individuals first initiate use, have met with modest success in most jurisdictions (see Fraser and Moore 2011; Reznicek

C. Duff, *Assemblages of Health: Deleuze's Empiricism and the Ethology of Life*,
DOI 10.1007/978-94-017-8893-9_5,

2012). Everywhere drug use appears as endemic as ever. I argue throughout this chapter that much of the failure of contemporary drug policy can be attributed to the habit of framing drug problems in conventional ontological terms, reifying an ostensibly autonomous subject, along with the equally discrete objects that comprise its social context (Keane 2002; Valverde 1998; Moore and Fraser 2006). Efforts across the health and social sciences to explain problems like addiction thus proceed from the calculating subject, whose predilection for the irrational choice of consumption must itself be explained ahead of any consideration of the biological, social, structural, economic and political forces that may bear upon that subject in the course of its consumption habits. This approach has succeeded brilliantly in revealing the array of forces, structures and processes that may be said to *mediate* consumption, even though it struggles to account for such forces in the pragmatic reckoning of the *real experience* of drug use in everyday settings. The problem, as I have noted in earlier chapters, is one of linking 'context' with 'practice', the 'macro' with the 'micro', 'structure' with 'behaviour', such that one may meaningfully connect the web of social, experiential, economic, cultural and affective forces present in the event of AOD use. Placing the subject at the centre of a social context – situating drug use within a matrix of social processes, political conditions, economic forces and collective norms – doubtless accords with the great axioms of social science, of 'man' and 'world', the 'individual' and 'society'. Endorsing these axioms, most accounts of AOD use reveal little of the actual experience of drug use in context. All that is repeated is the familiar refrain that cultures mediate consumption, that contexts matter, and that effective interventions must reflect these cultures and contexts if they are to succeed in reducing the harms associated with AOD use.

The point is that one is left with the familiar problem of *connecting* individual and society, practice and context, behavior and culture, consumption and norms in an effort to explain how cultural, political, economic and social forces mediate AOD use in producing problems like addiction (Fraser and Moore 2011). At issue is how to adequately explain the role of social contexts in shaping AOD use. Or, to pose the problem with recourse to a rival vocabulary, how to explain the social and structural determinants that produce consumption (or addiction)? That these forces are active in the expression of AOD use is rarely contested, even though compelling accounts of the terms of this mediation are as elusive as ever. Yet what if one were to start with the *connection*, rather than the *subject* (or its behaviours) as the basic unit of analysis? What if one were to prioritise the analysis of the *drug assemblage* rather than the drug user? This I wager is the principal advantage of an approach to the study of drugs and culture modelled on transcendental empiricism. Such an approach should permit novel analyses of varied social and structural aspects of AOD use and misuse, revealing more of the force of context, without at the same time assuming a subject who comes to culture only to affect, and be affected by it, in the course of behaviours like AOD use. Following Deleuze, I would argue that drug use may be explained not in terms of the human subject and its choices, mediated in a web of social, economic and political structures, but rather in terms of *an assemblage of forces* that produces both the subject of drug use and the effects of this use (see also Oksanen 2013). This is to insist, moreover, that conventional epistemological distinctions such as structure/agent and subject/object impede, rather than facilitate, the work of producing empirically nuanced accounts of AOD use and the problems associated with it (Wilton and Moreno 2012: 99–101). While the practice of empirical inquiry *absent, after or beyond* the subject/object dyad may appear almost perverse, this chapter advances from the claim that novel ontological investments are urgently required in light of the imbrications of culture, technology, government, communication and power that generate or enable contemporary problems like addiction (see Demant 2009; Fraser and Moore 2011; Gomart 2002).

I will develop this argument by analysing qualitative data collected in Melbourne, Australia and Vancouver, Canada among individuals (bodies and spaces) involved in the use of alcohol and other drugs. On the basis of this analysis, I will argue that AOD use draws together affects, relations, bodies and spaces in open extended events by which bodies are connected in a drug assemblage (see also Fitzgerald 1997). Each event of consumption combines spaces, bodies, affects and relations in the expression of drug effects – pleasure, humour, anxiety, camaraderie, hostility, euphoria, fear, violence, intimacy, alienation – in the *experience of intoxication* expressed by an order of degrees. In turn, each such event assembles fragments of subjectivity that are distributed in and among the bodies human and nonhuman that amass in that event. Concerned foremost with the logic of the event, the aim of transcendental empiricism is henceforth to trace the means by which assemblages are composed, the range of forces they combine, and the kinds of subjects, actions and affects each assemblage may be capable of enacting. Such aims invite an *empirical* investigation of the forces immanent to each consumption event, suggesting grounds for revitalising social science in the service of explaining AOD use. By doing away with the reification of subjects and objects, humans and nonhumans, structures and agents as particular kinds of things, Deleuze enables researchers and practitioners alike to become more sensitive to the array of relations entities, spaces, bodies, affects and signs involved in each actual event of AOD use.

Advancing this goal, the present chapter offers an empirical analysis of the *drug assemblage* in an effort to clarify the ways health is affected by AOD use, including the ways health problems of the kind associated with the misuse of alcohol and other drugs may be more effectively addressed. Looking ahead to the next two chapters, I will close with a consideration of an ethics of the drug assemblage, sensitive to the range of human and nonhuman bodies, forces, affects and spaces active in each event of consumption. The goal will be to determine how drug assemblages may be transformed (or reterritorialised) so as to reduce the harms associated with AOD use. I will start by clarifying the organisation of the drug assemblage, and the ways such assemblages may be studied. Only with such an empirical understanding in place may an ethics of the event – an ethics of the drug assemblage – be possible.

5.1 An Empiricism of the Drug Assemblage

My aim in adopting Deleuze's methods is to radically reframe assessments of the *social aspects* of AOD use, providing tools for the analysis of the full range of bodies, forces and spaces assembled in each event of consumption. Grounded in the logic of the social determinants of health, existing assessments of the social contexts of drug use tend to treat 'social' and 'structural' factors at some remove from the local circumstances in which consumption is experienced (Rhodes 2009). And so the economic conditions, gender norms and class distinctions that may potentially mediate use and related harms in particular places at particular times are almost always construed as having their proper locus elsewhere, outside the 'place' of consumption. This, indeed, is the basic rationale by which most empirical studies of drugs have been able to sustain the theoretical and methodological disjuncture of the 'macro' and the 'micro', 'context' and 'place' alluded to above. The problem of course is that while 'structure' is increasingly understood as an authentic feature of social conditions, it is spatially and temporally abstracted from these conditions in its reification in empirical research (see Latour 2005). In adopting Deleuze's methods, I intend to return social forces to 'real experience', to the actual conditions by which behaviours like AOD use are experienced in place. Such innovation will require a radical reconceptualisation of *social context* in terms of an assemblage of affects, spaces, relations, bodies and events (Duff 2012; Oksanen 2013; Rhodes 2009). Reframing context in this way should shed light on the experiential, social, political and economic conditions active in each event of AOD use, thus advancing my goal of transforming the study of the social determinants of health. This approach should also provide an alternative causal logic for assessing how distal and more proximate forces and processes intervene in events of AOD use. So what then is 'context'?

To study social contexts according to the logic proposed by transcendental empiricism entails the identification of the specific moments of connection and association by which social effects are produced; an explanation of how these relations come to comprise discrete assemblages; and a tallying of the varied efforts by which these assemblages are maintained or transformed (Brown 2010: 112–116). Analysis of this kind ought to reveal more of the ways contexts are materially, socially and affectively produced and reproduced in individual spaces or territories, providing in turn, a means of determining how specific contextual objects, processes and spaces mediate AOD use in specific settings. With these aims in mind, contexts may be defined as assemblages of local and non-local bodies, spaces, affects, objects, technologies, signs, habits and forces that participate in, or otherwise meditate, the use of alcohol and other drugs in specific territories. Social contexts comprise discrete processes that facilitate the creation of novel relations between bodies, objects, forces and spaces, and the distribution of diverse affects between them. Taking all these aspects into consideration, I would emphasise the constitutive role of *spaces, bodies and affects* in the formation and reformation (territorialisation and deterritorialisation) of the assemblages that express or produce a social context. I will clarify each domain before applying tools derived from Deleuze's empiricism to the analysis of data drawn from studies of AOD use in Vancouver and Melbourne.

5.1.1 Assembling Social Contexts: Spaces, Bodies, Affects

Contexts are an expression of an assemblage of forces. In Chap. 2 I noted that assemblages may be regarded as qualitative relations of force, affect and becoming, actualised in connections and flows and composed on planes or territories. De Landa (2008: 253) adds that Deleuze and Guattari characterise assemblages "along two dimensions": one identifying the "role which the different components of an assemblage may play, a role which can be either material or expressive"; and a second axis comprising varied processes which determine either "the emergent identity of the assemblage" or its destabilisation "opening the assemblage to change". In each respect, assemblages have *material* dimensions, forces or components (spaces, objects, technologies, bodies), and *expressive* ones (identities, signs, meaning, affects, desires). For my own purposes, De Landa's analysis suggests that social contexts assemble spaces, bodies and affects in a "constellation of singularities and traits", giving to each assemblage a provisional identity such that contexts may be distinguished from one another according to the specificity of their spatial and temporal arrangements (Deleuze and Guattari 1987: 406). Distinguishing contexts in this fashion is critical if one is to overcome the problem noted above in which contexts take on a kind of pan-spatial, structural hegemony, seemingly operating at all places, at all times with the same relentless mediating power. Yet the specificity of context also requires that one pay heed to the discrete arrangement of spaces, bodies and affects by which the assemblages that comprise context are composed in material and expressive dimensions. The active power of contexts lies in the force of these connections and flows. It is why one must conceive of contexts as an *assemblage of spaces, bodies and affects* rather than as a complex or composite of these forces (see also De Landa 2006; Deleuze and Guattari 1987).

With regard first to the spatial aspects of assemblages, and their expression in the modulations of context, space and matter alike are continuously constructed and reconstructed "through the agency of things encountering each other in more or less organized circulations" (Thrift 2003: 96). Space is not discovered but rather is socially mediated or enacted in the play of events, flows and encounters between bodies, affects, objects and territories. And so, space is less a natural property of the world, an inert substance, and more a means of making sense of the world, of negotiating movement and passage and organising relations and cultural practices. Above all though, matter and space are continuously evolving and becoming, being made and unmade, contested and settled, territorialized and deterritorialized. What is critically important for the reconceptualisation of context proposed here is the manner in which matter, objects, technologies and space are made meaningful in these processes of territorialisation and deterritorialization (Buchanan and Lambert 2005). How matter is used, how objects are deployed, how technologies are involved in activity, how space is made meaningful; each process inflects the ways assemblages come to denote a social context for the varied bodies active within a given assemblage. The spatial and material dimensions of context must, therefore, be construed in terms of the manifold connections, pathways, circulations and encounters that organise a territory in and for the assemblage (Thrift 2003: 98). Conceiving of context in this way draws attention to the ways spatial and material components are produced, or made sense of, in and through the specific uses bodies adopt for them. It further suggests the importance of "spatial relations" (Thrift 2008), and the ways relations between objects, bodies and forces are structured in and through distinct territories. The territorialisation of the assemblage organises and distributes relations, affects and bodies, like those common to the event of AOD use.

The manner of the assemblage's implication in the territorialisation of space, objects and affects provides an indication of the second, *expressive*, dimension of the assemblage. It also suggests something of the lived or embodied aspects of the assemblage, and the ways bodies are territorialised in a social context. Deleuze and Guattari (1987: 405–406) primarily conceive of the expressive, embodied dimensions of the assemblage in terms of the myriad affects, habits, practices and expressions deducted or contracted from the flow of intersecting ethologies (behaviours, actions, affects, practices) circulating on a given plane or territory. The varying ethologies evinced in any particular assemblage give that assemblage a certain expressive quality, consonant with an identity, 'sense' or specificity. It gives to each body within the assemblage an "emergent identity" (De Landa 2008: 253). Yet as I have stressed, Deleuze dismisses the subject/object binary distinguishing bodies and the material world in arguing that bodies represent "series of flows, energies, movements, strata, segments, organs, intensities; fragments capable of being linked together or severed in potentially infinite ways" (Grosz 1994: 167). What is striking about this position given the aims of this chapter is its emphasis on the situated character of all relations of embodiment. The materiality of embodiment entails the "infolding" of space, affects and practices at particular "local points" (Grosz 2011: 28–34). And so, the "specific skills, sensibilities and dispositions, sedimented into the body, are incorporated (implicated) contexts" (Harrison 2000: 508). At his most radical, Deleuze rescinds the distinction between space, matter and bodies in claiming that space and matter are constantly folded into bodies as the boundaries distinguishing matter, space and body are breached (Buchanan and Hughes 2011). As such, the body can no longer be understood as separate, or prior to the spaces around it; rather, the two are mutually embedded one within the other. The spaces and contexts that are coextensive with the body fundamentally matter *as they are folded into the body* in relations of movement and rest, in practice and reaction.

The folds by which spaces and bodies are territorialised in assemblages are equally implicated in the distribution of affects and relations between these spaces and bodies, suggesting another of the ways contexts are expressed in an assemblage. Affects are critically important insofar as they denote what bodies actually do in assemblages, establishing the third material and expressive domain of context in the model devised here. Nonetheless, as generations of social theorists have attested, what bodies do most certainly does not in every instance pertain to what bodies 'will' or 'desire' (see de Certeau 1984: xi–xiii). The great empirical purchase of Deleuze's understanding of affect lies in his suggestion that affects describe what bodies become in their encounters with other bodies, human and nonhuman. Encounters modulate the array of affects that 'pass through' bodies, determining in and for the moment of their encounter what each body may be capable of doing, enacting or being. This affective modulation involves, of course, a transfer of power, capacities or action-potential between bodies. Regardless of the nature of this body, whether human or non-human, all bodies are potentially affected by a panoply of other bodies in any particular encounter. It is in this sense that one may argue that the affects generated or experienced in space, in spatial relations, in encounters with place, are dynamically involved in the production and reproduction of context. It is to stress that the body's encounters in space involve affective resonances far beyond those experienced between discrete individuals. Just as bodies affect one another *in place*, bodies are inevitably affected *by place,* such that "place seems to be a vital element in the constitution of affect" (Thrift 2004: 60). Affects are experienced in bodies but emanate or emerge in diverse encounters; encounters between bodies and between bodies and contexts, bodies and events (Massumi 2002). Critically, each encounter generates unique affective capacities in that no two encounters ever produce the same affective modification in a body's power of acting. Bodies are affected by place in each instance anew, with each unique encounter with place. The experience of place might in this way, be said to differ affectively with each occasion in context.

All of which suggests that affective engagement with place, and with the "affective atmospheres" (Anderson 2009) this engagement supports, is another of the primary mechanisms by which social contexts are territorialised and deterritorialised in an assemblage of forces. Affective engagement creates a zone of indeterminacy, an *intensity* that transforms space in the very instance of creating place (McCormack 2007: 369–372). Affects are autonomous in this sense, in that they reside neither in individual places, nor in individual bodies, but rather in the dynamic and relational interaction of places and bodies, contexts and subjects (Massumi 2002). It follows, therefore, that the affective function of context – the extent to which contexts may transform or mediate the things bodies 'do' in place – can never be discerned in advance of empirical analysis of encounters in and with context. Refusing to posit context as *a determinant of encounters* in place is critical if the more active, aleatory and affective aspects of context are to be adequately understood. Contexts certainly mediate encounters, but only insofar as they contribute to the affective valence of the events or encounters that happen in and with context. It is the particular spatial and temporal assemblage of spaces, bodies and affects (enacted in the event of their encounter) that mediates the force of context not the other way around. Context is as much an event as it is a coherent pattern of spatial, temporal and affective relations.

Conceiving of context as an assemblage of spatial relations, modes of embodiment and 'affective atmospheres', provides a compelling new logic for the interrogation of individual drug use settings, and the broader contextualisation of drug related harm. The effort to reconceptualise (or better *reterritorialise*) context, should be understood as an attempt to move beyond conventional macro-structural understandings of context in order to clarify the active, local and contingent role of contexts in the mediation of what bodies do 'on' and 'with' drugs. My aim is to return context to the focus of empirical research, rather than to retain it as a heuristic shorthand for the vagaries of power or culture. Indeed, the problem with so much of the existing literature on context is that its heuristic value has fallen away sharply as context has congealed into a static, hypostasised synonym for power, structure or society. In the drugs field, structuralist understandings of context mostly frustrate its operationalization as an object of empirical research, given the bewildering array of group norms, economic processes, social traditions and political relations now regarded as properties of context (see Rhodes 2002: 88–89). Granted such expansive purview, structural approaches obscure the specificity of context and the particular means by which contexts shape local drug use behaviours. In response, I have argued that context should be characterized as an assemblage of spaces, bodies and affects, whereby the 'grouping together' of these elements inevitably mediates the ways contexts shape AOD use and related harms. The challenge now is to articulate how this approach may inform the development of new types of drug policy research and practice. Such has been the aim of the studies introduced below.

5.2 Making Use of Context: Methods and Procedures

The model of the drug assemblage set out above has, in part, emerged in the course of varied studies exploring the links between culture, context and the experience of AOD use in particular spaces in Melbourne and Vancouver (see Duff 2005a, b, 2008, 2009, 2010; Duff and Rowland 2006; Duff et al. 2007; Ivsins et al 2012). These studies have each in their own way revealed the shortcomings of macro-structural approaches to context, while suggesting the need for a model alert to the imbrications of space, bodies and affects in place. As such, my notion of the drug assemblage is intended to yield a set of discrete conceptual and methodological tools for the redesign of studies of the social contexts of AOD use. Before canvassing the results of research employing these tools, a number of methodological points are worth clarifying. It is particularly important that I clarify how drug assemblages were formally studied in Melbourne and Vancouver in order to properly introduce the results of this empirical inquiry.

Consistent with the theoretical understanding of context introduced above, the empirical investigation of drug assemblages in Melbourne and Vancouver pursued two related research aims. The first concerned the identification of the specific spatial features, modes of embodiment and affective relations discernible in particular settings. Importantly, this step also involved the determination of the *limits* of context for the purpose of analysis. The second broad aim required assessment of how spaces, bodies and affects coincide in the *expression of context*. How, for example, does the experience of space affect the embodiment of drug use practices, and how does space moderate the ways bodies affect (and are affected by) each other in place? These aims called attention to the role of spaces, bodies and affects in the modulations of context, and hence suggested the basic focus of dedicated empirical assessments of individual drug assemblages in Melbourne and Vancouver.

With more specific reference to the *empirical procedures* required of these three domains (spaces, bodies and affects); first, the analysis of space and its impact on AOD use suggested the need for investigation of the ways drug use spaces are experienced, both in terms of the embodied consumption of drugs, as well as the spatial mediation of the varied affects associated with intoxication. To the extent that spaces are selected by design, it was also important to consider how and why spaces are deemed appropriate for AOD use, over and above other settings. Once the spatial constituents of the drug assemblage had been identified, their specific physical and material characteristics were clarified. This inquiry also revealed something of how the geographical, affective and/or cultural limits of consumption spaces are determined, how these limits are identified and how they are crossed or negotiated. Attending to these spatial limits also involved some consideration of the ways encounters are structured in and through space, and the ways AOD use mediates these spatial interactions. Of further interest were the different ways space is made inhabitable, and the specific meanings spaces inspire in the territorialisation of the drug assemblage. How, in other words, are spaces and contexts 'made' in the event of AOD use, and how are different kinds of spaces and contexts encountered or transformed in the affective and relational negotiation of effects like intoxication?

The examination of embodiment required similar methodological innovation, particularly in relation to a body's immersion in space, and the different ways AOD use impacts this immersion (see Vitellone 2010). Once the specific spatial and cultural limits of individual drug assemblages had been assessed, it was crucial that the affective and relational modulation of bodies within these contexts be considered also. This entailed some analysis of how different drug using bodies are caught up in the local operation of power, and how power relations affect the range of things that bodies can and cannot do in such contexts. The examination of interactions between different drug using bodies, and the ways such corporeal connections are regulated and made meaningful in local contexts, was equally vital. Such focus called attention to the types of social, cultural and/or economic interactions observable or made possible in different drug assemblages, but also the types of affective encounters and symbolic engagements bodies were able to enter into (to the extent that this could be discerned in the research settings). The goal was to understand how drug use transforms the ways bodies connect with other bodies, with objects and spaces in the formation of drug assemblages. How different contexts make particular kinds of embodied or affective connections possible, while foreclosing other encounters.

Finally, the study of affect highlighted the *activity* of drug use in context. Such inquiry concerned the different ways drugs are used in specific contexts, how different consumption techniques and routes of administration emerge and how these practices take on particular meanings or significance. It pertained to the range of practices and activities observable in specific drug assemblages; of the things bodies do while affected by consumption, or while in the vicinity of bodies affected by drugs. The examination of these practices shed some light on the ways drug use frames the identification or articulation of specific drug assemblages and the actual physical and/or perceptual experience of these contexts. Yet the obverse was also true in that contexts were found to frame and transform drug use practices, while also affecting the physiological and psychological experience of AOD use. Of related importance was the manner in which bodies come to make sense of drug use practices, how drug use conveys symbolic meanings and how these meanings are mediated in context. Analysis of each ultimately revealed much of the way drug use practices are framed in and through a "disjunctive synthesis" (Deleuze 1994) of norms, habits, signs, affects and power relations enacted between bodies (human and nonhuman).

Turning from the research aims and procedures to methods, each study employed techniques described in Sarah Pink's (2009) sensory ethnography. This approach is primarily concerned with the generation of research methods open to the myriad affective and material textures of everyday life (Pink 2009: 23–25). Understood in terms of method, sensory ethnography is alert to the activity of the objects, spaces and bodies assembled in events like those that mediate AOD use. It relies on the sensitivities of the various bodies (both human and nonhuman) assembled in the course of empirical research, harnessing these sensitivities in the generation of novel kinds of research data. Sensory ethnography treats the body as a discrete research instrument, responsive to the contexts it inhabits, and retaining the traces of this habitation in unique ways. As an empirical method, it provides unique means of recording the traces of the body's inscriptions and its imbrication in the spaces and contexts of its affective encounters. Foremost among the tools furnished in sensory ethnography are various visual and communication technologies (Pink 2009: 97–99). In the studies described below, the use of film, photography, auto-ethnography, creative writing, interview methods and walking tours, among other more conventional techniques, provided a basis for documenting more of the interactive and indeterminate aspects of context. Each revealed the materiality of place along with the affective; the activity of objects and bodies in place, and their role in the production and reproduction of context. Each was employed in the projects canvassed in the next section to highlight more of the spaces, bodies and affects active in the formation of drug assemblages, and the contexts they manifest.

5.3 Drug Assemblages in Melbourne and Vancouver

Each of the studies described below sought to position the event of consumption (and the varied assemblages enacted therein) as the basic unit of analysis, rather than the subject of AOD use (see Duff 2004, 2005a, b, 2008, 2009, 2010; Duff and

Rowland 2006; Duff et al. 2007; Ivsins et al. 2012). The goal was to uncover as many of the forces involved in each event of AOD use as possible, so as to begin to trace the ways such forces, human and nonhuman, contribute to the expression of AOD use. In their own way, each study has sought to explain how social contexts come to shape the use of alcohol and other drugs. Despite the challenge of operationalising transcendental empiricism as method (noted above) the dividends of this struggle have been significant, elucidating the array of bodies active in each event of use, while hinting at the ways these bodies might be coaxed to act differently in the expression of a novel harm reduction praxis. Most importantly, this research has revealed that each event of AOD use is crowded with bodies, spaces and affects, just as the subject of this consumption remains the "moving target of a vast array of entities swarming toward it" (Latour 2005: 46). As such, the event of AOD use does not involve a meeting of bodies in a context, which then interact with one another. Rather the event enables, unleashes, folds and entangles the spaces, affects and bodies effected in a context. Reflecting the characteristic features of social context as depicted in the model of the drug assemblage outlined above, research in Melbourne and Vancouver revealed an array of specific *spaces, bodies and affects* active in each event of consumption.

5.3.1 The Drug Assemblage (Spaces)

The significance of spaces and settings in shaping the character and experience of AOD consumption has long been recognised (Zinberg 1984). Much of this analysis emphasises the importance of social, economic and political structures, and the everyday impact of norms and cultural values, in organising the spaces of AOD use (Durrant and Thakker 2003). In contrast, the studies in Melbourne and Vancouver emphasised the more immediate features of space and the ways they inform the *relational, affective and embodied experience* of AOD use. The diverse settings described in these studies – the chillout rooms, dance floors and bars, the private homes, parks, ski-slopes and street corners – make an important difference in the social, affective and physiological experience of consumption (see also Malins 2004; Jayne et al. 2008). Far from merely furnishing the material aspects of social context, research in Melbourne and Vancouver indicated that space must be understood as an active component of context, central to the varied drug assemblages enacted in each event of use. Space provides a context for consumption to the extent that it provides one of the primary mechanisms by which structural forces are made present (or active) in drug assemblages. The materiality of space evinces something of the way contexts are 'folded' into drug use events, rendering active the varied structural forces that shape the drug assemblage. Yet this is not to say that structure dictates the manner in which space is used, or the ways in which power relations may be said to flow through it. Space bears the mark of the production and reproduction of power, yet its activity is a function of territorialisation and reterritorialisation; of the ways space is made active in events. Space is involved, therefore, in the modulations of context, but rarely in the ossifications of structure. Space is a recurrent expression of context to the extent that it enables affects and power to flow in and through bodies in place. It is an active constituent of drug assemblages in this regard, modulating every event of AOD use.

In the studies conducted in Melbourne and Vancouver spaces were almost always described as active conditions of any event of AOD use, with different spaces having a significant bearing on the affective experience of intoxication. Confirmed in observational research, many participants indicated that preferences regarding the specific features of individual settings were keen factors in determining where and when AOD use should take place. As a participant in Melbourne said:

> The high is all about what you're doing and your surroundings. I mean like you never just drop a pill and sit in your room by yourself right because it probably won't work and it would just be a waste of a pill. So it's best to wait for the right time and the right place with drugs so you know it's all going to be good.

Other participants emphasised the particular energetic (or affective) appeal of particular spaces like clubs and bars, private homes, parks and other public places, stressing that AOD use provides a means of more effectively connecting with space:

> Mostly I think the high with drugs is the way it enhances the environment you're in, like if it's a club or someone's house or the beach whatever. Drugs just help you to connect with your surroundings which a lot of clubs, um like the décor is really set up for that you know. So its like the place you're in, what it feels like, can make a big difference to what kind of high you get.

A number of respondents also spoke of this idea of connecting with space in relation to outdoor and/or natural environments:

> I love being outside when I'm high, you know just dropping a pill with some friends and then exploring the gardens, climbing a tree, playing frisbee or smoking a joint and staring at the garden for a while.

Describing the use of cannabis while snowboarding, a man in Vancouver added:

> The thing with weed is that it really enhances your feeling for the snow and the mountain, the terrain you know? Like you feel more attuned to the board and your muscles feel more responsive to the snow somehow. I mean I know it sounds pretty hippy but weed just makes that connection so much stronger.

Others spoke about private spaces in the same fashion:

> I mostly use drugs at home now. I love that you're familiar with the environment, but everything can just change and you can find so much, like different things that you've never really noticed.

Another youth in Melbourne noted;

> Sometimes my flatmates and I will stay home on a Saturday night, like when we're all too poor to go out, pool whatever we have and get high. We'll wander round the neighbourhood, just walking and hanging out and it's amazing how different everything is, like the little things that you'll notice all of a sudden, like you're in a whole new city. Sometimes those are the best nights on pills, when you're just exploring your home, discovering things.

Indeed, for many participants, the use of drugs at home was said to profoundly enhance one's sense of comfort and connection in and with that space:

> (Using) at home is great because like it's a safe environment and it can be a really fun environment too. Drugs just make the place interesting again I guess, like you're bored of the same four walls, all the stuff you do at home and then you all have lines on a Saturday night and move all the lamps to the court-yard and turn it into a chill out space, play some music, smoke a joint.

Salient in each of these quotations is the sense of connecting differently with space, of experiencing space in a new way. The effects associated with AOD use were thus reported to far exceed the merely physiological, to include a kind of *spatialisation of intoxication*, a means of inhabiting space more affectively. While physiological pleasures were certainly reported to be important, too great a focus on the pharmacology of the drug high misses the range of affects associated with the use of different drugs in different contexts and spaces. This attention to space also goes some of the way to explaining why the same drug can produce such different pleasurable and/or sensory effects in different spaces. The narratives reported above suggest the need for an affective and relational account of the 'actual experience' of AOD use that downplays the material properties of the substance itself in favour of the *relational construction* of drug related effects. It is as if these effects are embodied, spatialised responses that may be manipulated or transformed according to the dynamic possibilities presented in the setting itself. Space may, in this way, be said to behave like a body in its encounters with other bodies in the assemblages expressed in the event of AOD use. There are of course a range of bodies, human and nonhuman, active in the drug assemblage in each event of use.

5.3.2 The Drug Assemblage (Bodies)

The force of human bodies is routinely elaborated in studies of AOD use, so it is arguably more interesting to commence with the nonhuman bodies active in the formation of drug assemblages, like the 'body' of alcohol and other drugs. Research findings in Melbourne and Vancouver, confirmed in participant reports, observational analysis, film and photographic elicitation, indicated repeatedly the force of alcohol and other drugs to alter the spatial and temporal course of individual and group activities, leading individuals to consume more than was planned, or throwing the day/night's itinerary into more random and unexpected encounters. It was especially common for participants to speak as if alcohol and other drugs were themselves active determinants of their consumption habits. As a participant in Melbourne noted,

> The drugs definitely take over right, like you'll be planning just a so so night, hang out with your friends, have a few drinks, home by 3 am know what I mean? And then you'll get to the club and get on it (ecstasy) and you're feeling great and you think well one more will feel better yeah and that's when the night just gets random, like you'll be walking back home at 10 am thinking how the fuck did that happen (laughs).

Other participants in related studies in Melbourne spoke in similar ways about alcohol, noting the courage and spontaneity they felt once intoxicated and the kinds of unexpected experiences this courage enabled. Describing the perceived benefits of mixing amphetamines and alcohol, one young man said, "it's like having the drinking power of ten men where all these things happen that are just so fun and so unexpected, that's the best part for sure". Without denying the physiological pleasures associated with AOD use, participants in Melbourne and Vancouver reported that these corporeal pleasures are matched by the activities, connections, encounters and experiences that intoxication facilitates or enables; with the array of bodies, human and nonhuman, that intoxication enables one to connect with. Ingestion of alcohol and/or other drugs was said to change the array of things bodies can, or will do, introducing novel (or 'random') encounters, while soliciting unexpected activities or behaviours. As a participant in Vancouver memorably put it:

> You know there are all those anti-drug ads, like this is your brain on ecstasy. Fuck that, there should be ads for tablets (ecstasy) that are like "press play". Just take one and press play, let yourself go with all the crazy random shit that happens, crazy conversations, doing dumb shit with your friends, how you never get home the same way, all that stuff. Nights get so scrambled.

These kinds of reports reflect findings published elsewhere indicating that AOD use is rarely the focus of either individual or group activities, but rather that drugs are consumed in order to facilitate or enhance some other activity like dancing, social interaction, conversation or sex (Aldridge et al. 2011; Hubbard 2005). A useful example concerns the significance of social interaction (connection between bodies) and the ways this interaction is mediated by alcohol and other drugs. Ecstasy was found to be particularly important in the Melbourne studies with many participants speaking of the ways ecstasy use "opens" one up with peers and strangers. When used among friends, participants agreed that ecstasy encourages deeper and more intimate conversations, sometimes on topics that friends rarely, if ever, discuss. It helps bodies connect. Speaking in Melbourne, a woman noted that:

> Yeah, it's a different type of connection, um, like a level that you're trying to get to which is why we take it (ecstasy). It's like that level where you're really in touch with your friends, cause everything is so connected you feel like you can really feel what your mates are feeling, what they are talking about you just understand it so much better. And that's where ecstasy can take you.

Other participants spoke of connecting with strangers in unexpected ways, stating that drugs like cocaine and alcohol transform the experience of social interaction in bars, clubs and private parties. A participant in Vancouver added:

> The part of it (drug use) that's really appealing is the idea that you have random connections, that's fun, you know I guess you're um, you feel able to go and talk to people at random. Like you'll be high and you'll go out into the street for a cigarette and it'll be raining crazy hard and you'll be talking to this random waiting for a bus or whatever and that'll be the best part of the night.

Sometimes, these kinds of encounters were described in terms of drug "effects", but studies conducted in Melbourne and Vancouver confirm that the most unpredictable aspect of drug use is precisely its corporeal or physiological effects. These effects emerge in context, in an assemblage of forces. As a participant in Melbourne noted,

> Like you can take the pill and just have this amazing feeling, this amazing time and your friend will be like "Jesus these are crap, I'm getting nothing". And I'll be like, "what do you mean? I'm on it!" So that's the level that you're trying to get to which is why we take it. It's like that level where you're really in touch with what's going on around you, but it doesn't happen every time.

Most research traces these kinds of divergent consumption experiences either to the unreliable pharmacology of "street drugs", or to the idiosyncratic psychology of the consuming subject (Levy et al. 2005). Drugs themselves may be granted some measure of causal efficacy but they are rarely admitted to the status of independent agent (Demant 2009). Transcendental empiricism however, suggests that drugs ought to be regarded as nonhuman bodies, inorganic life – packets of affects and relations – active in the formation of the drug assemblage, and the faltering course of the consumption event. As bodies, drugs combine with other bodies, spaces and affects in the encounters immanent to the drug assemblage; like the conversation with a stranger in the rain, or the "random" activities that leave the night "scrambled". Drugs effect a transition in the power of acting of the varied bodies they encounter, including those human bodies that both do and do not consume drugs. Consistent with Deleuze's account of affect, such transitions in the power of acting of bodies assembled in the drug event are a function of bodies acting together, rather than one body drawing an unrealised force out of another. Drug effects are not just pharmacological, much less physiological: drug effects are an event produced in an assemblage of forces where drugs themselves play an active, although rarely predictable role. To suggest that alcohol and other drugs serve as bodies of force in a drug assemblage is merely to acknowledge this power of acting, without imputing to such substances some mysterious volition. It is to argue, in turn, that drugs give form to the context of their own consumption. They are active constituents of the social contexts of AOD use, and not merely the objects of context. The challenge for health policy is to conceive of responses to AOD use more accommodating of the force of drugs. The task is to determine how the substances at work in the drug assemblage might be made to act differently in the development of a relational ethics of care and moderation. Such an ethics will need to accommodate the force of affect.

5.3.3 *The Drug Assemblage (Affects)*

Research participants in Melbourne and Vancouver spoke at length about the variety of ways in which one might be affected by drugs; in intoxication, pleasure, fear, aggression, intimacy, excitement, abandon, confusion and pain. What is perhaps most striking about respondent's accounts of these affects/effects is the difficulty most had articulating their precise nature and experience. Most were able to describe specific feelings and sensations peculiar to specific substances, yet there was little agreement about the relationship between consumption and effects, given how variable illicit drugs are both in terms of their composition and use. What was common, however, was the sense of experiencing the body differently; of being exposed to a radically new set of corporeal and psychological sensations. Speaking about his first experience with the drug ecstasy, one participant noted:

> I mean it (ecstasy) didn't hit me for about twenty minutes, and I was like 'this is crap anyway', right, and then suddenly, this thing happened that I can't describe. . .I can't explain the sensation, but you just, you go into this whole new world. I'd never felt like this before. . .it just felt so good.

Almost all participants in each city shared similar stories about their experiences with drugs such as ecstasy, amphetamines and cocaine and the way these drugs produced hitherto unknown sensations and feelings. Typically, these were described as physical or sensate pleasures experienced in and on the body:

> It's so hard to put into words. But the way your body feels, these waves and rushes, especially if someone touches you like runs their hands through your hair or something – I love it when my boyfriend does that – your whole body is so sensitive and every sensation is just this intense pleasure like you're a cat purring on someone's lap (laughs).

For other respondents, drug use was associated with a sudden heightening or enhancement of physical, sensate and perceptual functioning. Amphetamines in particular were said to enhance alertness and mental acuity, perception and endurance. This was experienced as a kind of optimal functioning; as if every sense was functioning at its highest capacity:

> When you're high like that it just feels like your body is so connected like every part is working perfectly, all coordinated and free. It's such an amazing feeling I love that part the most.

Although these sensations were not always experienced as pleasurable, what was most attractive to most participants was the experience of entirely novel sensations, of taking a drug in order to feel something unique. Indeed, many participants spoke about the desire to experience new sensations, new psychological and/or cognitive states as the primary ambition underpinning their specific drug use histories. Yet at the same time, drugs were not themselves the sole vehicles or mediators of this affective and corporeal novelty. As I have noted, the effects of intoxication were almost always described in relation to the *experience of connection*; connection to space, to other people, to objects, things and experiences. Moreover, these connections should be regarded as affectively charged to the extent that novel connections transform the particular kinds of things that bodies can do in and with context. What matters is the array of affective transitions enabled across the entirety of the drug assemblage. As a participant in Melbourne helpfully noted:

> Yeah, Summer Daze (festival event) last year was amazing, we had this really great coke. And it was sunny and the park looked so good with the city behind it and all my friends dancing around me. The DJ was playing these really great tunes and I felt just complete clarity listening to the music and hearing every detail of it, feeling it rush through my body, feeling everything.

It's not just the use of cocaine that describes or explains the nature of this young man's experience; it is clearly part of a richer and more intensive complex of affects and relations. The effect of AOD use is produced as a measure of the assemblage and the array of affects and relations it enables. The richer and more intense these relations, the greater the modulation in a body's power of acting in context, in the assemblage, will be. What matters is the capacity to enter into novel relations with diverse bodies, human and nonhuman. The role of substances themselves has already been noted, though participants in each city were quick to highlight a host of additional affective encounters critical to the expression of the drug assemblage.

Mobile (or cell) phones were identified in almost all of these studies, although their activity in drug assemblages varied considerably. Most participants spoke of mobile phones as indispensible to the coordination of consumption episodes, both in terms of the planning of events and throughout the evening as individuals tried to coordinate itineraries, to locate absent friends and to document the more memorable aspects of the night's events. SMS or text messages were especially important in facilitating interactions and spontaneous organisation, providing a means of locating and communicating with friends, even in instances when they were in the same building. A number of participants also spoke of the role of mobile phones in directing the experience of intoxication. A young woman in Melbourne noted:

> Like you'll be feeling amazing dancing, peaking and happy and you'll think I wish that Sarah and Madonna were here, where are they? So you'll just text them from the dance floor, you see loads of people do that so they don't have to go looking for people. You text them and wait for them to come over.

Communication technologies in this way facilitated a kind of *affective engineering* of the course and intensity of drug effects. Phones reportedly extended the array of affective encounters enactable within a particular drug assemblage, opening up relations, enhancing or transforming connections with friends and strangers and mediating the sensory experience of AOD use. This affective or sensory experience was further manipulated in the stylisations of the fashioned body. Clothing was typically considered "part of the whole package" necessary for the planning and coordination of a "big night out". Clothing was certainly important in portraying a particular side of oneself, "representing" one's designated tribe, yet it also provided a means of affectively preparing oneself for the consumption events to come:

> Yeah dressing up is a big part of it, getting ready, making sure we all look right. And we spend a lot of money on clothes for the big parties you know phat pants and other stuff. We try to organise it well in advance so we all have the best possible outfits, that we all look good together. So when you feel like you look hot that just puts you in the right mood right from the start of the night so you're really charged even before you take pills.

Without ignoring this effect, the most popular way of "getting in the mood to play" as one youth in Vancouver described it, was to turn the music up. Music was an unsurprisingly ubiquitous presence in each of these studies, providing inspiration during the pre-party 'warm up', uniting friends and strangers in common cultural tastes. Speaking in Melbourne, one participant reported that the best music enhanced the ecstasy high so that a "good pill can become a great pill when the music's right on". Another youth in Vancouver spoke of the critical importance of the hardware, a good PA, a powerful sound system and the right tunes:

> I'm a deejay so I am always listening, I'm really interested in the technical sides of things, you know how big PAs work in different rooms, the equipment, the audiophile bit I guess. Really it's about getting the most out of the music that you love so when you get a chance to work a big room you can take people somewhere amazing.

The affective urgency of music – a kind of contextual agency – was reported in each of these studies, with participants routinely attributing to music the power to alter one's consumption behaviours. So who, or what, then is responsible for this use?

5.4 The Drug Assemblage

Each of the studies reviewed above investigated the relationship between culture, context and the lived experience of AOD use in varied urban settings. To begin with, this research agenda proceeded from rather conventional ontological suppositions, tracing the interaction of bodies and spaces, and the ways cultures and contexts may be shown to mediate AOD use. Yet the more I observed these interactions, the closer I approached the 'real conditions' of AOD use in place, the more I noted the value of Deleuze's varied empirical pronouncements regarding the implication, or folding, of bodies, affects and spaces in an assemblage of forces. I realised that commencing with a relatively fixed understanding of 'bodies' and 'contexts', and proceeding to examine the manner of their interaction *missed the force of the event*; the actual transition in the power of acting of bodies in their assembling. Along with Deleuze and Guattari (1987), I discovered that one must not reify the subject who experiences events like drug use, for such reification merely privileges conditions such as will, intention, mediation, calculation, risk, pleasure, judgement and reason. I am sure that these conditions are active in drug events, but they are not primary. AOD use in 'real experience' does not involve a rational (or irrational) subject who comes to drugs as if in consideration of a problem; what to use, how much, when, where, with whom, for how long, why? *These judgements are a function of the event of drug use, rather than the subject of this event.* The subjectivities that are active in each drug event are distributed in and among an assemblage of human and nonhuman bodies, spaces and affects. Subjects, as such, are expressed anew in each consumption event, sometimes subtly, sometimes profoundly. The locus of action is equally distributed, such that attributions of judgement or responsibility for the carriage of consumption habits must include a wide cast of bodies and spaces.

The trouble with conventional approaches to drug use is that they ask rather too much of the drug user. The user bears responsibility for most of the dynamics of consumption, and subsequently remains culpable for any of the harm generated therein. In accordance with this logic, public health and harm reduction initiatives alike persist with the subject as the focus of health care interventions, either in terms of the prevention or treatment of AOD related problems. Among a panoply of forces, the subject is picked out merely because it is the most familiar, the one considered most amenable to intervention, if not transformation. Occasionally efforts are made to transform the "risk environments" in which events of AOD use transpire (Rhodes 2002). Some of these efforts, like needle and syringe programs and supervised injection facilities have been spectacularly effective despite the moral and legal controversies that have invited (Small et al. 2007). Otherwise, efforts are made to educate users, to encourage risk avoidance, to limit the supply of illicit substances in the community, or to transform the ways drugs are apprehended either in pleasure or despair (Fraser and Moore 2011). One might have a harder time faulting these approaches if they had been more successful in either reducing AOD use, or the harms associated with it. The fact is that alcohol and other drugs are now a 'normal' part of popular culture in most population groups in most societies (Aldridge et al. 2011). This does not mean that AOD use is common, much less pervasive, only that alcohol and other drugs are a part of the repertoire of habits or activities available to individuals among varied objects of cultural and material consumption, even if this consumption is occasionally enacted in the form of addiction (Keane 2002). Targeting the drug user, while attempting to minimise the availability of illicit substances, has not proven especially effective at reducing the prevalence of use or its more deleterious consequences, despite public investment on a scale which makes the rhetoric of a 'war on drugs' wholly warranted. It is against this backdrop of diminishing practical and intellectual returns that I, along with colleagues, have sought to examine alternative ontological and empirical tools for the interrogation of AOD use in context. Subsequent to this research, I would argue that while the subject offers much scope for the modification of the assemblages that enact AOD use, other forces, other spaces, bodies and affects, are also potentially modifiable in the work of reducing harmful encounters with drugs.

Realising such a goal will require more nuanced accounts of the 'real experience' of AOD use, and more sophisticated models of the role of context in mediating this use. The principal advantage of the Deleuzian approach to the analysis of social contexts and their role in the mediation of AOD use offered here is the capacity to identify the specific spaces, bodies and affects by which contexts actually effect this mediation. Far from affording social contexts some mysterious causal force – ascribing a capacity to intervene in everyday life to an external structure or 'society' that remains everywhere and nowhere in particular – transcendental empiricism calls attention to the specific character of individual contexts and the assembled forces by which they are enacted or expressed. Indeed, Deleuze's work inspires a more dynamic account of context than hitherto available in the study of AOD use, one that helps to determine the array of bodies that are active in any event of use. Such a claim confirms the conventional view that 'contexts matter' in the study of AOD use, with the advantage of contributing a robust explanation of the ways that places and contexts transform consumption in real experience. As the studies in Melbourne and Vancouver canvassed above demonstrate, spaces, bodies and affects mediate the character and experience of AOD use in complex ways, primarily by transforming the range of things that bodies can do in their encounters with one another in context.

Such an understanding of context arguably effects a kind of rapprochement between 'structure' and 'agency', the 'macro' and the 'micro' in the work of describing AOD use in individual settings. What matters is how bodies, spaces and affects are arranged in the event of AOD use, not where they come from. There are, as such, no purely 'structural', 'macro' or 'contextual' bodies, spaces or affects, only forces in their encounters in an assemblage. This is not to say that all action is local, or that power and structure don't matter in AOD use. Of course they do, yet the value of Deleuze's empiricism may be found in the tools it avails for the analysis of how forces combine in the event of consumption (see also Oksanen 2013). It follows, for example, that while the settings of drug use are involved in the modulations of use, and while these settings are themselves shaped by various structural forces (such as economics, local investment decisions, town planning regulations, law enforcement, architecture and design trends) the extent to which these structural forces *actually participate* in individual events of AOD use, in real experience, cannot be definitively determined in advance of careful empirical assessment of that experience. Spatial forces expressive of a social structure may well be important, but they cannot be assumed to act uniformly in events of AOD use, nor in relation to individual bodies therein. The same goes for the other bodies that abound in the event of AOD use.

The last section described the role of mobile phones, fashion, music, drugs themselves, public transport arrangements, gardens, beaches, bars and more besides. Each of these 'bodies' may conventionally be said to manifest power relations and the press of structural forces. The mobile phone for example is doubtless composed in the force of economics, telecommunications regulation, design, fashion, taste, subjectivity, communication and privacy (see Crawford 2009). None of these forces is exclusively local, nor are they remote from structural and/or social processes. Still the extent to which such forces implicate themselves in the event of AOD use can never be assumed as some kind of axiomatic *a priori*. This means that the heuristics that have governed so much contextual analysis of AOD use – the sense that contextual factors like class, gender, economics, poverty, power and governance inevitably mediate consumption – very rarely explain the dynamics of AOD use in context (see Moore and Fraser 2006; Rhodes 2009). They cannot explain the 'real experience' of AOD use because they each remain abstractions that have been isolated from experience in their reification as scientific objects (see also Law 2004: 70–74). Objects, as such, are assumed to be stable and easily transported from one setting to another. And so the structural forces that inform context in the analysis of drug use – such as the force of class, gender, power and governance – are treated like stable entities that everywhere behave the same way. Their effects can be predicted because their ontologies are thought to be settled.

Transcendental empiricism seeks to return context to experience, to bridge the gap between 'structure' and 'place' by focusing on the machinations of the assemblage and the specific means by which forces distal and proximate encounter one another in context. No contextual force is static; much less does it entail uniform effects. Non-local forces, distal and structural forces, are always involved or folded into drug assemblages. Even so, it is the manner of this folding that matters in events of AOD use; that 'determines' how distal forces affect use, not some set of properties held to be immanent to each structural entity. Gender is involved in drug use, for example, but its involvement entails, in each instance, the production of gender not the imposition of some structural fiat. Class, power, economic relations too can never be said to simply impose themselves on events of AOD use like a reagent added to a medium in a petri dish. What matters is not how a force is situated, whether it is regarded as bearing a more 'structural' or 'local' hue, but how it is folded into the assemblage. In privileging the figure of the assemblage, I have sought to prioritise the empirical analysis of events of AOD use in order to shift the focus of contextual analyses to the forces immanent to the instantiation of context in each event of use. The context of AOD use is coextensive with each event of consumption, rather than lingering at a distal remove, waiting to impose itself 'from above' to local interactions.

The logic of the assemblage thus overcomes the fissure between 'macro' and 'micro', 'structure' and 'behaviour' not in some grand dialectical gesture, but rather in a simple empirical commitment to 'real experience'; to the manner in which bodies converge in experience. And so, the task for further empirical studies of AOD use is to identify in each event of consumption *deemed worthy of analysis* (and this qualification is utterly central) what kinds of spaces, bodies and affects are involved in consumption, and then to trace how such forces came to 'be present' in the event. As I noted in Chap. 2, Deleuze's account of the event emphasises the spatial and temporal antecedents of each event, the sense that each event 'picks up' or is affected by a potentially infinite series of prior activities or 'states of affairs'. However, far from treating all activity as a function of some grand, all encompassing web of inter-related phenomena, Deleuze insists that what matters in the event is discerning which forces may be manipulated in order to "counter-actualise" the event, to transform it. The same logic holds, I would argue, for the notion of context devised here. A potentially limitless set of contextual forces may be said to be present in events of AOD use, some of which will be uniquely local, and some which may be traced to more 'social' or 'distal' antecedents. The extent to which one may wish to identify these forces in empirical analysis is always a matter of deciding what such analysis is for; for what reason may one wish to intervene in events of AOD use to counter-actualise them, to have them unfold differently? One must start with 'real experience', with the event of AOD use, employing the tools of transcendental empiricism in an effort to identify as many of the spaces, bodies and affects implicated in the drug assemblage as possible. This assembled cast is of course, the context of the event of AOD use. Deciding how far one advances in the analysis of context will depend on the reasons one wishes to intervene in the event of AOD use.

One obvious reason may be to counter-actualise the event of AOD use in the interest of promoting safer use and/or reducing harmful use. This introduces the problem of determining how the contexts and places of AOD consumption may be transformed in the interests of reducing AOD related harms. How might the diverse spaces, bodies and affects involved in a drug assemblage be harnessed in novel health promotion initiatives? This chapter has sought to identify some of the most significant of these bodies and spaces in drug assemblages in Melbourne and Vancouver as a critical first step in the design and implementation of such initiatives. The analysis offered above suggests that efforts to reduce the harms associated with AOD consumption *ought to address the entirety of the drug assemblage*. This will require greater recognition of the distributed and relational forces active in AOD use such that assemblage-wide strategies to transform these forces may be identified. It should also involve a shift away from the over-reliance evident in many AOD interventions on highlighting and sometimes exaggerating the risks associated with AOD use, and the subsequent attempt to transform individual attitudes and behaviours (Duff 2003). Positing AOD use as a simple product of human choice ignores the additional forces involved in this consumption, while restricting the onus for transforming AOD use to individual subjects. Focus should shift instead to specific consumption contexts or drug assemblages. This move may well facilitate the identification of the various forces involved in AOD use, and the development of tailored strategies to modify or reterritorialise these forces in local AOD interventions.

Yet it may also provide a way out of interminable debates regarding the causes of problems related to AOD use, such as the suggestion that methamphetamine and/or cannabis use causes psychosis (Dwyer and Moore 2013), or that alcohol use causes violence (Demant 2013). The problem with this kind of causal attribution is the temptation to quantify and ascribe causal responsibility to individual bodies, objects or forces, such that one might identify the degree of variance attributable to these factors (Hacking 2001). Such work is premised on the assumption that individual factors may be statistically abstracted from their contexts in order to probabilistically determine their contribution to the particular state of affairs under investigation (Law 2004). Ever more sophisticated statistical techniques have emerged to support (or express) this logic, leading researchers to apportion causal significance to identifiable variables involved in the temporal and spatial production of phenomena like psychosis or alcohol related violence. Without ignoring the significance of these kinds of studies, they haven't fared especially well in the treatment of counterfactuals, like those instances in which methamphetamine misuse does not cause psychosis, or where alcohol intoxication fails to produce violent (male) subjects. The model of context presented throughout this chapter would assert, in contrast, that all action, all phenomena, are an effect of contexts (or assemblages) rather than individuals bodies (or forces). The assemblage generates the cause just as it expresses the effect. It makes little sense, in other words, to attempt to determine the degree of causality attributable to any one body, space or object within an assemblage, because the assemblage produces activity as an emergent effect of all affects and relations immanent to it. Activities like psychosis or violence (understood *precisely as activities* because of the array of forces at work in their production) are the function of a 'disjunctive synthesis' incorporating diverse human and nonhuman forces, some of which are present 'in the event' just as others reach back in temporal and spatial folds to reveal a host of antecedent activities.

According to this logic, alcohol related violence, for instance, ought to be regarded as a relational effect of particular assemblages, rather than a simple conjunction of (male) bodies and alcohol (in volume). Alcohol and human bodies are but two forces in a broader assemblage, which necessarily incorporates additional forces including (but never limited to) transportation infrastructure; the behaviour of staff and patrons in drinking venues; policies, procedures and protocols for training security and bar staff; liquor licensing arrangements; policing and law enforcement practices; cultural norms regarding the expression of alcohol intoxication in public; information and communication technologies; alcohol advertising; objects and devices that enable the consumption of alcohol (later repurposed as weapons, for example); the spatial design of entertainment precincts in the night-time economy, and so on (see also Fitzgerald 2009; Moore and Fraser 2006). Each of these bodies and processes may or may not be involved in the production of violence in a particular assemblage, at a particular time. Hence, it is never simply a case of alcohol acting on a receptive set of human organs. Nor is violence a function of the additive accumulation of known risk factors. Violence is produced in a particular configuration of affects and relations where it is the *character of this configuring* that causes violence rather than any one body or force within that assemblage. This is because bodies are determined in the specific affects and relations they express by the array of bodies (human and nonhuman) around them, and the varied encounters that support this expression. Virtually all of the most significant insights derived from Deleuze's empiricism and applied to the study of AOD use follow from this logic.

It follows, indeed, that neither alcohol, nor the human body consuming it, may be said to produce stable actions, which can in turn be reliably predicted without regard for the context of their enactment, because transcendental empiricism refuses to regard either alcohol or the human body as stable. This suggests that alcohol is not the same thing from one context to another, or from one event of consumption to another. Alcohol is a 'multiplicity', whose activity within a particular assemblage always modifies its characteristic properties. It is simply nonsensical in this regard to say that alcohol causes violence, because alcohol is not some discrete, stable and knowable entity. Put another way, it is not clear what the proper referents of the terms 'alcohol' and 'drinker' may be for the purpose of assessing the merits of studies purporting to establish the causes of alcohol related violence. For the alcohol (force/body/affect) that 'causes' violence in one context is not the same object that may or may not 'cause' violence in another. This, finally, is the reason why it makes little sense to argue about whether alcohol causes violence, or whether or not methamphetamine use causes psychosis. The empirical assessments offered in this chapter would suggest that neither alcohol nor methamphetamine is the same thing from one context to another, from one assemblage to another. Alcohol may indeed be active in an assemblage that produces violence, just as methamphetamine may be present in an assemblage that generates or expresses psychosis. Yet the 'alcohol' and/or 'methamphetamine' that is active in these assemblages is unique to these contexts. The extent to which alcohol configured as a particular kind of force may produce violence in another assemblage is entirely dependent on the cast of spaces, bodies and affects assembled in that context. Configured in a different way, alcohol use may produce euphoria, relaxation, humour, excitement, reflection *or* violence; or indeed endless philosophical debate about the character of alcohol itself. Alcohol is not stable and it does not produce stable effects; simple empirical observation is sufficient to carry this contention (see Law and Singleton 2005: 337).

What all this means is that ascribing causal responsibility to individual bodies or forces, rather than assemblages or contexts, is bound to produce errors. More charitably, one might say that it simply fails to explain enough of 'real experience'. What needs to be explained is how problems related to AOD use emerge in particular kinds of relations. Another key question is to enquire into what kinds of associations, between what kinds of spaces, bodies and affects, are involved in the amelioration of these problems. The first step in addressing these questions ought to involve careful empirical study of particular assemblages in particular contexts in order to generate robust empirical accounts of the specific affects and relations at work in the production of harms like violence or psychosis. I would add that such analysis has important implications for the ongoing development of harm reduction policy. The model of social context developed above would suggest that as much of the assemblage must be understood as possible if effective interventions are to be described for transforming contexts in ways that limit the expression of harm. Rather than identifying the relative responsibility of individual spaces, bodies or forces, the goal ought to be to understand the range of affects and relations active in the production of harm. Another goal should be to transform the ways different spaces, bodies and forces *affect one another* in the event of their association, such that the production of harm may be reduced across the entire assemblage. Taking up this challenge, this chapter has sought to put Deleuze's empiricism to work in an attempt to avail fresh insights into the ongoing effort to transform drug assemblages in the promotion of health. The next two chapters seek to derive an ethics from this effort.

References

Aldridge, J., F. Measham, and L. Williams. 2011. *Illegal leisure revisited: Changing patterns of alcohol and drug use in adolescents and young adults*. London: Routledge.

Anderson, B. 2009. Affective atmospheres. *Emotion, Space & Society* 2(2): 77–81.

Brown, S. 2010. Between the planes: Deleuze and social science. In *Deleuzian intersections: Science, technology and anthropology*, ed. C. Jensen and K. Rödje. Oxford: Berghahn.

Buchanan, I., and J. Hughes (eds.). 2011. *Deleuze and the body*. Edinburgh: Edinburgh University Press.

Buchanan, I., and G. Lambert (eds.). 2005. *Deleuze and space*. Edinburgh: Edinburgh University Press.

Carter, A., W. Hall, and J. Illes (eds.). 2012. *Addiction neuroethics: The ethics of addiction neuroscience research and treatment*. London: Academic.

Crawford, K. 2009. Following you: Disciplines of listening in social media. *Continuum: Journal of Media and Cultural Studies* 23(4): 525–535.

De Certeau, M. 1984. *The Practice of Everyday Life*. Trans. Steven Rendell. Berkeley: University of California Press.

De Landa, M. 2006. *A new philosophy of society: Assemblage theory and social complexity*. London: Continuum.

De Landa, M. 2008. Deleuzian social ontology and assemblage theory. In *Deleuze and the social*, ed. M. Fuglsang and B. Sørensen, 250–266. Edinburgh: Edinburgh University Press.

Deleuze, G. 1994. *Difference and repetition*. London: The Athlone Press.

Deleuze, G., and F. Guattari. 1987. *A Thousand Plateaus: Capitalism and Schizophrenia*. Trans. Brian Massumi. Minnesota: University of Minnesota Press.

Demant, J. 2009. When alcohol acts: An actor-network approach to teenagers, alcohols and parties. *Body & Society* 15(1): 25–46.

Demant, J. 2013. Affected in the nightclub: A case study of regular clubbers' conflictual practices in nightclubs. *International Journal of Drug Policy* 24(3): 196–202.

Duff, C. 2003. The importance of culture and context: Rethinking risk and risk management in young drug-using populations. *Health, Risk & Society* 5(3): 285–300.

Duff, C. 2004. Drug use as a 'practice of the self': Is there any place for an 'ethics of moderation' in Contemporary Drug Policy? *International Journal of Drug Policy* 15(6): 385–393.

Duff, C. 2005a. 'Charging' and 'blowing out': Patterns and cultures of GHB use in Melbourne, Australia. *Contemporary Drug Problems* 32(4): 605–653.

Duff, C. 2005b. Party drugs and party people: Examining the 'normalization' of recreational drug use in Melbourne, Australia. *International Journal of Drug Policy* 16(3): 161–170.

Duff, C. 2008. The pleasure in context. *International Journal of Drug Policy* 19(5): 384–392.

Duff, C. 2009. The drifting city: The role of affect and repair in the development of enabling environments. *International Journal of Drug Policy* 20(3): 118–129.

Duff, C. 2010. Towards a developmental ethology: Exploring Deleuze's contribution to the study of health and human development. *Health* 14(6): 619–634.

Duff, C. 2012. Exploring the role of 'enabling places' in promoting recovery from mental illness: A qualitative test of a relational model. *Health & Place* 18(6): 1388–1395.

Duff, C., and B. Rowland. 2006. 'Rushing behind the wheel': Investigating the prevalence of drug driving among club and rave patrons in Melbourne, Australia. *Drugs: Education, Prevention and Policy* 13(4): 299–312.

Duff, C., J. Johnston, D. Moore, and N. Goran. 2007. *Dropping, connecting, partying and playing: Exploring the social and cultural contexts of party drug use in Victoria, Australia*. Melbourne: Premier's Drug Prevention Council.

Durrant, R., and J. Thakker. 2003. *Substance use and abuse: Cultural and historical perspectives*. Thousand Oaks: Sage.

Dwyer, R., and D. Moore. 2013. Enacting multiple methamphetamines: The ontological politics of public discourse and consumer accounts of a drug and its effects. *International Journal of Drug Policy* 24(3): 203–211.

Fitzgerald, J. 1997. An assemblage of desire, drugs and techno. *Angelaki: Journal of the Theoretical Humanities* 3(2): 41–57.

Fitzgerald, J. 2009. Mapping the experience of drug dealing risk environments: An ethnographic case study. *International Journal of Drug Policy* 20(3): 261–269.

Fraser, S., and D. Moore. 2011. *The drug effect: Health, crime and society*. Melbourne: Cambridge University Press.

Gomart, E. 2002. Methadone: Six effects in search of a substance. *Social Studies of Science* 32(1): 93–135.

Grosz, E. 1994. *Volatile bodies: Towards a corporeal feminism*. Bloomington: Indiana University Press.

Grosz, E. 2011. *Becoming undone: Darwinian reflections on life, politics and art*. Durham: Duke University Press.
Hacking, I. 2001. *An introduction to probability and inductive logic*. Cambridge: Cambridge University Press.
Harrison, P. 2000. Making sense: Embodiment and the sensibilities of the everyday. *Environment and Planning D: Society and Space* 18(4): 497–517.
Hubbard, P. 2005. The geographies of 'going out': Emotion and embodiment in the evening Economy. In *Emotional geographies*, ed. J. Davidson, L. Bondi, and M. Smith. London: Ashgate.
Ivsins, A., C. Chow, S. Macdonald, T. Stockwell, K. Vallance, D. Marsh, W. Michelow, and C. Duff. 2012. An examination of injection drug use trends in Victoria and Vancouver, BC after the closure of Victoria's only fixed-site needle exchange. *International Journal of Drug Policy* 23(4): 338–340.
Jayne, M., G. Valentine, and S. Holloway. 2008. Geographies of alcohol, drinking and drunkenness: A review of progress. *Progress in Human Geography* 32: 247–263.
Keane, H. 2002. *What's wrong with addiction?* Melbourne: Melbourne University Press.
Latour, B. 2005. *Reassembling the social: An introduction to actor-network theory*. Oxford: Oxford University Press.
Law, J. 2004. *After method: Mess in social science research*. London: Routledge.
Law, J., and V. Singleton. 2005. Object lessons. *Organization* 12(3): 331–355.
Levy, K., K. O'Grady, E. Wish, and A. Arria. 2005. An in-depth qualitative examination of the ecstasy experience: Results of a focus group with ecstasy using college students. *Substance Use and Misuse* 40(12): 1427–1441.
Malins, P. 2004. Body-space assemblages and folds: Theorizing the relationship between injecting drug user bodies and urban space. *Continuum: Journal of Media and Cultural Studies* 18(4): 483–495.
Massumi, B. 2002. *Parables for the virtual: Movement, affect, sensation*. Durham: Duke University Press.
McCormack, D. 2007. Molecular affects in human geographies. *Environment and Planning. A* 39 (2): 359.
Moore, D., and S. Fraser. 2006. Putting at risk what we know: Reflecting on the drug-using subject in harm reduction and its political implications. *Social Science & Medicine* 62(12): 3035–3047.
Oksanen, A. 2013. Deleuze and the theory of addiction. *Journal of Psychoactive Drugs* 45(1): 57–67.
Pink, S. 2009. *Doing sensory ethnography*. London: Sage.
Reznicek, M. 2012. *Blowing smoke: Rethinking the war on drugs without prohibition and rehabilitation*. Plymouth: Rowman & Littlefield Publishers.
Rhodes, T. 2002. The 'risk environment': A framework for understanding and reducing drug-related harm. *International Journal of Drug Policy* 13(2): 85–94.
Rhodes, T. 2009. Risk environments and drug harms: A social science for harm reduction approach. *International Journal of Drug Policy* 20: 193–201.
Small, W., T. Rhodes, E. Wood, and T. Kerr. 2007. Public injection settings in Vancouver: Physical environment, social context and risk. *International Journal of Drug Policy* 18(1): 27–36.
Stortia, C., and P. De Grauweb. 2009. Globalization and the price decline of illicit drugs. *International Journal of Drug Policy* 20(1): 48–61.
Thrift, N. 2003. 'Space': The fundamental stuff of human geography. In *Key concepts in geography*, ed. S. Holloway, S. Rice, and G. Valentine. London: Sage.
Thrift, N. 2004. Intensities of feeling: Towards a spatial politics of affect. *Geografiska Annaler* 86B(1): 57–78.
Thrift, N. 2008. I just don't know what got into me: Where is the subject? *Subjectivity* 22(1): 82–89.

Valverde, M. 1998. *Diseases of the will: Alcohol and the dilemmas of freedom*. New York: Cambridge University Press.

Vitellone, N. 2010. Just another night in the shooting gallery? The syringe, space and affect. *Environment and Planning D: Society and Space* 28: 867–880.

Wilton, R., and C. Moreno. 2012. Critical geographies of drugs. *Social and Cultural Geography* 13(3): 99–108.

Zinberg, N. 1984. *Drug, set, setting: The basis for controlled intoxicant use*. New Haven: Yale University Press.

Chapter 6
The Ethics of an Assemblage of Health

Health and illness are a function of encounters; good and bad encounters, the salubrious and the insalubrious. Encounters may, in turn, be understood in terms of the events that sustain them, and the affects and relations that all encounters express. As a lived transition in a body's power of acting, health is forever moderated, maintained, threatened or diminished in the relations that obtain between bodies in specific territories or milieus. Taken in its positive valence, health may be said to entail an increase in a body's power of acting as it becomes more capable of affecting (and being affected by) the various entities it encounters. Illness, in contrast, effects a specific diminution in these capacities, limiting a body's affective sensitivities. The principal advantage of such a formulation lies in the attention it calls to the factors, processes or conditions by which a body may be said to *become healthy or ill* in 'real experience'. Just as the encounter between flesh and virus may in certain propitious circumstances produce influenza, other encounters, more conducive to a body's capacitation will engender health in their own auspicious happenstance. It follows that very few encounters can be said to be intrinsically healthy or unhealthy, given the indeterminacy of the affects and relations that pass between bodies in their encounters. While taking a poison or leaping from a bridge may be objectively dangerous or unhealthy, the majority of encounters require an "experimental ethos" (Foucault 1984: 41) by which their impact on a body's health or wellbeing may be discerned. Those specific encounters which affect a body with the felicitations of health will differ from body to body and event to event. Each body in its assembling with other bodies must determine the character of those encounters that promote health as a particular kind of affective or relational capacity.

Understood in this way, health is converted from a physiological condition into a distinctive "mode of existence" reflecting the particular events, affects and relations that sustain health in encounters between bodies (Deleuze and Guattari 1994: 75). This suggests moreover, that health ought to be regarded in ethical terms – requiring an evaluation of what bodies 'can do' in their encounters with one another – and not as an effect of the observance of particular principles or rules. This more ethical understanding of health, and the events, affects and relations by which health and

C. Duff, *Assemblages of Health: Deleuze's Empiricism and the Ethology of Life*,
DOI 10.1007/978-94-017-8893-9_6,

illness are moderated, accords with the analysis described in the case studies presented in the last two chapters. It further reflects the shortcomings of a binary conception of health and illness in which one state necessarily advances at the expense of the other (Blaxter 2004). Neither recovery from mental illness, nor the use of alcohol and other drugs, can be understood in these terms. The notion of recovery completely dismisses the logic of health *or* illness, of affliction and cure, in describing a process whereby an individual struggles to maintain some measure of wellbeing in the face of enduring illness. It is not the case that one is either sick or well; it is a matter of traversing the line in between, a line of becoming well that seizes on the affects, events and relations of a body's health in vitality. Health, in this regard, is neither the restoration of some 'pre-morbid' state or functioning, nor the result of a cure administered at the hands of an expert authority. Experienced as a *practice of health and its maintenance*, recovery advances and retreats in relation to the advances and retreats of mental illness itself. What matters is the range of practices, relationships, activities, affects and experiences individuals may draw from to maintain their recovery. Even the most conventional understandings of recovery hint at the centrality of this kind of ethical praxis, conceived in terms of the 'work' a body undergoes in the course of recovering from mental illness (Leamy et al. 2011). As I noted in Chap. 4, recovery may be regarded as a process of becoming sensitive to the affects, relations, signs and forces by which bodies become healthy. Few of these forces may be identified as a matter of principle. Instead, they must be discovered, fashioned or invented in and through the ethical expression of an enhanced capacity to affect (and be affected by) other bodies and events. Recovery from mental illness requires the articulation of a distinctive *mode of existence* whereby a particular way of engaging with bodies, spaces and objects is asserted in the establishment of a therapeutic praxis within a broader assemblage of health.

The proper characterisation of alcohol and other drug (AOD) use, and its impacts on health and illness, suggest similar ethical considerations. Despite efforts to either prohibit use in the case of illicit substances, or to dictate safe drinking guidelines in the case of alcohol – efforts which each presuppose a clear demarcation between healthy and unhealthy use, between the safe and the harmful – the notion that the therapeutic consequences of consumption can be determined in the absence of any consideration of its social, physical or biological contexts has met with persistent scepticism and limited practical compliance (see Fraser and Moore 2011; Keane 2009). At issue is the suggestion that the outcome of an encounter with alcohol and other drugs can be determined in some axiomatic fashion, as if all bodies encounter drugs in the same way, in the same assemblage of bodies, spaces, forces, affects, objects, technologies and desires. Even as public health discourses acknowledge individual differences in the experience of AOD use and its consequences (Babor et al. 2010), the dictates of health promotion and the logical distinction of health and illness, safety and harm, seem to necessitate the universalisation of the encounter with drugs in the development of health and social policy. As such, all differences are erased in the presentation of a generic human subject and its encounters with a stable psychoactive substance. These encounters are then rendered knowable in terms of the limits of healthy and unhealthy consumption (Fraser and Moore 2008).

Within such limits, health is once again reified as a function of the adherence to norms; the norms of safe consumption, of healthy bodies and prudential self management. Actual encounters between bodies and drugs are less important than the reliable articulation of norms derived from studies of populations and their epidemiological coherence. Yet the fact that illicit drug use persists almost everywhere, along with the routine defiance of safe drinking guidelines (Durrant and Thakker 2003; Keane 2002; Race 2009), suggests that *actual encounters between bodies and substances* ought to be central to any attempt to regulate the use of alcohol and other drugs in the course of promoting health however it is conceived. Surely, it is the way in which bodies encounter drugs that is central to the social, personal and acute effects of AOD use. Expressed in the context of an assemblage of bodies, forces, relations, affects and signs, one encounter with drugs may produce overdose, violence, intoxication or injury, just as another induces pleasure, happiness, conviviality, reverie or repose. The analysis presented in the previous chapter indicates that the volume of consumption is less significant in determining which of these divergent outcomes transpires in any specific encounter with drugs, than the particular mix of bodies, forces, objects, signs and affects active in each event of use. Determining, in turn, which encounter may be regarded as healthy and which should be considered unhealthy requires *ethical judgement* in each instance.

This chapter posits a set of ethical, affective and aesthetic criteria to guide such judgements derived from Deleuze's discussion of the ethical systems proposed by Michel Foucault and Baruch Spinoza. Applied to the real experience of mental health and substance use, I will argue in each case that the promotion of health demands a kind of *ethics of the assemblage* inasmuch as recovery from mental illness and the reduction of harms associated with AOD use may each be regarded as functions of particular encounters between bodies, forces and spaces. It is a question of reorganising one's encounters within an assemblage of bodies, spaces and forces in order to express a mode of existence consonant with the lived experience of health. Yet for such practices to be regarded as properly ethical endeavours, one must determine *how* encounters may be reorganised within an assemblage of forces; *why* certain encounters ought to be regarded as conducive or inimical to health; and *what* can be done to transform unhealthy encounters in the further extension of a body's scope of activity. That is to say that an ethics of the assemblage must be capable of endorsing distinctive normative criteria to guide the practical, everyday experience of health and recovery (see also Fox 2011). I argued in the first chapter that Deleuze is unique among contemporary philosophers for his commitment to just this kind of normative orientation in ethics, politics and aesthetics (Patton 2000; Smith 2012). While the normativity one finds in Deleuze's mature philosophy is not the kind that one finds in Kant, Mill or Rawls – that is to say that Deleuze is not interested in describing a set of universal rules or "categorical imperatives" by which all lives ought to be led at all times – Deleuze nonetheless proposes a set of "heterogenetic" norms capable of informing ethical practice in real experience (Smith 2012: 339–345). What Deleuze's work does not provide however, and this is perhaps the greatest weakness in Deleuze's treatment of ethical problems, is a *clear and systematic sense* of how the norms derived from transcendental empiricism may be applied in "real experience" (Buchanan 2011: 7–11). One finds hints regarding such applications scattered throughout his writings, although Deleuze fails to describe the 'ethical life' in anywhere near the detail that his contemporary Michel Foucault did.

Much, indeed, has been made of the consonance between Deleuze's and Foucault's ethical writings (Buchanan 2011). Addressing this debate, the present chapter proposes an ethics of the assemblage derived from each thinker's work. I argue in particular that reading Deleuze's and Foucault's ethics in concert enables one to begin to overcome shortcomings discernible in each approach. Foucault, for example, has long been criticised for failing to provide normative criteria to guide the practice of an "ethics of the self" (Koopman 2013). Critics stress that the absence of these criteria makes it difficult to discern ethical from unethical practices of the self, and difficult to determine the goals to which such practices ought to be oriented (Fraser 1981: 272–275). In refusing to articulate normative criteria, Foucault has been rebuked for reducing ethics to a naive "dandyism" incapable of informing an emancipatory politics (Simons 1995: 54–57). Foucault, of course, refused to endorse normative positions because he was wary of how the normative criteria provided by intellectuals may be co-opted in the design of novel forms of power and control (Foucault and Deleuze 1980: 207–209). Foucault (1988: 265) added that "the role of an intellectual is not to tell others what they have to do. By what right would he do so?" He was equally insistent that the absence of normative criteria was essential in "the search for styles of existence as different as possible from one another" (Foucault 1988: 253). Norms, in Foucault's (1983: 212) view, merely reinforce the "government of individualisation" such that an anti-normative ethics must be regarded as central to the design of viable practices of resistance and novel forms of subjectivity.

Even so, the argument I want to make in this chapter is that an ethics of health and illness does indeed require normative foundations in light of the *normativization of health* described by critics like Nikolas Rose (2001) and Monica Greco (2004). Each thinker stresses that contemporary health policy involves novel apparatuses of government, surveillance and power in the articulation of norms regarding the 'ideal' body, and the ways wellbeing, happiness and development may be maximised. The "will to health" (Rose 2001: 17) invoked in this governmentality is expressed in almost every facet of contemporary health care. It follows that any attempt to establish a novel ethics of health must either endorse this governmentality or propose an alternative set of normative criteria to guide ethical practice. While Foucault's last works suggest a means of resisting the *normalisation of health* (and the subjectivation required of it), his failure to consider the *normative* orientation of resistance has limited the more widespread adoption of his work (Koopman 2013). It is in this respect that Deleuze's explicit commitment to norms is all the more attractive. All the same, while Deleuze provides normative criteria to guide ethical practice (Patton 2008), he largely fails, as I have noted, to clarify how his ethics might be lived or *practised*, something that Foucault addresses much more directly (Nealon 2008). When read together, therefore, it is arguable that one may derive the normative criteria necessary to fashion a novel ethics of health from Deleuze's work, while Foucault's far more systematic treatment of an ethics of the self furnishes the requisite pragmatic and experiential framework for the design of such an ethics in everyday life. It is for this reason that I would conclude that reading each thinker's ethics in concert enables one to address shortcomings discernible in each approach.

Working through the consonances and antinomies of these ethical systems, the present chapter seeks to articulate how a healthy life might be lived according to a distinctive ethics of the assemblage. I would add that the question of the 'healthy life' and how it ought to be lived, is central to a number of contemporary health debates as resistance to the "government of health" proliferates (Greco 2004: 1–3). One key concern is how to maintain health and alleviate illness without succumbing to the *normalisation of health* and the strictures of the 'healthy subject' (Fox 2011; Metzl and Kirkland 2010). Deleuze's heterogenetic approach to norms suggests a means of negotiating this challenge, advancing an ethics of the assemblage that is not prepared to normalise health or its subjects. For only in 'real experience' can a body determine those encounters likely to yield some increase in its affective sensitivities and so promote its health and wellbeing. This is not to argue, however, that the practice of organising one's encounters in 'real experience' should not be guided by certain principles, norms or rules (Foucault 1984: 345–360). The present chapter proposes such principles, first reviewing the central features of an ethics of the assemblage, and its antecedents in the work of Deleuze and Foucault, and then considering how an ethics of the assemblage may inform the everyday practice of health and its maintenance. This should clear the way for the analyses to follow in the concluding chapter regarding the prospects of an ethics of recovery from mental illness, and the relative merits of the ethical consumption of alcohol and other drugs.

6.1 Deleuze's Ethics

Echoing Foucault's final works, Deleuze's (1995: 100) mature philosophy casts ethics as a set of "optional rules that assess what we do, what we say, in relation to the ways of existing involved". Underpinning this perspective is a sharp distinction between ethics and morality. Deleuze (1995: 100) argues that morality relies on "a set of constraining rules. . .that judge actions and intentions by considering them in relation to transcendent values (this is good, that's bad)". Ethics, in contrast, entail a series of "facultative" principles that enable evaluations of rival "modes of existence" in terms of their amplitude, or the extent of their power of acting (Deleuze and Guattari 1994: 75). The ethical life, as such, involves an "ethos, a style, a mode of thinking and living" (Flaxman 2012: xix) capable of yielding "an amplification, an intensification, an elevation of power, a growth in dimensions and a gain in distinction" among those forces, powers or capacities that define life (Deleuze 1993: 73). It is a question of identifying particular encounters, affects or relations within a particular assemblage that may extend the force of life to the limit of its power of acting. This process may be regarded as ethical insofar as it is primarily concerned with the question of how life ought to be lived (Buchanan 2011: 8). Nonetheless, Deleuze's ethics differ sharply from most established ethical systems by refusing to ground ethical practice in a particular moral code, just as he refuses to conflate the ethical life with the experience of a self-identical ethical subject. In effect, Deleuze rejects conventional understandings whereby ethics is presented as the application in practice (or experience) of a set of received moral principles (Audi 1995). Much less is it a problem of realising some set of innate human virtues in the contingencies of experience (Smith 2012: 146–149). Ethics do not express a more refined moral order, nor do they establish in practice the means by which human beings may be 'liberated' to reflect this order. In Deleuze's hands, ethics entail a creative, experimental and always provisional *praxis* by which immanent criteria are devised for the creation and evaluation of distinctive 'modes of existence' or 'styles of life'. The most significant of these immanent criteria is "novelty" (Jun 2011: 102–105).

Despite characteristic discrepancies in tone and orientation, Deleuze's varying treatments of the ethical life emphasise at every turn the "conditions of the new" (Smith 2012: 235–237). If difference ought to be regarded as the principal genetic condition for life in its emergent heterogeneity, then novelty (or creativity) must be regarded as the ethical principle that best accords with this condition (Deleuze and Parnet 1987: vii). Just as life differs from itself in the becomings that are its most distinctive ontological feature, Deleuze prioritises the role of creativity in ethical life as a means of harnessing the actual force of becoming. The goal is to render life "reasonable, strong and free" (Deleuze 1992: 262). Understood in this way, creativity is most clearly discernible in the efforts bodies make to "organise their encounters" (Deleuze 1992: 260). This organisation demands a creative ethos – an ongoing experiment in and with life – such that the most "compatible relations" for extending a body's power of acting may be identified (Deleuze 1992: 262). All bodies rely on other bodies (and the relations they are capable of enacting with these bodies) for the realisation of "what is most useful" in life (Deleuze 1992: 261). Only those relations of "proper and true utility" will provide the resources, support or alliances necessary for a body to "persevere in its being" (Deleuze 1992: 259–261). As such, all bodies must experiment with their relations, affects and associations in order to fashion a set of encounters most conducive to their power or utility in life. It is only by creatively organising its encounters that a body may achieve a "totality of compatible relations" equal to the "full possession" of its power of acting (Deleuze 1992: 262). Each resulting 'totality' is completely novel, insofar as the specific combination of affects and relations expressed therein embodies a new and distinctive form of life.

Paul Patton (2008) argues that Deleuze's valorisation of novelty introduces a uniquely normative orientation to his ethics. This normativity may be observed most directly in Deleuze's enduring commitment to deterritorialisation and the creativity and inventiveness required to promote it (Patton 2000: 2–3). Deterritorialisation effects discrete 'lines of flight' in the folding and unfolding of bodies, forces and affects within a particular milieu or assemblage. The force of deterritorialisation is exemplified in the disruption of relations between bodies, economies, semiotic systems and state forms common to all social, affective and political struggles. The notion of deterritorialisation thus provides a *conceptual and empirical logic* for tracing lines of becoming in political, corporeal, affective and economic life. This includes lines of transformation and empowerment, as well as lines of 'capture', stultification or oppression (Deleuze and Guattari 1987). However, Patton (2000: 83–85) stresses that deterritorialisation takes on a more normative hue in Deleuze's ethics to the extent that it traces those lines that enable novel movements, greater creativity, new capabilities, greater 'scope of activity', new modes of existence, more progressive forms of organisation, new affective resonances between bodies, more articulate expression, and so on. Regarded as such, 'deterritorialisation' furnishes the necessary normative criteria to "describe and evaluate movements and processes" by which novelty is produced (Patton 2000: 136). The work of evaluation is critical in determining which particular forms of creativity – and which specific expressions of novel social, corporeal, affective, economic or political organisation – should be regarded as important or useful, and which should be resisted or ignored. Even so, the risk with this approach is that the very idea of novelty takes on a kind of normative value, such that any novel deterritorialisation may be regarded as valuable in and of itself. Indeed, the problem with much of Deleuze's treatment of the relationship between novelty and deterritorialisation is the sense that the 'production of the new' is *innately valuable* regardless of the circumstances of this novelty, or its consequences. Yet surely not all novelty should be regarded as useful or significant?

Certainly, much of Deleuze's discussion of ethics leaves the impression that all novelty and all practices of creativity should be regarded as valuable to the extent that they enable resistance to prevailing regimes of power, political organisation and/or economic exploitation (O'Sullivan and Zepke 2008: 1–4). Notwithstanding the more sweeping endorsements of novelty that pepper Deleuze's writing, it is arguable that he does in fact provide immanent criteria for evaluating the particular modes of existence expressed in creative practice. Indeed, a given mode of existence may be regarded as 'ethical', 'good' or 'useful' to the extent that the deterritorialisations by which that mode is expressed enable it to become "reasonable, strong and free" (Deleuze 1992: 262). Of course, each term ('good', 'useful', 'reasonable', 'strong', 'free') assumes a distinctive valence in Deleuze's account of the ethical life (see Smith 2012: 345–350). Each term serves primarily to establish the conditions or criteria by which a particular event of deterritorialisation, a particular line of flight or instance of creativity, may be regarded as ethically significant or useful in terms of the "amplification", "intensification" or "elevation of power" that it enables (Deleuze 1993: 73). Patton (2000: 80–84) concludes that 'freedom' serves as the most significant of those conditions by which individual modes of existence (or processes of deterritorialisation) may be evaluated, inasmuch as freedom functions as both the *condition* and the *effect* of all 'good', 'useful' or 'strong' encounters between bodies.

While the idea of freedom appears incidentally in much of Deleuze's writings, both alone and in his collaborations with Felix Guattari (see Patton 2000), his book length discussion of the work of Michel Foucault provides the clearest indications of the place of freedom in Deleuze's ethics. Deleuze (1988a: 99–100) presents Foucault's oeuvre as a "counter-history" of the "doubling" of self and other, power and resistance, inside and outside, constraint and freedom, which enables the modern "government of individualisation". Whereas Deleuze suggests that Foucault's earlier works were primarily concerned with how the forces of the 'outside' (power, truth, justice, right, order) evoke the 'inside' or interiority of 'subjected' (human) life, Foucault's later works explore how the forces of the outside are refolded in life, in subjectivation, in a practice of freedom. Insofar as power, knowledge and truth function in the modern episteme to produce 'man' as a living, speaking and labouring subject, the discourses of biology, philology and political economy in which this subject appears enact a "doubling process" by which a line to the outside, a line of freedom, is preserved (Deleuze 1988a: 97–98). This is because 'modern man', precisely by virtue of 'his' "living, speaking and labouring ... (gives) rise to a life that resists power" (Deleuze 1988a: 94). Following Foucault, Deleuze (1988a: 100) characterises this resistance in terms of a "relation to oneself"; a folding of the force of power and truth back upon itself in a reconstitution of the 'inside' of subjectivity. Enacted in a series of "practical exercises", the subject comes to wield the forces of the 'outside' rather than being subjected to them in relations of constraint or duty (Deleuze 1988a: 100). The exercises by which power is folded constitute "*a relation which force has with itself, a power to affect itself, an affect of self on self*" (Deleuze 1988a: 101 emphasis in original). Deleuze (1988a: 101) describes this affective relation as a practice of freedom insofar as the folding of force enacts a "dimension of subjectivity derived from power and knowledge without being dependent on them".

Freedom must be understood, therefore, as the capacity subjects obtain by virtue of their very subjection to fold the forces of life, power and truth in the expression of a 'relation to oneself'. For this reason, freedom can only ever be achieved by being practiced or enacted: "just as power-relations can be affirmed only by being carried out, so the relation to oneself, which bends these power relations, can be established only by being carried out" (Deleuze 1998: 102). So how is this relation to oneself 'carried out' or practiced such that Foucault (and Deleuze after him) may describe it as a properly ethical endeavour? Deleuze (1988a: 104) identifies four distinctive folds by which freedom is expressed in ethical conduct. The first fold "concerns the material part of ourselves" (Deleuze 1988a: 104), such as the body and its material environs, its habits, desires and conduct, each of which may be modified or manipulated in a practice of freedom. The second "is the fold of the relation between forces" whereby power is doubled back on itself in a practice of resistance or transgression (Deleuze 1988a: 104). Each such fold creates novel forms of subjectivity by modifying the self's "auto-affection" (Deleuze 1988a: 118). The third fold by which freedom may be enacted "is the fold of knowledge, or the fold of truth insofar as it constitutes the relation of truth to our being, and of being to truth, which will serve as the formal condition for any kind of knowledge" (Deleuze 1988a: 104). Truth and knowledge are always plagued by what Foucault (1978: 100) called the "tactical polyvalence of discourses"; by inconsistencies, antinomies or "reversals" between rival knowledge claims that present "a point of resistance and a starting point for an opposing strategy". Each of these points avails an opportunity for freedom by exposing a weakness in truth, and a site of possible resistance to power. The final, enigmatic, fold concerns "the fold of the outside itself. . .from which the subject, in different ways, hopes for immortality, eternity, salvation, freedom, death or detachment" (Deleuze 1988a: 104). The fold of the outside conjures a line of flight, the lived pursuit of one's becoming free, healthy, immortal or eternal, whereby the subject is "created on each occasion, like a focal point of resistance, on the basis of the folds which subjectivize knowledge and bend each power" (Deleuze 1988a: 105).

This, finally, reveals the more normative aspect of freedom inasmuch as each of the four folds by which freedom is enacted "presents itself. . .as the right to difference, variation and metamorphosis" (Deleuze 1988a: 106). Henceforth, freedom must be characterised in terms of a "struggle for subjectivity" oriented in defence of the right to difference or variation in life (Deleuze 1988a: 106). Conditioned by the four folds described above, freedom involves a practice, or an 'auto-affection' of self by self whereby novel expressions of subjectivity may emerge. Understood in this way, freedom provides the overarching normative orientation for Deleuze's ethical system insofar as the various 'modes of existence' enacted or expressed in ethical conduct must be evaluated according to the degrees of freedom they enable. In each case, the effort to organise one's encounters in an attempt to live a more 'reasonable, strong and free' life must be assessed according to the normativization of a right to difference, found first, Foucault insists, by the ancient Greeks, but rendered all the more urgent in the context of the contemporary relation to oneself formed amid the "constraints of power" and the potency of "recognised identity, fixed once and for all" (Deleuze 1988a: 106). Freedom takes on normative weight for Deleuze (1988a: 114) to the extent that it leads subjects to ask of their ethical conduct "(w)hat can I do, what power can I claim and what resistances may I counter? What can I be, with what folds can I surround myself or how can I produce myself as a subject?" These questions suggest the criteria by which rival modes of existence should be assessed in weighing up the merits of different instances of conduct, practice or experience.

For all of the normative conflation of freedom and the 'right to difference' in Deleuze's ethics, it is not yet clear how freedom is actually produced in encounters between bodies. I would venture that freedom is experienced or maintained in those encounters in which bodies are (or become) *strong and reasonable* in their conduct. Each condition, strength and reason, provides further indications of the kinds of immanent criteria required by Deleuze for the proper evaluation of modes of existence in practice. To begin with, strength must be construed in terms of a body's power of acting, extended to the limits of its scope of activity. Yet strength cannot be understood as the power bodies wield over one another (a power to dominate, control or direct the conduct of other entities) for this kind of power is merely an expression of a body's force and not a means of extending or enhancing it. Recall that Deleuze, following Spinoza, regards a body's power of acting to be the result or effect of bodies *acting together* in their encounters. A body's strength is only ever enhanced in encounters which extend the power of acting of bodies acting together. Action is always relational inasmuch as activity is only ever possible in encounters between bodies. No action is solitary, not even the relation to oneself, which is always a matter of a particular set of simple bodies acting on other simple bodies within the assembled 'body proper'. A body's strength, therefore, is enhanced in those encounters which extend its power of acting, understood or expressed as an increase in each body's capacity to affect and be affected by their encounters. Strength can never be reduced to brute force if understood in this way because it refers to a body's capacity to connect with, or relate to, the bodies both human and nonhuman that it acts with in practice. In this sense, strength measures a body's receptiveness to new encounters and connections rather than its quantum of force.

It follows that a body's strength may be observed in those encounters which enable the acquisition of simple parts; parts which 'agree' with that body, affecting it with joy and an increase in its power of acting. A body *becomes strong* to the extent that it can organise its encounters in ways that enable it to create richer, more numerous relations with other bodies, resulting in an increase in the simple parts assembled in and for each body in the encounter. Each encounter by which a body becomes strong leaves that body better equipped, as it were, to further extend its encounters in order to acquire additional simple bodies, to either improve its understanding, to increase the array of bodies it may affect and be affected by, or both. Indeed, a body becomes strong to the extent that it is able to multiply the array of forces assembled within it. This includes the forces of knowledge, understanding and empathy; the force of acting with, or relating to, other bodies; the force of auto-affection and the relation to oneself; and the force of directing or manipulating the material entities that compose a body's territory or milieu (Smith 2012: 153–159; also Buchanan 1997: 79–81). Regarded as such, a body may be considered more capable, stronger or more powerful than another body when it might be said of that body that it is "more capable than others of doing many things at once, or being acted on in many ways at once, so its mind is more capable of perceiving many things at once. . .(and) more capable of understanding distinctly" (Spinoza, cited in Deleuze 1992: 256–257). This suggests that a body's power of acting is directly proportionate to, if not a function of, its capacity to affect and be affected by the various bodies it encounters. Yet it also suggests that a body's strength is relational as it is distributed across an assemblage of forces, signs and territories. Strength is held in common among the varied bodies, human and nonhuman, simple and complex, organic and inorganic, assembled in a given territory. This is why strength cannot be conflated with power as is it typically understood, as a force one actor exerts over another. Power over another body is never strength in the Spinozist sense because the exercising of power over another actually reduces each body's strength by closing off the prospects of sympathetic relations between those bodies in a recombination of forces. Exercising power over another body actually curtails the strength of the 'dominant' body in this sense.

While it follows that Spinoza's valorisation of strength should not be regarded as some nascent 'will to power', Deleuze (1992: 257) observes that Spinoza's ethics elevate a body's power of acting to the status of a "natural right". He adds that a body is forever "seeking what is useful in terms of the affections that determine it. . .a body always goes as far as it can, in passion as in action; and what it can do is its right" (Deleuze 1992: 258). With this gesture, Spinoza transforms the problem of strength from one of duty, and the proper limits of one's power, into a "law of nature", concerned not with the "rule of duty, but with the norm of a power, the unity of right, power and its exercise" (Deleuze 1992: 258). If a body 'naturally' seeks what is right, advantageous, good or useful, and if this effort should itself be understood as natural, even normative, then the task for ethical practice is not to curtail a body's rights in accordance with some moral conception of power and its discharge, but rather to establish a means of determining which encounters extend a body's power of acting within a broader society of bodies, and which in fact reduce this scope of activity. Such endeavours suggest to Deleuze (1992: 255) a properly "ethical vision of the world". Consistent with this vision, "we" should always "strive to unite with what agrees with our nature, to combine our relations with those that are compatible with it, to associate our acts and thoughts with the images of things that agree with us" (Deleuze 1992: 261). As a function of the efforts one makes to organise one's encounters in this way, one has a "right. . .to expect a maximum of joyful affections (as) our capacity to be affected will be exercised in such conditions that our power of action will increase" (Deleuze 1992: 261). Yet the problem with this conclusion is that it is not yet clear how one may decide which of one's encounters enable the combination of relations necessary to increase one's power of acting, and which 'decompose' these relations in the diminution of one's scope of activity. Solving this problem requires the use of *practical reason* in the 'valuation' of affects and relations.

Practical reason is not, however, the reason of 'God', 'man', 'nature' or the transcendental; it is neither natural, nor received. Reviewing Spinoza's account of the 'reasonable' life, Deleuze (1992: 262) notes that "(n)obody is born free, nobody is born reasonable; and nobody can undergo for us the slow learning of what agrees with our nature, the slow effort of discovering our joys". Reason is evinced in practice as a dawning realisation of what 'agrees' with one's 'nature'. It follows from the identification of those events, affects and relations that enable the greatest utility, understood in terms of an increase in one's power of acting. Just as it is impossible to determine in some axiomatic way which encounters, events, affects or relations are likely to impart the greatest increase in a body's scope of activity, reason cannot be derived from a set of transcendental principles but must instead be invented or discovered in the vicissitudes of 'real experience'. There is no such thing as 'universal' or innate reason in Spinoza's ethics; no categorical imperative or due process that may finally deliver the rudiments of reasonable conduct. Reason is expressed in practice, in a body's encounters, and in the identification of what accords with its strengths, joys and affections. Yet this does not mean that reason may be reduced to a kind of solipsistic fancy. Practical reason is always relational (or processual) insofar as it is concerned with 'sympathy', congruence and the transmission of capacities (or simple parts) between bodies. Such a process has nothing to do with what might satisfy individual bodies in their isolation. It is in fact concerned to delimit what benefits a society of bodies acting in their sympathetic relations to extend the powers of acting of each body so assembled. Reason is always contingent in this sense, as it manifests in the conduct of bodies acting together in an assemblage of forces. It is for this reason that Deleuze (1992: 262) concludes that reason is a function of "development, a formative process, a culture".

A body *becomes* reasonable (or unreasonable) in other words. The unreasonable person, the "child", the "weak man" or the "fool" remains unreasonable for as long as he or she remains incapable of determining the character of the encounters he or she experiences, and the ways these encounters shape the affects and relations he or she commands (Deleuze 1992: 262–263). The unreasonable person is "left to chance encounters" (Deleuze 1992: 263), unable to discern good from bad encounters, and unsure of the "actual causes" of the fluctuations in one's power of acting that these encounters effect. The reasonable person, in contrast, submits to a "long formative process…a very slow empirical education" (Deleuze 1992: 263–265) whereby one considers one's encounters, reflects on their causes and effects, and determines the fluctuations in one's power of acting that each entails. This process does not, however, involve a kind of isolated, heroic struggle conducted in quiet repose. The process of becoming reasonable is always, already developmental and cultural, transpiring in the midst of a society of bodies acting together. It involves a collective experiment as it were, as bodies struggle in their encounters to identify the specific affects, events and relations that are most likely to enhance their collective power of acting with an assemblage of forces. If it is true that no one body ever acts alone, then it is equally apparent that no one body ever discovers reason on its own. Reason is the achievement of a collective intelligence (both human and nonhuman) that proceeds by way of a "natural combination of relations" (Deleuze 1992: 264).

Reason resides, therefore, in "compatible" relations or "reasonable association(s)" (Deleuze 1992: 265). Each of these associations coheres in the empirical education by which bodies move from passive, chance encounters – encounters which are as likely to result in sadness and a diminution in one's powers as joy – to active and deliberate encounters. Such an education depends on what Latour (2004: 208) memorably calls a "supplement of attention"; a kind of training or experimentation with the character of one's relations to oneself and others so that one may realise what agrees with one's self in its affective modulations. Reason is the 'supplement of attention' that is added to the encounter in a body's determination of those affects and relations that most effectively enhance its powers of acting. Attention, or reason, like Whitehead's prehensions introduced in the second chapter, are not the exclusive preserve of the human body. Humans are, nonetheless, capable of very specific kinds of attention, which may each be trained, modified, enhanced or expanded in ethical conduct (Robinson 2009). Attention, I would argue, is the mechanism within practical reason that permits bodies to reflect on their encounters in the movement from chance encounters, with all the aleatory modifications in one's capacities they entail, to more active encounters, replete with a more reliable increase in one's scope of activity. Following Spinoza, Deleuze (1992: 273–276) argues that one's attention should be trained, in the first instance, on *joyous encounters*. That is because the positive affects that such encounters entail yield the first indications of the agreement or sympathy of bodies, and their potential for *compatible association*.

One slowly acquires the capacity for practical reason – and a capacity over the longer term for more active affections in the realisation of one's powers in life – by first noting the circumstances, if not the causes, of one's joyous encounters and the affects and relations therein that most agree with one's nature. Such a process requires that one ask of oneself "what must (I) do in order to be affected by the maximum of joyful passions" so that I might "become reasonable" (Deleuze 1992: 274). Joy is the essence of practical reason in this sense, and it is why the realisation of positive affects lies at the heart of Deleuze's 'ethical vision of the world'. Positive encounters lead one to reason by availing the first, tenuous indications of the particular affects, relations and associations that extend one's power of acting within an assemblage of forces. Joy is the earliest manifestation of practical reason in other words, providing a sense of how active affects may be realised. Joy avails an 'adequate idea' of how and why certain affects enhance one's power of acting. It does this by revealing "common notions" among the bodies assembled in any positive or joyous encounter (Deleuze 1992: 275). The idea of 'common notions' is central to the practice of Spinoza's ethics because it describes the very mechanism by which joyous encounters enhance a body's scope of activity. A common notion is simply the "idea of a similarity of composition in existing modes" or bodies (Deleuze 1992: 275). Positive encounters, which express joyous or compatible relations in the transfer of simple parts in and between complex bodies, extend a body's power of acting by equipping it with novel parts or capacities. In entering such relations, bodies begin to form a new "community of composition" that practically, affectively, cognitively and/or experientially extends what a body can "do. . .say, believe, feel (or) think" (Deleuze 1992: 269). If positive encounters entail an 'agreement' between bodies (experienced as a positive commingling of forces, affects and relations) then common notions establish the *reason for this agreement*. Common notions "find in a similarity of composition, the necessary internal reason for an agreement of bodies" (Deleuze 1992: 276). Common notions, in turn, confirm the actual cause, or the 'adequate idea' of this agreement, identifying the ways forces combine in a 'community of composition' tantamount to a more powerful body.

Common notions furnish adequate ideas of the ways body combine to form more powerful communities, extending a body's scope of activity. Once a body has an *adequate idea* (correct, accurate, true or sound) of how and why particular encounters affect it with joy and an increase in its power of acting, that body is finally able to move from passive to more active affections. This transition from passive to active affections is the primary goal of Spinoza's ethics (Deleuze 1992). Spinoza argues that a body may be said to experience passive affections when its affects (either positive or negative, joyous or sad) are determined by external causes. This happens as a consequence of the *inadequate ideas* (wrong, partial, misguided or fanciful) that body has of the character and causes of its encounters. Constrained by the inadequacy of its ideas, such a body is subject to the chance and tumult of its encounters, unable to direct its encounters to maximise its joyous affections, and unaware of the causes of its recurrent sad passions. With the development of *adequate* ideas, a body slowly acquires the capacity to form active affections as it establishes itself as the (internal) cause of its encounters. It is for these reasons that Deleuze (1992: 280) states that the "forming of a common notion marks the point at which we enter into *full possession* of our power of acting" (emphasis in original). In taking possession of our power, "we become reasonable beings" capable of directing our encounters in the formation of mutually agreeable communities of bodies that further extend or express our power of acting (Deleuze 1992: 280). Such a process is ethical insofar as it is concerned with the organisation of one's conduct in order that one might live a stronger, freer and more reasonable life. This is a life governed by two overarching imperatives. First, a body must strive to "exercise (its) capacity to be affected in such a way that (its) power of action increases". A body must then "increase this power to the point where (it) produces active affections" (Deleuze 1992: 269). All of which requires the active organisation of one's discrete encounters.

If, ultimately, all of Deleuze's ethical precepts may be said to concern the nature of encounters, and the importance of their more active or deliberate organisation, it is difficult, nonetheless, to derive from these precepts much sense of the *practical means* by which one's encounters may be reorganised in 'real experience'. The goals or purpose of this activity are certainly clear enough even if the means are not. With reference first to goals, Deleuze emphasises the importance of individuals becoming strong, reasonable and free in and through the active manipulation of encounters within an assemblage of forces, bodies, spaces, signs and affects. Such work entails a slow, developmental process, an empirical education, as individuals discover those encounters, associations or communities which enhance their power of acting, their understanding and awareness, just as they learn to avoid or temper the impact of 'bad' associations. In strength as in reason, a body traces a line of becoming free in its activity within the assemblages, territories, cultures or milieus in which it is subjected. Deleuze is far less convincing, however, when addressing the means by which an ethics of becoming might actually be lived or practiced. Despite affirming the importance of novelty, the creative reorganisation of one's encounters, deterritorialisation and practical reason, Deleuze provides only vague indications of how each of these practices unfolds in life, in a community of bodies acting together.

At worst, Deleuze seems to describe a body acting at a kind of scholastic remove, slowly acquiring a reasoned sense of its passions and relations, reflecting at leisure on the proper means of affecting the various bodies (human and nonhuman) that it encounters. For all of Deleuze's insistence on the empiricity of the encounter, and the importance of 'real experience' in the conduct of ethical life, it is not always clear how a body may begin to modify its encounters in order to identify 'common notions' and so acquire a measure of practical reason, strength and freedom. Close readings of Deleuze's varied accounts of the 'ethical life' certainly yield a number of practical insights regarding the conduct of an ethics of becoming, although it is difficult to argue that such insights amount to a coherent model for the organisation of ethical conduct. Perhaps this kind of systematicity is undesirable; it may even be inconsistent with the ethos or spirit of Deleuze's ethics (Smith 2012: 158–159). Even so, I would argue that systematicity is essential if Deleuze's ethics are to influence the design of ethical life in the ongoing promotion of health and development in 'real experience'. As Buchanan (2011: 8–9) insists, if one cannot "decide what 'the right thing to do' is from a Deleuzian perspective", then it is likely that Deleuze's impact on the health and social sciences will be modest at best, and deservedly so. I share Buchanan's (2011: 8) interest in articulating a "Practical Deleuzism" capable of informing ethical conduct while promoting the resolution of concrete ethical problems like 'how might one live a more healthy life'. As I have noted, reading Deleuze's ethics in relation to the far more pragmatic and systemic model offered by Michel Foucault ought to provide the means of realising this more practical 'ethical vision'.

6.2 Foucault's Ethics

Foucault's (1997: 177) late interest in the articulation of an "ethics of the self" was motivated in part by the realisation that his earlier genealogies of the subject had "perhaps insisted too much on the techniques of domination". This emphasis had yielded accounts of the subject inattentive to the myriad techniques by which individuals actively engage in practices of 'self-fashioning'. In correcting this oversight, Foucault provided a more rounded genealogy of the subject, emphasising both practices of domination (or 'government'), and of the self (or 'freedom'). His later works also established stronger grounds for resistance to those modes of subjectivation that Foucault's earlier studies had systematically revealed. In turning to consider the subject's ethical conduct, Foucault was concerned to identify practices, techniques or strategies through which the individual might resist the form and limits of existing modes of subjection. Foucault, indeed, regarded the practice of an ethics of the self as a means of affirming new forms of subjectivity. Foucault provides the clearest account of this goal in the late essay "*What is Enlightenment?*"

Starting with an assessment of Kant's version of enlightenment, Foucault (1984: 34) proceeds to consider the prospects of an "exit" or "way out" of the individual's "subjection" to external modes of authority, power and morality. Foucault is especially interested in the extent to which the 'modern' individual might "escape" the ties of identity associated with the modern state and its institutions. For Miller (1993: 327) this objective betrays "a decisive will not to be governed"; an interest in resisting government, and the normalisation associated with it, in order to live a more "free", happy or exemplary existence. To this end, Foucault (1983: 216) proposes an ethical art of self-fashioning, an *aesthetics of existence*, whereby the individual may resist the "ruse" of power and knowledge in the realisation of "new domains for liberty". This goal primarily requires that one resist the limits identity imposes upon experience, such that one may come to experience greater freedom in the active fashioning of oneself, in the very realisation of enlightenment (Foucault 1997: 266–268). Nonetheless, the problem remains of identifying particular strategies through which relations of power, subjection and identity might be resisted. Foucault began to address this problem in his later writings, examining a range of historical practices through which freedom and resistance may be enacted in experience. The most important of which involves what Foucault called transgression or a ‘limit attitude’.

Transgression requires the interrogation of limits and the creative experimentation with their transformation; goals which certainly express something of the essence of Foucault’s late politics (see Simons 1995; Ransom 1997). In undertaking to work with limits, the subject “fashions new forms of subjectivity, thus attaining unstable and undefined freedom” (Simons 1995: 4). Transgression, in this sense, is the very essence of freedom understood as a careful and deliberate practice of resistance and creative self-fashioning. Foucault (1984: 50) further describes transgression in terms of “an attitude, an ethos, a philosophical life” aimed at overcoming the limits imposed upon experience through the reification of identities and the practice of subjection. It requires that one affirm the historical contingency of limits in an “experiment with the possibility of going beyond them” (Foucault 1984: 50). Foucault (1984: 44–48) goes on to describe this “philosophical ethos” as a “limit attitude” characterised by a “permanent critique of our historical era…oriented towards the contemporary limits of the necessary”. Such an attitude entails a “historico-practical test” involving the identification of that which “is no longer indispensable for the constitution of ourselves as autonomous subjects”. Consistent with this ‘test’, Foucault (1984: 46) regards ethics as “a work done at the limits of ourselves” in order to “open up a realm of historical inquiry…both to grasp the points where change is possible and desirable, and to determine the precise form this change should take”.

Indeed, it is Foucault’s insistence on determining the “precise form” ethical conduct should take that most sharply distinguishes his ethics from Deleuze’s sympathetic approach. Foucault (1985) pursues this pragmatic interest by assessing what he called “technologies” or “practices” of the self, and their role in the cultivation of a personalised ethical practice. By “practices of the self” Foucault (1985: 10–11) means those “intentional and voluntary actions by which men not only set themselves rules of conduct, but also seek to transform themselves, to change themselves in their singular being, and to make their life into an oeuvre that carries certain aesthetic values and meets certain stylistic criteria”. All of which requires very particular “relations with the self” (Foucault 1985: 30) whereby specific techniques are developed such that the self and its proclivities may be known and if necessary modified. In this way, Foucault’s (1985: 29) ethics are grounded in specific “relationships with the self, for self-reflection, self-knowledge, self-examination, for the decipherment of the self by oneself, for the transformations that one seeks to accomplish with oneself as object”. These relationships establish the self as both the object and subject of one’s ethical and aesthetic practices (Foucault 1983: 236–237). Accordingly, only the individual can know for themselves how to bring to their own existence particular qualities or values that may exemplify a more beautiful, free, hopeful or righteous existence. Of what, however, does such a process consist, and how might one practice an ethics of the self in everyday life? Foucault explicitly addresses these questions in his study of classical Hellenic and Roman ethics.

6.2.1 Aesthetics of Existence

Conventionally, ethics is understood as "the philosophical study of morality" (Audi 1995: 244) whereby attempt is made to discern universally verifiable codes of moral and social conduct. It is concerned, more directly, with the application of "human rationality" to the problem of deciding "how one ought to act" (Audi 1995: 244). Foucault (1988: 247), of course, remained consistently hostile to such a model of ethical conduct, stressing in a late interview that "the search for a form of morality that would be acceptable to everyone – in the sense that everyone would have to submit to it – strikes me as catastrophic". In contrast to such an ethics, Foucault was interested in articulating a model that might *guide or inspire* the individual's ethical practices without dictating them. Foucault discovered a historical precedent for this approach in the ancient Greek practice of *askesis*. Though admitting of no entirely accurate contemporary translation, *askesis* described a form of moral exercise or training (Foucault 1985: 72–77). It was devised by the Stoic philosophers as a means of providing moral training for the young noblemen destined to one day rule the great city-states of the classical period. The practice of *askesis* typically consisted of exercises considered "indispensable in order for the individual to form himself as a moral subject" (Foucault 1985: 77). This included "training, meditations, tests of thinking, examination of conscience, control of representations...dietary regimens (and) the interpretation of dreams" required for self-mastery or self-control (Foucault 1985: 74). To this end, individuals were subjected to specific tests in which various desires or appetites were to be mastered and particular temptations averted. The successful completion of which enabled the individual to form himself as an ethical subject, as the bearer of a virtuous and free existence. Summing up these regimens, Foucault (1997: 282) described ascetics as an "exercise of self upon self in which one tries to work out, to transform oneself and to attain a certain mode of being".

In late interviews, Foucault offered a contemporary perspective on this ancient practice, suggesting that the classical definition of asceticism ought to be retrieved in favour of the Christian version which, in his view, exaggerated the importance of renunciation and self denial. Foucault (1988: 264) was greatly attracted to the classical understanding of ascetics, particularly the "elaboration of self by self" in the work of "transform(ing) oneself in one's singular being". Yet for all of his enthusiasm, it is important to stress that Foucault was not at all interested in reviving classical ethics in the contemporary period. He stressed that "you can't find the solution of a problem in the solution of another problem raised at another moment by another people" (1984: 343). In the same interview he even goes so far as to express some disgust at the specific content of classical ethics in terms of the individual practices and techniques of a Greek arts of existence (Foucault 1984: 346). Notwithstanding these reservations, Foucault suggests that while the specific features and practices of the ethical systems developed by the ancients may not be amenable to contemporary revival, the *principle* of the aestheticisation of existence is. As Foucault (1988: 259) puts it "this is what I tried to reconstitute: the formation and development of a practice of the self whose aim was to constitute oneself as the worker of the beauty of one's own life". Mitchell Dean (1994: 199) offers a slightly more illuminating assessment of Foucault's purpose in noting that "the core of the present relevance of these later volumes may be discerned in a certain diagnosis of contemporary life, how to construct oneself ethically in the face of the failing assurance provided by moral codes, generalisable norms, or universal values".

Of equal importance, however, is Foucault's view that the ethical practices of ancient Hellenic and Roman culture avoided the pervasive normalisation that remains such a strong feature of most contemporary ethical and moral systems. Foucault (1983: 230) noted that "I don't think one can find any normalisation in, for instance, the Stoic ethics. The reason is, I think, that the principal target of this kind of ethics was an aesthetic one. First, this kind of ethics was only a problem of personal choice...The reason for making this choice was the desire to live a beautiful life, and to leave to others memories of a beautiful existence. I don't think that we can say that this kind of ethics was an attempt to normalise the population". Classical ethics was not the subject of "civil law or religious obligation" but was rather the expression of certain voluntary choices within the individual's "conduct of conduct" (Foucault 1983: 244). The practice of an aesthetics of existence was considered a moral choice made by certain individuals in order to bring certain values to their life. It was a "question of making one's life into an object for a sort of knowledge, for a *techne,* for an art" (Foucault 1983: 245). This, in fact, is the reason why Foucault speaks of the ancients and their ethics in explicitly aesthetic terms, as an aesthetics of existence, for the self's *rapport à soi*, its relations to self, involve the creative and aesthetic elaboration, cultivation or transformation of oneself. In the late interview Foucault (1997: 131) observed that "this transformation of one's self by one's knowledge, one's practice is, I think, something rather close to the aesthetic experience. Why should a painter work if he is not transformed by his own painting?" More than this, however, Foucault, like Deleuze, regards creative endeavour as the very foundation of agency and empowerment, providing an enduring basis for ethical transformation.

The *aestheticisation* of the ethical subject concerns, more directly, what Foucault came to call practices of the self; those ordinary, everyday activities through which the subject regulates its own conduct and develops its own 'personality'. Importantly, such practices entail a range of strategies through which the individual might resist the forms of individualisation or identity imposed upon the self by culture and power. Yet these strategies are not invented by the self; rather, the subject modifies and develops techniques already available to it in order to more profoundly individualise the experience of subjectivity (see Foucault 1997). It is, indeed, this modification, this adaptation and development, that Foucault regards as an aesthetic practice. It is worth noting that all individuals make some attempt to fashion their subjective existence through their own ethical conduct and, hence, all individuals are self-fashioning to some extent. However, this engagement is rarely an entirely reflexive or conscious practice, in that most individuals rarely bring to their ethics a comprehensive *aesthetics* of existence. Foucault (1984: 362) stresses that "we find this is the Renaissance, but in a slightly academic form, and yet again in nineteenth century dandyism, but those were only episodes". Foucault (1988: 1–21) laments the absence of a more contemporary practice of an aesthetics of existence, arguing that such an ethical framework presents great potential for the practice of freedom today.

Foucault is thus compelled to return to the study of classical Hellenic and Roman ethics in order to draw out the features of an ethical practice that might enable greater liberty in the experience of subjectivity and the body. To this end, Foucault develops a model or taxonomy of classical ethics that observes the structure and ethos of the ancients without replicating its content. This model has four dimensions, each of which forms part of an ethical relation to oneself constitutive of an aesthetics of existence. Foucault (1985: 26) describes the first element as the *determination of the ethical substance*. This involves the isolation of that part of the self in its ontology, behaviour or constitution that becomes the "material" of one's ethical practice. The ethical substance is, indeed, the very subject matter of one's personal ethics. One might here draw examples from the experience of certain of the new social movements and their struggles against sexism, homophobia and racism. For example, if one's decides that one wants to overcome the 'learned habits' of sexism or racism, then one may elect to focus on that aspect of one's own ethical behaviour through which such discrimination is inadvertently perpetrated. This may well involve a greater reflexivity of self, and greater consciousness of how one interacts with others. Taking up such themes, Foucault (1984: 353) argues that many of the liberation movements of the 1960s focused upon sexuality itself as an "ethical substance" in their attempts to "liberate" a true or deep sexuality free of the repressions associated with modern societies and certain bourgeois sensibilities.

The second dimension of an ethical relation to oneself involves a distinctive *mode of subjection*. Modes of subjection concern the practices through which individuals establish their particular responsibilities in relation to existing moral codes. It invokes "the way in which people are invited or incited to recognise their moral obligations" (Foucault 1984: 353). This process requires the identification of specific practices through which a more ethical life might be realised. It involves some sense of the appropriate mode of ethical transformation and the forms of subjectivity produced therein. Foucault (1984: 353) argues that ancient Greek ethics were characterised by a mode of subjection grounded in the practice of an aesthetics of existence. Elsewhere, Foucault (1984: 45–50) examines the Kantian model of universal rationality, and its associated mode of subjection, in which the individual is required to recognise oneself as a subject of reason and thus transform one's ethical and political practices to enhance reason, or to manifest it more perfectly or completely.

The *practice* of an ethics of the self is grounded in what Foucault calls the *mode of asceticism,* referring to those self-forming activities through which the subject seeks to transform its existence in order to obtain certain spiritual, aesthetic or ethical states. This is, properly speaking, what Foucault is referring to when discussing technologies of the self (see 1985: 27). Foucault also describes such practices as an exercise in *askesis* or ascetics. As I have noted, the Greeks understood ascetics as the promotion of a certain way of life, founded in critical self-reflection, in which the individual engages in a practice of self-transformation, of invention, creativity and discovery. In this way, the mode of asceticism engages the critical problem of what is to be done. It asks what self-forming activities must the self practice in order to transform itself, to transgress the limits of the self as it is currently constituted in order to attain a certain, more aesthetic state? The identification of the specific qualities of this "aesthetic state" concerns the fourth element of an aesthetics of existence; the realisation of the ethical goal or *telos*. Foucault (1985: 29) stresses that ethical relations to oneself are always oriented towards a specific mode of being, which forms their goal or end. What, in other words, is the subject attempting to *become* through its ethical practices. This may be as nebulous as a more beautiful, happy or wise existence; it may be the realisation of freedom and a self unfettered by the interdictions of one's social milieu; or one's telos may aspire to the purification of the soul through various abstinences and privations. Ethical practice is always oriented towards the ongoing refinement of a particular state of being, or a particular quality of the self. It requires the explicit identification of the specific aims informing one's ethics, in terms of one's understanding of the self, its manifestations and limits.

In observing these four principles (the determination of the ethical substance, the mode of subjection, the mode of *asceticism* and the telos of one's ethics) the self engages in a practice of self-fashioning; an ethical relation to oneself characteristic of an aesthetics of existence. However, the particular manner in which these four elements are practiced in the conduct of an ethics of the self – including the specific ways in which the various techniques, combinations and priorities associated with it are actually employed in ethical conduct – are dependent on the specific goal of one's ethical practice. The means of actually *practising or developing* an aesthetics of existence may be clarified through closer reference to the ethical practices of the ancient Greeks, with particular focus on how each of the four domains of ethical life described above were enacted in the individual practice of an ethics of the self.

6.2.2 "The Use of Pleasure": The Practice of an Aesthetics of Existence

What Foucault discovered in his analysis of the Ancients and their ethics was the development of a set of personalised practices concerning the everyday deployment *of pleasure* across four main sites or regions. First, this "ethical surface" featured the practical regulation of one's pleasure in relation to *dietetics*, or "the management of the health and life of the body" (Foucault 1985: 98). It was considered important for the 'free man' to regulate the practice of his sexual pleasure in order to maintain the 'proper functioning' of the body-organism. Second, one must manage one's household in terms of the proper relations with one's wife, slaves and children. While there existed in antiquity no particular juridical interdictions prohibiting extra-marital relations, these were considered to be an "excess" or hubris, and were thus "inappropriate" for the habits of an ethical man. Such moral teachings formed a key component of the ancient Greek study of *economics* and the proper management of the household (see Foucault 1985: 143–146). Third, Greek ethics considered the use of pleasure in terms of the free man's relations to *erotics*, or the love and courtship of boys (a relatively common practice among the great nobles of the ancient city-states). Here the focus was not the virtue or otherwise of sexual relations with members of one's own sex, but rather the specific type and nature of those relations. What, for example, was the nature of any sexual contact? Who initiated it? Who occupied the more 'active' role? The fourth domain concerned the ethical relation to *truth,* in which sexuality or the use of pleasure was considered to be a particularly important source of wisdom. The ancient practice of philosophy involved considerable reflection upon the nature of 'true love', and its practical manifestations, as a means of accessing truths thought to be otherwise prohibited or unattainable. It was argued that one must conduct one's use of pleasure according to specific ethical principles if one hoped to access that domain of truth manifested within intimate relationships. Love was, in this way, considered a divine state that admitted of many of the most inaccessible and arcane "secrets of existence" (Foucault 1985: 229–233).

Turning to consider such an ethics in light of the general taxonomy developed by Foucault and briefly summarised above, pleasure or *aphrodisia* and its proper deployment, served for the Greeks as the *ethical substance* of an aesthetics of existence. Ancient Greek ethics were primarily concerned with the proper use of pleasure; with how the ethical subject might moderate his pleasures in order to manifest a more exemplary existence. This moral preoccupation did not, for the ancients, concern particular acts or practices, but rather, established how the free man should moderate his pleasures in terms of their frequency and intensity in order to master his more base appetites. Importantly however, the absence of moderation was not itself punishable for it was considered the virtue of men of rare ethical strength. As such, self-mastery in the use of pleasure brought to the individual a certain aesthetic quality; it made the self a more beautiful thing. For the Greeks therefore, the *ethical substance* of an aesthetics of existence concerned the proper use of pleasure. The *mode of subjection* associated with this ethics concerned the management of pleasure, or the problem of *chresis*, defined as utility or deployment. However, 'utility' was not simply a matter of function, for it had more to do with the stylistics of sexual conduct and the ongoing stylisation of one's lifestyle and personal habits. Moreover, the great Greek philosophers of morals argued that the stylisation of pleasure should prioritise moderation of the *quantity* of one's sexual acts. Sexual pleasure should be experienced only as the satisfaction of one's innate needs and never indulgently pursued for its own sake. This view translated into detailed reflection upon the most appropriate time to engage in sexual relations, the frequency of such relations, the status of one's partners, and reciprocity of activity and passivity in the proper conduct of one's sexual relations. The noble practitioner of an aesthetics of existence controlled the practice of his sexuality, and the use of his pleasures, according to these prudential principles. It is for these reasons, moreover, that Foucault refers to such relations as a specific *mode of subjection*, for their practice involved voluntary subjection to a particular set of aesthetic principles.

Practices of self-mastery underscored the specific *mode of asceticism* characteristic of the ancients and their ethics. This concerns those self-forming activities through which the subject actively seeks to transform its existence. For the Greeks the practice of *enkrateia*, or self-mastery, was considered among the most virtuous of personal qualities. It required profound ethical effort or struggle and was thus understood to enable the expression of divine qualities within the self. Self-mastery was directed most immediately at the regulation or control of one's erotic desires, fantasies, drives and proclivities. The goal was complete victory over oneself understood in terms of the permanent control of one's desires and the attainment of a state of moderation "impervious to the violence of those desires" (Foucault 1985: 65). The ancient Greeks understood this as a permanent expression of struggle within the self in which "one part of the self (the nobler part) was expected to defeat the other part (the weaker and baser part)" (McHoul and Grace 1993: 101). One could rarely expect to eliminate the desire for immoderate pleasures, in that such desires arose within the body of its nature. Rather one must master one's desires through diligent practice and eternal vigilance. It is in this sense, moreover, that the Greeks regarded ethics as a form of moral training in which the individual attempted to prepare himself for the temptations of desire and the immoderate pleasures of the flesh. As a result of this training, the ethical individual was able to control the body and its 'invading desires' and so avoid becoming enslaved to them.

This, in turn, introduced the *telos* of a Greek ethics of the self. The 'teleological' component of Greek ethics was concerned with the realisation of *sophrosyne*, or the moderation of desire and its satisfaction. The practice of moderation was believed to bring to the individual a certain freedom, understood as the liberation of oneself from one's own constraining desires. As Foucault (1985) observes, the problem of slavery was paramount in the ancient world, not only in terms of a contract of labour or ownership, but also in terms of the enslavement to one's own desires. Indeed, to give in to one's desires, to lack self-restraint, was to become a slave to, rather than a master of, oneself. It was considered impossible to be truly and completely free if one remained beholden to one's temptations. As Foucault (1985: 79) notes "of all the dangers carried by the *aphrodisia*, dishonour was not the most serious; the greatest danger was bondage to them". Thus "immoral people were slaves of their desires" (Foucault 1985: 79), while the free man exercised complete mastery over them. Hence, the practice of moderation was understood to be fundamental to the enjoyment of freedom. Freedom guaranteed the self's quantum of power, which vouchsafed, in turn, the self's ongoing enjoyment of freedom. Freedom, so experienced, enabled one to resist the "tyranny within the self", the tyranny of immoderate desire (Foucault 1985: 80). This is also the sense in which the ancients regarded ethical virtue as a condition of leadership, for how could a man enslaved to his own passions be expected to resisted tyranny both within and outside the city? The practice of political power was thus conditional upon control over oneself in the practice of an aesthetics of existence. This required a careful practice of moderation in the use of pleasure; the goal of a Greek ethics of the self. Having illustrated how ancient Hellenic and Roman ethical practices were organised in relation to the four great axes of an aesthetics of existence, my goal now is to imagine how a contemporary ethics of health may be similarly organised in aesthetic practice.

6.3 The Ethics of an Assemblage of Health

Throughout this book I have sought to articulate a positive account of health, more alert to the 'real experience' of bodies in their everyday encounters. The need for such an account is surely apparent in light of the contemporary *normativization of health* and the associated effort to regulate the body in its conduct, practices and interactions. The risk with this ascendant normativity is that health is reified in a grim index of the body's homeostatic functioning. In conflating health and biology, the human sciences, biomedicine and public health alike conjure an 'ideal body', efficient in its metabolic performance, prudent in its self-management, and confident in its 'natural' capacities (Fox 2012). Yet as the resurgence of interest in wellbeing, function, freedom and the 'quality of life' demonstrates, health conceived in terms of physio-psychological performance captures but a fraction of the 'real experience' of bodies in their associations, struggles and ambitions. This is to say nothing of the pervasive normalization associated with the contemporary 'will to health', with its manifold injunctions regarding the virtues of a 'healthy life' and the proper comportment of 'healthy' bodies (Petersen and Bunton 1997). Wherever health is first conceived as the absence of disease, the temptation to convert health into a measure of the body's 'natural' biological order inevitably appears (Canguilhem 1989). Left to its 'nature', health is whatever is good, therapeutic, beneficial or sustaining for the body. This conception leads, often enough, to the generation of injunctions regarding the healthy life; rules by which health in its vitality may be sustained. Whatever supports this natural vitality must be healthy, just as anything that harms it, even risks the incidence of harm, must be avoided for its obvious folly.

The problem with this 'naturalisation' of health, as Foucault (1988: 49) observed, is that adherence to a universal morality such as one discovers undergirding the codes, interdictions and moral prescriptions advanced in contemporary biomedicine is "now disappearing, has already disappeared" from modern cultural and political life. Indeed, the moral foundation on which the contemporary 'health society' ostensibly rests no longer commands the consensus it once enjoyed, inspiring the search for new approaches more accommodating of difference and personal liberty (see Greco 2009). This is also the reason why the presentation of a more 'heterogenetic' definition of health is critical. As the instruments of governmentality cast more and more of the everyday work of states and markets in the service of health and its maintenance, a more positive understanding of health is essential for the evaluation of good and bad policy. That is to say that one must have some basis for distinguishing policies or practices that enable bodies to become "strong, reasonable and free" from those that leave individuals "weak, base and enslaved" (Smith 2012: 147). Just as the notion of health now exceeds the proper functioning of the body to include the mediation of lifestyles, contexts and values, health must be converted from a moral into an ethical consideration. For there can be no morality of the body if the body is as much a function of its contexts or interactions as it is a natural or biological given. Indeed, there can be no morality of health given the indeterminacy of the myriad encounters, affects, events and relations by which health is realised in an assemblage of forces. This, in turn, suggests the need for an *ethics of the assemblage*, rather than the individual human actor, given the role of nonhuman forces in the modulations of health in experience. As Foucault (1988: 263) put it "the problem of an ethics as a form to be given to…life has arisen once more".

The question of how life may be 'given form' in the course of ethical practice further indicates the need for a more positive conception of health. Indeed, the elision of health and life in the contemporary workings of biopower suggests that the aestheticisation of health may well become one of the most striking means of resisting this power (Greco 2009; Rose 2007). Resistance may therefore entail renewed assessment of the risks and benefits of the contemporary 'will to health' along with the various human and nonhuman forces active in the mediation of health. It is with these interests in mind that I have described health and illness as a function of encounters, such that one may trace the measure of a body's becoming well (or ill) in an assemblage of forces. As a function of encounters, I would conclude that both the promotion of health, and recovery from illness, necessitate the identification of affects, relations, events, bodies, forces, spaces and signs that enable a body to maintain or recuperate its strength, reason or freedom in real experience. The question of how this process transpires in experience suggests the need for an appropriate ethics of and for an assemblage of health. Conceived as a distinctive 'mode of existence', it is critical that one consider how health may be promoted, sustained or recovered in practice, in an assemblage of forces, in life. Consistent with the analysis offered in the last two sections, I would like to close this chapter with an attempt to integrate the heterogeneous ethical approaches proposed by Deleuze and Foucault in order to sketch an ethics of the assemblage. I will do this by corralling Deleuze's 'heterogenetic' ethics into the more systemic confines of Foucault's aesthetics of existence. Yet before this may be done, it is important that I address the degree of complementarity between these two approaches; one addressed to a 'compound of forces', the other concerned with 'practices of the self'.

6.3.1 A Compound of Forces

As I have noted, Foucault's ethics are primarily concerned with practices of the self; those intentional activities by which individuals seek to transform themselves, their personality, character, qualities or capacities. Some commentators have taken issue with the apparent "return to the subject" intimated in Foucault's final writings, suggesting that an ethics of the self all but reinstates a conventional subject (Dews 1989: 37–41). Deleuze (1995: 97–99) emphatically rejected this view, arguing instead that Foucault's ethics introduce a "play of forces" (the "folding" or "doubling" of power relations) into the study of the individual's subjection. Deleuze (1995: 98) adds that the "process of subjectification, that is, the production of a way of existing, can't be equated with a subject, unless we divest the subject of any interiority and even any identity". It is not the subject that returns in Foucault's ethics, with all the apparent reassurance of a foundation at last for the resistance of power and force. Rather, Foucault's late interest in ethics was inspired by the realisation that power always equips the subject with a capacity to bend or fold force in the creation of a variable relation to itself (Deleuze 1988a: 104–105). The capacity to fold power, to manipulate the 'play of forces' at work within the subject gives rise to an ethics because it introduces the problem of determining the particular 'mode of existence' or 'style of life' that should direct the subject's ethical praxis (Smith 2012: 146). For Foucault, it is a question of determining the ethical substance of one's practice, and the specific ends or goals to which these practices ought to be oriented. This is not so far from Deleuze's own discussion of ethical matters, and his interest in the ways a body may manipulate its encounters in the practice of becoming strong, reasonable and free.

Even so, it seems clear that Deleuze's ethics are primarily concerned with a 'compound of forces', an assemblage of spaces, bodies, affects and signs, whereas Foucault is more interested in the forces active within the subject. That is to say that the account of subjectivity presented in Foucault's work is not the same as the account provided by Deleuze, either alone or in his writing with Felix Guattari. Foucault draws attention to the capacities subjects obtain as a result of their subjection to power in order to clarify how individuals may bend or displace force in a deliberate, patient and reflexive praxis. Deleuze, however, was more interested in the zones, spaces, flows or milieus in which bodies (simple and complex, human and nonhuman) converge in an assemblage of forces. This move distributes or spatializes subjectivity, construing it as an 'intensive event' expressed within a community of relations, bodies and spaces acting together. For Deleuze, subjectivity ought to be regarded as a dense point, a zone of intensity within a wider assemblage of forces, bodies, spaces, territories, objects, signs and processes. The experience of the healthy subject is surely the perfect example of this process, given the array of material, spatial, structural, intensive, affective and organic forces involved in the production of health and illness in experience. The well (or ill) subject is produced as a nexus of indeterminate forces; a moment in the folding of power, affect, matter, relationality, organic and inorganic life. This suggests, finally, that a Deleuzian ethics of health and illness must concern itself with this assemblage of forces, as much as it attends to the ethical proclivities of the assembled subject. Far more so than Foucault, Deleuze is interested in the ontology of the 'forces of the outside', and not merely in the ways these forces are folded within the subject in practice. This leads Deleuze into the flux of force – an immanent field of 'pre-personal' affects, relations, and events – that gives form to the becoming body, becoming subject of 'germinal life'. It is perhaps no wonder that the ethics of germinal life should be so mysterious.

I should expect that this mystery will be greatly diminished in its reconfiguration in the guise of an aesthetics of existence. For all of their discrepancies, I would argue that Foucault's and Deleuze's treatment of the subject and subjectivity offer merely divergent emphases; a difference of degrees rather than a difference in kind (Deleuze 1988b: 14–16). It is worth repeating, in this context, that Foucault's ethics ultimately emphasise the practice of askesis or 'auto-affection' in the bending of force relations rather than the subject of this practice as such. While Deleuze shares this interest in force, it is nonetheless important to prioritise the figure of the assemblage in any consideration of Deleuze's ethics, rather than the subject per se for all of the reasons articulated above. I would also wager that when applied to the experience of health and illness, an ethics of the assemblage will remain sensitive to the mix of social and structural factors, the biological and the cultural forces, active in a body's becoming well (or ill). So how might such an ethics 'work' in practice, in the varied becomings that determine a body's health and illness? It is in response to this question that I would assert the merits of presenting Deleuze's varied ethical pronouncements within the frame of Foucault's ethics of the self. The four folds of Foucault's aesthetics of existence would appear just as well suited to the folds of the assemblage as they are the self. Reorganising Deleuze's ethics in this way should also provide insights into the nature of an assemblage of health, and the ways this assemblage may be manipulated in the ongoing promotion of health in experience.

6.3.2 The Four Folds of an Ethics of the Assemblage

The first of Foucault's folds, or ethical precepts, concerns the 'determination of the ethical substance'. I would like now for my own purposes to conceive of this ethical substance in terms of health itself, and the ways health is expressed in an assemblage of forces. Throughout this book I have characterised health as a process of becoming strong, reasonable and free. Such becomings entail a series of affective and relational transitions in a body's power of acting at the reach of its scope of activity. Always, already a function of an assemblage of human and nonhuman forces, a body's scope of activity determines the array of entities it may affect and be affected by, along with the sum total of relations that body may enter into. As such, any body (or assemblage of forces) may be regarded as healthy to the extent that it can "(do) many things at once, or (be) acted on in many ways at once", just as "its mind is...capable of perceiving many things at once...of understanding distinctly" (Spinoza, cited in Deleuze 1992: 256–257). And so, to the extent that health may be regarded as a function of encounters, health conceived in more ethical terms requires for its maintenance the active manipulation of encounters in order to render a body more capable of 'doing', 'affecting', 'perceiving' and 'understanding distinctly'. This, indeed, ought to serve as the ethical substance of an ethics of the assemblage.

More directly, health conceived as an 'ethical substance' should provide a focus for folding relations of force in the manipulation of encounters within an assemblage of spaces, bodies and signs. It provides an orientation for a body's becoming strong, reasonable and free to the extent that strength, reason and freedom actually extend, promote or enhance a body's health. To be more clear, I would suggest that when conceived in relation to health, freedom may be construed as a right to variation in the transformation of the body; strength may be construed as the measure of a body's power of acting, or the extent of its scope of activity within a field of forces; and reason ought to be construed as an 'adequate' understanding of 'what agrees' with a body in the accrual of those specific associations that enable its 'active affections'. Each achievement, freedom, strength and reason, accords with any useful, substantive definition of health. Each provides a sense of the substance of an ethics of the assemblage; or the objects of a more ethical understanding of health.

Foucault would insist that such an ethics must also feature a distinctive 'mode of subjection'. While the mode of subjection suggested in a Deleuzian ethics is likely a stranger beast than the one found in Foucault's more genteel aesthetics, Deleuze as I have noted, is not opposed to the notion of subjectivity. He does, all the same, prefer to speak of a "mode of intensity" (Deleuze 1995: 99), a field, zone or plane in which subjectivity accrues or converges. It is always a question of determining how particular 'pre-personal' affects, relations, signs, events and forces are folded into an assemblage in the expression of subjectivity (Tucker 2012: 774–776). As such, the 'mode of subjection' (or 'intensity') suggested for a Deleuzian ethics of the assemblage may well resemble the more aesthetic model promoted by Foucault. Indeed, there seems no reason to think that aesthetics cannot be applied to an assemblage of forces, just as it may be applied to a subject, body or practice. However, I would add that an equally useful guide may be observed in Deleuze's discussion of practical reason, introduced above. If health may be regarded in part as a function of the realisation of practical reason, and if reason ought itself to be understood as the product of a slow cultural and empirical education, then it would seem that reason may provide a suitable mode of subjection to guide ethical conduct in pursuit of health and wellbeing. Indeed, Deleuze's discussion of reason suggests diverse justifications as to why a body may elect to *subject itself to reason* in an attempt to maintain or restore its health. Following Spinoza, Deleuze (1992: 265) argues that bodies strive to invent or discover a method of practical reason in order that they may come to understand the causes and consequences of their own encounters. As a body comes to reason, either as a result of its immersion in a 'formative process, a culture', or as a result of a more 'experimental ethos', that body is able to direct its encounters, its affects and relations, in order to maximise its joyous passions. Joyous passions, of course, provide the first hint of the 'adequate ideas' necessary to recognise common notions, which themselves presage the realisation of active affections. *Reason thus describes a logic of 'real experience' by which the causes of particular health promoting encounters may be determined.* One may elect to subject oneself to practical reason, therefore, in order to identify those associations by which one may become strong and free, healthy and well in life.

This leads to the question of activity, or the particular mode of asceticism required of an ethics of the assemblage. Borrowing from Foucault, I would suggest that *practices of the encounter* ought to be sufficient to the task. Encounters are clearly central to a Deleuzian ethics and they must, for this reason, be central to an ethics of the assemblage too. Following Deleuze (1992), the focus of such an ethics should in the first instance remain with the body itself. The body in 'real experience' is ideally placed to judge or evaluate the character of its encounters, and their impact on its health and wellbeing. Naturally, individualism is central to the ethical remit of the contemporary 'will to health', yet the difference is that the 'body' of Deleuze's ethics is an assemblage rather than an isolated, atomic entity. Practices of the encounter must, in this regard, consider as many of the affects and relations immanent to the encounter as possible, and not merely those which pertain to the body (or subject) of the encounter. My point is that encounters draw together an array of bodies, spaces, affects, relations and signs, the human and the nonhuman, and so any practice of the encounter must evaluate as many of these forces as possible in determining the consequences of a given encounter for a body's health and wellbeing. This is not to suggest, however, that bodies need to become masters of their own encounters, studiously observing the vicissitudes of events, affects and relations in painstaking application. Reason, as I have indicated, is central to an ethics of the encounter (and the identification of their varied effects on a body's health and wellbeing), although reason is as much a function of culture and knowledge as it is the outcome of an 'empirical education'. What I mean to say is that the effects of encounters, and their impact on one's health and wellbeing, may be learned in culture as much as they are experienced in practice. Like Foucault's practices of the self, practices of the encounter can be adopted and modified from techniques and strategies already existing in culture in the course of reorganising one's encounters. Some encounters will be well known in culture and knowledge as potentially injurious to health, and so the means of their avoidance will likely be clear enough. Other more novel encounters will, nonetheless, require equally novel practices for their manipulation, requiring the kinds of strength and reason in practice described in Deleuze's ethics. The task is to organise or refashion one's encounters in order to maximise one's joyous passions, and so enjoy the full measure of health associated with them.

This suggests, finally, something of the telos or goal of an ethics of health, and the assemblages in which health is expressed. This goal, simply enough, ought to be the maintenance of health and wellbeing experienced "in such a way that a body's power of action increases...to the point where it produces active affections" (Deleuze 1992: 269). The *activeness* of a body's affections may be said to enhance its health to the extent that it increases the array of entities that body may establish relations with. These relations, in turn, enable a body in its freedom, strength, adaptability, responsiveness or poise to determine what it can do, what powers it may claim, what resistances it may enact, what folds it may surround itself with, and how it may produce itself as a 'healthy' subject (see Deleuze 1988a: 114). A body's *health in activity* opens up a line of becoming well, a line outside power and control whereby existence itself may be transformed. Yet as Deleuze (1988a: 129) notes "it is obvious that any form is precarious, since it depends on relations between forces and their mutations". It follows that health is precarious too because it relies on practices and ethical relations that are vulnerable to change, disruption or reversal. This vulnerability must become central to one's ethical practice, insofar as the mitigation of vulnerability ought to form something of the goal of one's ethics. The question to ask of any practice related to the maintenance or promotion of health is simply "has it helped to enrich or even preserve the forces within (the body), those of living, speaking or working?" (Deleuze 1988a: 130). Living, speaking or working, *the affecting, understanding and doing* of a body in its health and vitality; a health that is not an order of the living, but an infinite play of forces, a "diversity of combinations" of affects, events and relations in and for life in its being lived (Deleuze 1988a: 131–132).

The four folds of Foucault's ethics of the self thus suggest a structure, an organising logic, for the conduct of a Deleuzian ethics of the assemblage and its application to the problem of health and its maintenance or promotion. Health, as it is lived from day to day in the modulations of practice, affects, events and relations, should serve as the substance of such an ethics. A practical reason of encounters, effects and transitions suggests a suitable mode of subjection inasmuch as a body may elect to subject itself to the rigors of practical reason in the organisation of its encounters. The very practice of the encounter yields a convenient mode of asceticism, with its related practices of strength, reason, freedom, reflection and activity. It is a question of becoming sensitive to one's encounters such that one may come to understand the forces at work within them and the means of their manipulation. The goal of this manipulation, of all of these technologies of the encounter, may figure simply as the promotion of health itself, or the realisation of a body at the limit of its power of action, its 'natural right', and the enjoyment of its joyous passions. So stands an ethics of the assemblage, of health itself. The concluding chapter will deploy this ethics in reassessing the experience of recovery from mental illness and the 'healthy' consumption of alcohol and other drugs. I will seek to indicate how a Deleuzian ethics of the assemblage may suggest novel ways of promoting recovery, and new responses to the problems associated with the misuse of alcohol and other drugs. My purpose will be to take the full measure of Deleuze's ethics in order to finally assess its value in the production of a line of becoming strong, reasonable and free.

References

Audi, R. (ed.). 1995. *The Cambridge dictionary of philosophy*. Cambridge: Cambridge University Press.

Babor, T., R. Caetano, S. Casswell, G. Edwards, N. Giesbrecht, K. Graham, J. Grube, L. Hill, H. Holder, R. Homel, M. Livingston, E. Österberg, J. Rehm, R. Room, and I. Rossow. 2010. *Alcohol: No ordinary commodity: Research and public policy*. Oxford: Oxford University Press.

Blaxter, M. 2004. *Health: Key concepts*. London: Wiley.

Buchanan, I. 1997. The problem of the body in Deleuze and Guattari, or, what can a body do? *Body and Society* 3(3): 73–91.

Buchanan, I. 2011. Desire and ethics. *Deleuze Studies* 5(S1): 7–20.

Canguilhem, G. 1989. *The normal and the pathological*. New York: Zone Books.

Dean, M. 1994. *Critical and effective histories: Foucault's methods and historical sociology*. London: Routledge.

Deleuze, G. 1988a. *Foucault*. London: The Athlone Press.

Deleuze, G. 1988b. *Bergsonism*. New York: Zone Books.

Deleuze, G. 1992. *Expressionism in Philosophy: Spinoza*. Trans. Martin Joughin. New York: Zone Books.

Deleuze, G. 1993. *The fold: Leibniz and the Baroque*. London: Athlone Press.

Deleuze, G. 1995. *Negotiations: 1972–1990*. Trans. Martin Joughin. New York: Columbia University Press.

Deleuze, G. 1998. *Essays Critical and Clinical*. Trans. Daniel W. Smith and Michael Greco. London: Verso.

Deleuze, G. and F. Guattari. 1987. *A Thousand Plateaus: Capitalism and Schizophrenia*. Trans. Brian Massumi. Minnesota: University of Minnesota Press.

Deleuze, G., and F. Guattari. 1994. *What is philosophy?* London: Verso.

Deleuze, G., and C. Parnet. 1987. *Dialogues*. London: Athlone Press.

Dews, P. 1989. The return of the subject in the Late Foucault. *Radical Philosophy* 51(2): 37–41.

Durrant, R., and J. Thakker. 2003. *Substance use and abuse: Cultural and historical perspectives*. Thousand Oaks: Sage Publications.

Flaxman, G. 2012. *Gilles Deleuze and the fabulation of philosophy*. Minneapolis: University of Minnesota Press.

Foucault, M. 1978. *The history of sexuality. Vol 1: An introduction*. London: Penguin.

Foucault, M. 1983. Afterword: The subject and power. In *Michel Foucault: Beyond structuralism and hermeneutics*, 2nd ed, ed. H. Dreyfus and P. Rabinow. Chicago: University of Chicago Press.

Foucault, M. 1984. *The Foucault reader*, ed. Paul Rabinow. London: Penguin.

Foucault, M. 1985. *The history of sexuality. Vol. 2: The use of pleasure*. London: Penguin.

Foucault, M. 1988. *Politics, philosophy, culture: Interviews and other writings 1977–1984*, ed. L. Kritzman. New York: Routledge.

Foucault, M. 1997. *Michel Foucault ethics: The essential works*, vol. 1, ed. Paul Rabinow. London: Allen Lane/Penguin.

Foucault, M., and G. Deleuze. 1980. Intellectuals and power: A conversation between Michel Foucault and Gilles Deleuze. In *Language, counter-memory, practice: Selected essays and interviews*, ed. M. Foucault and D. Bouchard. Cornell: Cornell University Press.

Fox, N. 2011. The ill-health assemblage: Beyond the body-with-organs. *Health Sociology Review* 20(4): 434–446.

Fox, N. 2012. *The body*. Cambridge: Polity Press.

Fraser, N. 1981. Foucault on modern power: Empirical insights and normative confusions. *Praxis International* 3(2): 272–287.

Fraser, S., and D. Moore. 2008. Dazzled by unity? Order and chaos in public discourse on illicit drug use. *Social Science & Medicine* 66(3): 740–752.

Fraser, S., and D. Moore. 2011. *The drug effect: Health, crime and society*. Melbourne: Cambridge University Press.
Greco, M. 2004. The politics of indeterminacy and the right to health. *Theory, Culture and Society* 21(6): 1–22.
Greco, M. 2009. Thinking beyond polemics: Approaching the health society through Foucault. *Oesterreichische Zeitschrift fuer Soziologie* 34(2): 13–27.
Jun, N. 2011. Deleuze, values, and normativity. In *Deleuze and ethics*, ed. N. Jun and D. Smith, 89–107. Edinburgh: Edinburgh University Press.
Keane, H. 2002. *What's wrong with addiction?* Melbourne: Melbourne University Press.
Keane, H. 2009. Intoxication, harm and pleasure: An analysis of the Australian National Alcohol Strategy. *Critical Public Health* 19(2): 135–142.
Koopman, C. 2013. *Genealogy as critique: Foucault and the problems of modernity*. Indiana: Indiana University Press.
Latour, B. 2004. How to talk about the body? The normative dimension of science studies. *Body & Society* 10(2–3): 205–229.
Leamy, M., V. Bird, C. Le Boutillier, J. Williams, and M. Slade. 2011. Conceptual framework for personal recovery in mental health: Systematic review and narrative synthesis. *British Journal of Psychiatry* 199: 445–452.
McHoul, A., and W. Grace. 1993. *A Foucault primer: Discourse, power and the subject*. Melbourne: Melbourne University Press.
Metzl, J., and A. Kirkland (eds.). 2010. *Against health: How health became the new morality*. New York: New York University Press.
Miller, J. 1993. *The passion of Michel Foucault*. London: Flamingo.
Nealon, J. 2008. *Foucault beyond Foucault: Power and its intensifications Since 1984*. Stanford: Stanford University Press.
O'Sullivan, S., and S. Zepke (eds.). 2008. *Deleuze and Guattari and the production of the new*. London: Continuum Books.
Patton, P. 2000. *Deleuze and the political*. London: Routledge.
Patton, P. 2008. Becoming democratic. In *Deleuze and politics*, ed. N. Thoburn and I. Buchanan, 178–195. Edinburgh: Edinburgh University Press.
Petersen, A., and R. Bunton (eds.). 1997. *Foucault, health and medicine*. London: Routledge.
Race, K. 2009. *Pleasure consuming medicine: The queer politics of drugs*. Durham: Duke University Press Books.
Ransom, J. 1997. *Foucault's discipline: The politics of subjectivity*. Durham: Duke University Press.
Robinson, K. (ed.). 2009. *Deleuze, Whitehead, Bergson: Rhizomatic connections*. New York: Palgrave MacMillan.
Rose, N. 2001. The politics of life itself. *Theory, Culture & Society* 18(6): 1–30.
Rose, N. 2007. *The politics of life itself. Biomedicine, power, and subjectivity in the twenty-first century*. Princeton: Princeton University Press.
Simons, J. 1995. *Foucault and the political*. New York: Routledge.
Smith, D. 2012. *Essays on Deleuze*. Edinburgh: Edinburgh University Press.
Tucker, I. 2012. Deleuze, sense, and life: Marking the parameters of a psychology of individuation. *Theory & Psychology* 22(6): 771–785.

Chapter 7
Conclusion: A Line of Becoming Well

Health in its meaning, form and experience is forever conveyed in a positive valence. It is surely present in each of the virtues, joys and capacities of being embodied. Accounting for the positivity of health demands substantive theoretical reflection, for the preservation of health necessarily requires clear ontological, experiential and affective goals (Metzl 2010). It demands some sense of the ends or purpose to which the promotion of health – which after all commands a handsome share of available public and private investment – might meaningfully be oriented. Throughout this book, I have drawn from Deleuze's transcendental empiricism in an effort to elaborate the social, affective and material experience of health at is it lived in the midst of a social context; in an assemblage of forces. Consistent with Deleuze's understanding of (human) life canvassed in earlier chapters, health cannot be said to pertain solely to a remote physiological entity. For all the achievements of public health, for all of the attention to the social, structural and environmental determinants of health and illness, the primacy of the atomic human agent still holds great sway over the theoretical and empirical imagination of the health and social sciences. This book has attempted to conceive what the study of health might look like were the focus of analysis to shift from the 'human' and its preferences, capacities and vulnerabilities to the study of 'life' itself. My goal has been to articulate a posthuman account of health, more attentive to the imbrications of matter, affect, biology, technology and politics that characterise so much of contemporary life (Rose 2007). If health may no longer be taken to be the preserve of a discrete biological agent – if it must instead be distributed among an assembled throng of human and nonhuman forces – then health should be regarded, in its turn, as a relational achievement, as the effect of bodies acting together in force and sympathy.

Health is a function of the assemblage in other words. Deleuze's notion of the assemblage has, indeed, provided compelling theoretical and empirical support for prising open the workings of health as it is produced at the nexus of social, biological, political, economic, affective and material forces. Taken first in relation to mental illness, and then with respect to the use of drugs and the problems associated with them, I have sought throughout the book to demonstrate the utility

C. Duff, *Assemblages of Health: Deleuze's Empiricism and the Ethology of Life*,
DOI 10.1007/978-94-017-8893-9_7, © Springer Science+Business Media Dordrecht 2014

of Deleuze's empiricism for a radical rethinking of health by way of the assemblage itself. This thinking suggests, as I have noted several times, that health ought to be regarded as a function of encounters between bodies, between forces and between practices. As such, the human body cannot be regarded as naturally healthy, any more than any particular mix of human encounters can be said to be either innately healthy or innately dangerous, excepting only the most obvious predicaments. It must be said that the human body is sustained in its encounters, which deliver its most basic needs while satisfying its more elevated ambitions, its baser ones too of course. From nutrition, shelter, warmth, security and sociality, to love, empathy, understanding and wonder, all of the body's needs are contingent upon the affects, relations and materials it may secure in its encounters. All of this is obvious, even though the most obvious corollary, the need to distribute health within an assemblage of human and nonhuman forces, has mainly eluded the health and social sciences, which seem universally reluctant to offend the ontological primacy of 'human nature' (see Buchanan 1997; Fox 2011; Metzl 2010). This is another of the reasons why Deleuze's posthumanism is of such critical utility for the health and social sciences. Not because it somehow erases the 'human', relegating it to ontological obsolescence, but because it ushers in a thought of the "not yet human", "more than human" becomings that may finally establish in the study of life, becoming, health and vulnerability a "superior human nature" (Ansell Pearson 1999: 59). Moving beyond an anthropocentric understanding of health has permitted greater elucidation throughout the book of the nonhuman forces at work in the modulations of health and illness, including the various structural factors long described in established accounts of the social determinants of health (Baum 2008).

Conceiving of health as a function of social, material and affective encounters has lead, in turn, to the attempt to furnish a more positive definition of health, one that is alert to the cast of human and nonhuman forces involved in the experience of health. Taken in its positive guise, health is normally regarded as whatever is 'good', 'proper', 'enabling' or 'beneficial' for the body in its active vitality. It should retain this valence, if only as a counter to the more morbid preoccupations of the contemporary health and social sciences, which seem singularly focused, most of the time, on whatever threatens to harm the body in its 'natural' plenitude. I am not arguing that the health and social sciences should be unconcerned with the etiology of illness, the epidemiology of risk and harm, or the therapeutics of treatment and public policy. Since their inception, the health and social sciences have contributed immeasurably to the mitigation of human suffering and the promotion of human wellbeing. It is just that the focus on cataloguing and redressing human suffering has so often been accompanied by an enduring indifference to the dynamic experience of health at the limits of its power of acting. Even as, more recently, scholars have turned their attention to the character of human flourishing, to 'strengths' and 'capabilities' (see Peterson and Seligman 2003), the focus of this attention has mainly rested with the idea of extracting from human nature the full measure of its potential. The idea that the 'human' might not be natural at all, that it might be the contingent achievement of biological, cultural, social and political forces has lingered only at the margins of research activity in the health and social sciences. In this sense, *Assemblages of Health* rests on a hunch, a feeling that we are entering a posthuman age where the advances of science and technology, commerce and creativity, media and aesthetics, culture and practice are all but erasing any necessary ontological distinction between 'man' and 'world', 'agent' and 'structure', 'subject' and 'object'. Many in the health and social sciences are well advanced in the work of cataloguing this epistemological dissolution (see Latour 2005; Law 2004; Mol 2002; Rose 2007; Wolfe 2010; Zammito 2004). *Assemblages of Health* has contributed to this effort by tallying the conceptual and empirical resources available in Deleuze's oeuvre for the ongoing articulation of a posthuman science of health and illness.

The posthuman account of health and illness that has emerged in these considerations emphasises the 'openness' of the body and its susceptibility to ever more dynamic articulations of affects and relations in its compositions and decompositions in life. Regarded as such, health may be construed as the net effect of each of those affects and relations that extend a body's scope of activity, its power of acting within a given assemblages of spaces, bodies, events, signs and technologies. As I have noted, a healthy body is one which can affect and be affected by a multitude of bodies and forces around it, just as it is able to understand distinctly the character of its encounters, and the affects and relations generated therein. *This is a body that is strong, reasonable and free*. Free to act widely within the insuperable constraints of its environment; reasonable in the manner in which it understands and organises it encounters, in its 'acting with' the bodies and forces it enters into community with; and strong in its capacity to bend the relations of power that structure its milieu. These are, moreover, the reasons why health ought to be conceived in relation to affects, events and relations, for it is a question of identifying the processes by which bodies *become healthy* (strong, reasonable and free) within an assemblage of forces. As I noted in Chap. 3, this position is not so far from many existing theoretical approaches to the study of health and human development, even if the conceptual vocabulary is occasionally mystifying. For example, Amartya Sen's (1999) capabilities approach shares with Deleuze a reluctance to specify the values, goals or capacities that might characterise the 'good' or 'healthy' life. This suggests that the problem of determining the *quality of life* isn't likely to be settled in a long catalogue of virtues, as if a list of norms and values may ever say anything of importance about how virtue may be realised in life. Along with Sen (1999), I would argue that the problem of determining the experiential content of health – or the specific meaning of strength, reason and freedom in life, in the realisation of health and the mitigation of illness – should always be left to individuals and groups, to the assemblage itself, to determine. This is why I have sought to describe a process by which bodies may become healthy, as much as I have sought to characterise the heterogenetic norms (strength, reason and freedom) to which this process ought to aspire. All of which is simply another way of saying that the study of health and illness ought to shift from a moral to an ethical register.

Thinking about health in more ethical terms arguably cuts to the heart of the contemporary preoccupation with health in a "therapeutic society" (Wright 2010; also Rieff 1966). Within this society, interest in the role of technological innovation in the palliation of disease, and a concern for the social and structural determinants of health and illness, converge in the *governmentality of human conduct*, and the attempt to determine what bodies do, say or think in the work of maintaining their health more directly (Greco 2009). Public health is the most explicit of the health and social sciences in this attempt to modify conduct, knowledge, attitudes and behaviour, although the ambition is pervasive (Lupton 1995). Foucault (1991) observed that the problem of conduct lies at the heart of contemporary practices of governmentality, even though the subjection that this government necessarily induces instils in subjects the capacity to resist the 'conduct of conduct' in a practice of freedom. Conduct is both the object of power and the means of its necessary resistance in this sense. This is why ethics may indeed present new "strategic possibilities" for the design of novel practices of health (Veyne 1986: 1–11). If health may be characterised in terms of strength, reason and freedom, then it is arguable that the promotion of health will require the ongoing modification of one's conduct in pursuit of these states. In the last chapter, I detailed a model for the generation of an ethics of health grounded in Deleuze's treatment of a 'compound of forces' amid Foucault's more systematic 'practices of the self'. The ethics that emerged in this analysis specified a series of heterogenetic norms (and a suggestive form) to guide the practice of an ethics of health without specifying the content of this ethics given the difficulty of determining the rules or encounters that may reliably inform ethical practice in every instance. This is why, despite identifying strength, reason and freedom as ethical goals, Deleuze does not indicate the content of a practice of becoming strong, reasonable and free. How strength, reason and freedom contribute to the promotion of health in real experience is contingent on the play of forces in an assemblage of health. Only in the trial and error of conduct may a body discover the encounters, affects and relations that most reliably enhance its health in experience.

Having described the philosophical underpinnings of this argument in the previous chapter, along with the form of a novel ethics of the assemblage, I would like now to apply this ethical schema to the health problems canvassed in Chaps. 4 and 5. My analysis should go some way towards clarifying what an ethics of the assemblage may look like in 'real experience', in its application to concrete health problems. I will focus first on an ethics of recovery from mental illness, before turning to consider a novel ethics of consumption, and the character of 'healthy' encounters with alcohol and other drugs more directly. I will close with a discussion of how Deleuze's empiricism may inform ongoing innovation across the health and social sciences.

7.1 An Ethics of Recovery

In Chap. 4 I concluded that recovery from mental illness may be characterised in Deleuzian terms as a process of learning to manipulate the affects, signs, territories and events of a body's 'becoming well'. Recovery is an open extended event by which the recovering body becomes sensitive to an array of affects and relations evinced in diverse social, material and affective milieus (see also Tucker 2010: 436–439). As a body becomes sensitive to its milieus, it necessarily learns to identify and manipulate select events, affects and relations within these milieus in a practice of becoming well. It follows that recovery ought to be reframed in terms of the broad assemblages of health that sustain recovery in particular territories or contexts. The ethological analysis of qualitative data collected among individuals recovering from mental illness, canvassed in Chap. 4, indicated that recovery occurs within an assemblage of human and nonhuman forces as that assemblage's capacity to affect the varied forces it encounters grows. This capacity grows as the recovering body is able to organise its encounters in ways that yield a balance of supportive, positive or enabling affects in a novel assemblage of health. Recovery traces a line of becoming well in this organisation of encounters, and the increased power of acting it enables.

It is for this reason that I sought to emphasise the ethical aspects of recovery from mental illness at the conclusion of Chap. 4. Most contemporary models of recovery make a similar point, albeit for different reasons, in stressing that recovery necessarily proceeds in various life domains (such as employment, education, relationships and family life) as individuals endeavour to transform, or take control of their lives. This is likely why the language of *connectedness, hope, identity, meaning and empowerment* has become so central to recent discussions of the nature and experience of recovery (Leamy et al. 2011: 448–450). Recent studies indicate that recovery is promoted, at least to some extent, in the effort individuals undertake to reorganise their social, affective and material encounters in support of their 'becoming well' (Fox 2002; Parr 2007). I wish now to revisit this conclusion in sketching an ethics of recovery consistent with the analysis offered in Chap. 6. More directly, I would like once again to apply the template offered in Foucault's aesthetics to indicate what an ethics of recovery may look like in 'real experience'.

Consistent with the analysis offered at the close of Chap. 6, I should think that the *ethical substance* of a novel ethics of recovery ought to concern health itself. Conceiving of health as the sum effect of the social, affective and material encounters that promote a body's becoming 'strong', 'reasonable' and 'free' would seem entirely consistent with most existing understanding of recovery, and their emphasis on the importance of connectedness, hope, empowerment and change in particular. It follows that an ethics of recovery might profitably focus on enhancing or increasing the frequency and intensity of those encounters that extend a body's power of acting, understood with respect to a body's capacity to manipulate relations of force. This suggests that recovery may be advanced in a body's becoming strong, insofar as these becomings enhance a body's scope of activity within a particular social context. As the qualitative data presented in Chap. 4 indicates, recovery, along with the day-to-day management of the symptoms associated with mental illness, are each facilitated to the extent that individuals living with mental illness have a full repertoire of activities, practices, techniques or strategies they can draw from to sustain their 'becoming well' (see Tucker 2010: 446–448). From spending time with friends, finding a job, engaging in creative arts, volunteering in local services, browsing in shops, visiting green spaces, playing sport, or simply taking a journey on a train, the greater a body's scope of activity (its power of acting), the more likely it is to sustain its recovery, while coping with the demands of living with a mental illness. An ethics of recovery should, in this respect, take health itself, or the means of a body's *becoming strong, reasonable and free*, as its primary goal or substance.

In the previous chapter I suggested that the notion of 'practical reason' may provide a suitable *mode of subjection* to guide the everyday practice of an ethics of health. Assessed now in relation to recovery from mental illness, I would argue that 'reason' ought to furnish a pragmatic basis for determining which of one's encounters actually promote one's recovery (or 'becoming well') in an assemblage of forces, and which encounters frustrate or diminish this recovery. The qualitative reports presented in Chap. 4 suggest very strongly that the everyday experience of recovery does, indeed, entail a good deal of consternation regarding the kinds of associations, activities, pastimes or encounters that either promote one's recovery, or further mitigate the impact of the symptoms associated with mental illness. Most of the individuals whose experiences were reported in Chap. 4 seemed to describe an experimental process whereby the effects of particular encounters, activities or pastimes were progressively examined and reassessed over time. This includes decisions regarding the individuals or groups one may wish to spend time with; the extent to which one seeks to maintain close relationships with peers and family; how one elects to spend one's free time; the employment one may be in a position to pursue, including the prospect of unpaid or volunteer work; even how one engages in, or utilises, public spaces such as cafes, libraries, shops, parks or community centres. Each of these places, associations or encounters may potentially support the practice of 'becoming well', one's recovery in life, even though the challenge remains of determining how and why particular encounters support recovery at particular times, in particular contexts (or assemblages). It is important to add, of course, that mental illness itself and its associated symptoms, inevitably mediate any assessment of which encounters support one's recovery, and which undermine it.

Practical reason may, nonetheless, provide an additional basis for determining the mix of encounters, activities, associations and experiences that most effectively supports one's recovery within an assemblage of health. Drawing on various of the examples furnished in Chap. 4, this may include reflection on the reasons why a particular café, shop, park or public space serves to promote one's recovery, along with the events, affects and relations that are available in these encounters to extend one's 'becoming well'. It is to suggest that practices and experiences as diverse as travelling without any particular destination on a city train; getting one's hair cut in the company of sympathetic strangers; browsing for a film or a novel in a local store; launching into a handstand on a quiet street corner; enjoying the repose of the botanical gardens; or simply brewing a cup of tea in one's kitchen can avail social, affective and material resources for the ongoing formation of an assemblage of health. Each of the examples canvassed in Chap. 4 suggests something of the everyday affects, relations and events by which recovery transpires as a line of 'becoming well' in life. I recognise that the prospects of individuals living with mental illness adopting such a Deleuzian practice of 'becoming well' may seem far-fetched. Yet the evidence presented in earlier chapters would suggest that individuals in recovery do indeed reflect on the nature and significance of their relationships, activities and pastimes, insofar as recovery from mental illness is understood as something that one has to work very persistently at maintaining over time. I would suggest, therefore, that individuals in recovery are comfortable enough with the *practice of reason*, even if the characterisation of this experience is rarely offered in Deleuzian terms. Indeed, if the work of recovery should be regarded as an everyday labour advanced in the identification of the various activities, encounters and alliances that promote health in life, then practical reason would seem to be of vital importance in the course of reorganising one's encounters in support of recovery. It suggests, finally, why one may wish to subject oneself to reason in 'becoming well'.

Naturally, the application of practical reason introduces the problem of identifying a suitable *mode of asceticism* to guide ethical conduct in support of recovery. In the last chapter I argued that practices of the encounter ought to provide the measure of this mode, insofar as encounters may be said to govern the everyday modulations of recovery within an assemblage of health. I would add that Chap. 4 provided a suggestive suite of examples indicating how practices of the encounter function in support of one's 'becoming well'. One particularly striking example concerned the efforts some participants described to observe social interactions in public spaces, such as cafés, restaurants and shopping precincts, without necessarily participating in them. Akin to a kind of 'pedagogy of the sign', the direct observation of social contact gave way to a series of reflections regarding the 'proper' way of comporting oneself in public. This learning seemed to entail the identification of the various affects and relations released in each event of social interaction, and how these affects and relations may be 'put to work' in support of recovery. Just as hope and empowerment are increasingly regarded as central to the everyday experience of recovery, social interaction, or social connectedness are routinely highlighted in discussions of how the *feeling of hope* or empowerment may be cultivated in recovery from mental illness (Leamy et al. 2011). Connectedness should, in this sense, be understood as a vital part of the affective labour of maintaining one's mental health. The data presented in Chap. 4 confirm that this labour is routinely performed in encounters in and with particular social milieus. Social encounters are central to recovery, in other words, and yet *the cultivation of encounters* in an assemblage of health requires varied affective skills. These skills are acquired in observation and in practice, further illustrating the ways sociality supports (or fails to support) the experience of hope, empowerment, meaning and belonging in recovery.

While social encounters are no doubt central to much of the everyday experience of recovery, the evidence presented in Chap. 4 indicates that a wide variety of additional affective and material encounters may be important too. This includes encounters in (and with) public spaces such as parks and gardens; encounters in nature, with 'peace and quiet', the 'wild', 'silence' or 'solitude'; encounters with material objects including tools, artefacts and precious belongings, along with 'bric-a-brac' or ephemera; and in encounters with 'place', including places of belonging such as churches or community centres, as well as places that are *made meaningful* in the cultivation of 'place attachment'. Each of these encounters may potentially furnish the affects and relations necessary for the promotion of recovery, just as each suggests the centrality of an ethics of the encounter to the 'real experience' of mental health. What matters is that bodies come to connect with other bodies, both human and nonhuman, in the composition or expression of an assemblage of health. What matters is the *affective rhythm of the assemblage* in its proximity to the full measure of its power of acting. In each encounter, in each affective modulation, the recovering body takes on simple parts, both human and nonhuman, which enhance its scope of activity. These simple parts – the wall supporting a handstand on a quiet street; the bench in the cemetery overlooking the water; a poster gifted by a staff member at a local DVD library; the water, trees and sky in the park; the cookbook acquired in a second hand bookshop – are each folded into the assemblage, adding to its capacities, furnishing an incremental improvement in the health of the recovering body. Each thereby confirms the significance of a discrete art or practice of the encounter in support of an ethics of becoming well in an assemblage of health.

The *telos* of such an ethics ought to concern the promotion of a body's 'becoming well' to the limit of its power of acting observing only the constraints of resources, time and industry. If health may be regarded as a function of a body's power of acting, expressed in the balance of its active affections, then recovery too may be understood as a process (or 'line') of becoming-active in the organisation of one's encounters. As I noted in the last chapter, the activeness of a body's affections can be said to enhance its health given the ways this activity extends the array of objects, signs, forces and territories that body may establish relations with. Cultivated in its encounters, the full complement of a body's affects and relations expands its scope of activity while increasing the freedom, strength, adaptability, responsiveness or tenacity by which that body may affect (and be affected by) the bodies it enters into community with. Considered in terms of the affects and relations of its 'becoming well', a body's health in recovery opens up a line of flight beyond mental illness. In strength, reason and freedom, an ethics of recovery thus suggests a novel basis for the *practice of becoming well* in the midst of the contexts (or assemblages) which structure the everyday experience of mental illness. The next section considers encounters with alcohol and other drugs in an attempt to trace a novel ethics of consumption. The goal, once again, is to provide a concrete sense of how an ethics of the assemblage may serve to promote health in 'real experience'.

7.2 An Ethics of Consumption

Foucault's last works remind one of what the ancient Greeks apparently knew well, that the experience of pleasure is always shadowed by the antinomies of moderation and excess. Recognising that the resolution of these tensions is a matter of personal proclivity, the Greeks sought to cultivate an *aesthetics of moderation* in accordance with the more ethical 'use of pleasure'. In our own time, governments have often resorted to the machinery of law and policy in an effort to control those 'pleasures of the flesh' deemed too unruly, disruptive or unpredictable to be entrusted to individual fancy (Walton 2002). Even as the erstwhile regulation of sexual and corporeal expression, of questions of lifestyle and identity, has receded in recent decades, the use of (illicit) drugs for pleasure is still firmly prohibited in most places (Fraser and Moore 2011). This is despite the fact that prohibition has failed to prevent the pervasive use of illicit drugs, while arguably increasing the specific risks and harms associated with their consumption (Davenport-Hines 2002: 15–20). It is arguable that the failures of prohibition may be traced to the generic difficulties associated with the legislative regulation of 'private' conduct. Being largely unenforceable, such laws rely on the maintenance of a popular and supportive moral consensus. Once this moral consensus breaks down, enforcement becomes progressively more difficult. This, I would suggest, is precisely what has happened in most contemporary cultures with respect to the use of illicit drugs (see also Walton 2002). Particularly within youth cultures, the taboos proscribing illicit drug use have been steadily eroded in recent decades such that the use of alcohol and other drugs (AOD) has become 'culturally normalised' in many instances (Aldridge et al. 2011). Evidence collected in both the developed and the developing world indicates that many young people now regard illicit drug use as generic leisure activity to be enjoyed alongside other common pastimes (Cheung and Cheung 2006: Measham and Brain 2005).

Consistent with this evidence, it is arguable that the increasing availability of illicit drugs, coupled with falling prices and the emergence of more liberal attitudes regarding their use, have conspired to replace an older, more conservative consensus that once worked to mitigate illicit drug use, with a newer, more permissive compact (see Parker et al. 2002; Parker 2005; Pearson 2001). Characterised by a kind of "reasoned choice" (Williams and Parker 2001: 397), certain kinds of illicit drug use are increasingly tolerated (if not openly celebrated) in a range of contemporary cultural settings. While this tolerance is almost universally restricted to the "sensible" or "recreational" (Parker et al. 2002: 941) use of drugs like cannabis, ecstasy and cocaine – it does not extend to injection drug use for example – it may be argued in light of this cultural shift that drug policy, along with health and social policy too, ought to move from the embrace of prohibition towards an effort to manage or "live with" illicit drug use (Pearson 2001: 192). Central to such a stance ought to be an attempt to intervene in cultures of illicit drug use as a way of more directly mediating the ways illicit drugs are understood, argued about, consumed and managed. If drugs are here to stay, as it were, then it would seem that the proper focus of health and social policy ought to shift to the work of reducing the harms sometimes associated with their consumption. It is in this respect that one might argue for greater attention to the 'use of pleasure' in the design of a novel ethics of consumption (see Race 2008: 419–423).

In the language of *Assemblages of Health*, the endorsement of a more ethical approach to the use of alcohol and other drugs is primarily concerned to elucidate the character and experience of 'healthy' encounters with these substances. This approach proceeds from the self-evident fact that not all drug use can be regarded as innately harmful, dangerous or unhealthy. Just as throughout history alcohol has been regarded as a source of great conviviality, repose and enjoyment, if consumed in particular ways, it would seem that contemporary generations have arrived at a similar consensus regarded the use of other drugs, such as amphetamines, cannabis, ecstasy and cocaine (O'Malley and Valverde 2004). This is simply to point out, as recent studies have confirmed, that these substances can in fact be used safely, with few if any immediate (or longer term) consequences for one's health or social circumstances (DeCorte 2001; Malbon 1999; Pearson 2001). It is further the case that this partially explains the relatively steady increase in the incidence and prevalence of drug use in many nations since the mid 1960s (see Davenport-Hines 2002; Keane 2002; Fraser and Moore 2011). Indeed, if it were not possible for illicit substances to be used in *more controlled ways* – if it were not possible for these substances to be used relatively safely – then it is difficult to imagine how it might have been possible for the prevalence of drug use to have increased in the ways that it has in so many places in recent decades. Surely, this has only happened because people have found ways to use drugs more safely, in ways that maximise the myriad pleasures to be derived from their consumption, while working to minimise any associated harms. This would suggest, moreover, that a kind of practical or *de facto* 'use of pleasure' serves as a common feature of many existing cultures of drug use.

While drug use always takes place within a social context, it is also a matter of personal conduct, of choice and compulsion, practice and reflection. Drug use may for this reason, be described as a distinctive 'practice of the self', opening up the prospect of describing a more ethical relationship to drugs, to the encounter with drugs, consistent with the ethical model developed in the previous chapter. Reflecting Foucault's treatment of an aesthetics of existence, I would like to argue here for the relevance of the principles of *moderation* and *self-mastery* in the design of a novel ethics of the drug assemblage. Without ignoring the moral connotations that so readily attach to these principles, I would note that moderation, control and self-mastery are utterly integral to the conduct of healthy encounters with alcohol and other drugs (see Decorte 2001; Race 2008; Zinberg 1984). It ought to be easy enough, in this context, to imagine a kind of *aesthetics of the encounter* aimed at modifying the character of drug use in an attempt to entrench moderation, control and self-mastery in each event of consumption. Given how rare problems of drug addiction or dependency actually are – considered in relation to the sheer prevalence of consumption in most cultures – it is arguable that the principles of moderation, control and self-mastery already inform a great many existing practices of drug use (Race 2008). Moderation and control may, for this reason, be regarded among the principal norms governing cultures of drug use in most places. Notwithstanding the raft of cultural and contextual factors that mitigate the incidence of drug problems, the everyday assumption of moderation in the use of alcohol and other drugs suggests that the reflexive, controlled or *ethical consumption* of drugs is common enough, even if the characterisation of this practice in ethical terms is not.

No doubt some will demur that there is no such thing as responsible, safe or healthy drug use. Yet the great advantage of Deleuze's approach to these kinds of ethical questions is his rejection of moral distinctions such as 'right' and 'wrong', 'good' and 'evil', in favour of the consideration of *good and bad encounters*. Good encounters, as I have noted, involve the sympathetic union of bodies in ways that enhance their power of acting, while bad encounters tend to diminish this power. This is why Deleuze describes his ethics in empirical terms, for bodies must learn in life, as in practice, to distinguish between good and bad encounters. Learning arises either in experience or in the collective wisdom of one's social and political milieu. What matters is the encounter, not the perceived moral standing of the entities party to it. This is why one can speak of 'healthy encounters' with drugs, because they happen in 'real experience' all the time. Bodies often encounter drugs in ways that enhance their power of acting; this is likely the reason why drug use is as common as it is. The ethical question, as always, is how to fashion one's encounters with drugs in ways that release the maximum of active affections, while minimising 'sad passions'.

Following Foucault, it may be said that all encounters with drugs should be concerned with the determination of limits and the practice of moderation in the ongoing cultivation of an ethics of safe (or healthy) use. This could also serve as an effective means of reducing the harms sometimes associated with consumption. For some, the identification of safe limits may involve complete abstinence, for others it may involve abstaining from certain substances while enjoying others in moderation. I would add that the most satisfying insight advanced in a Foucauldian approach to the 'problem' of drugs in society lies in the recognition of the *benefits of moderation*. Typically, biomedicine and public health, among other organs of the 'health society', valorise moderation of drug use, if not outright abstinence, as inherently proper and virtuous. As if the 'healthy' body ought to desire abstinence in and of its nature. Perhaps one might have more success promoting moderation if one were also to identify its numerous benefits. Based on his assessment of the 'use of pleasure' in classical Roman and Hellenic ethics, Foucault (1985) makes the intriguing point that moderation was valued by the Ancients mainly because it enabled the *intensification of pleasure* on those rarer occasions in which it was experienced. Applied to the practice of drug use, it is arguable that the ethical moderation of use could serve a similar function in ensuring that each remaining episode of use is more distinctive, intensive, singular or pleasurable than might otherwise have been possible. This is to argue for an ethics of moderation aimed at intensifying the pleasures associated with consumption, as much as it is concerned to foster safer, healthier, more controlled encounters with drugs. Moderation may be advisable, in this regard, not merely as a virtue in and of itself, but also for the practical benefits it delivers for health as in life.

The practice of such an ethics of moderation could, moreover, seek to build on the indigenous or 'folk' expressions of safe, sensible, responsible or controlled drug use manifest in most existing cultures of consumption. As numerous scholars have observed (see Zinberg 1984; Moore 1993; Lupton and Tulloch 2002; O'Malley and Valverde 2004), most drug use takes place within distinctive social contexts that exhibit norms, practices and conventions that actively encourage moderation by discouraging excessive drug use. Sean Slavin (2004: 270) argues that "messy" or uncontrolled drug use is condemned in many drug using peer groups as the preserve of inexperienced and/or irresponsible users. Slavin (2004) goes on to argue that considerable cultural and social cachet often attends the cultivation of more refined and controlled personal habits, in the fashioning of a capacity to "handle" one's drug use (see also Measham et al. 2001: 124–129). While the observance of these kinds of social norms often reflects the desire to avoid the embarrassment or social stigma associated with "messy" drug use, messy or irresponsible use is usually regarded as embarrassing precisely because it conveys an inability to control one's use, to regulate one's pleasures in accordance with the ethical precepts of decorum, pride, maturity or reason (see also Decorte 2001; Pearson 2001; Zinberg 1984). It suggests, more directly, that the grounds for an ethical practice of moderation already exist in many drug using cultures, in the practices, values, norms and principles drug users have devised in an effort to discriminate between 'good' and 'bad' encounters with drugs. Sometimes referred to as "folk" harm reduction (see Southgate and Hopwood 2001: 322), or as a kind of "counterpublic health" (Race 2009: 161), it is plain enough that the rudiments of an ethics of the encounter, of an ethics of moderation, are present in the 'practical reason' that many users have devised both to intensify the pleasures derived from consumption, but also to ameliorate the harms occasionally associated with it.

All of which suggests that pleasure might serve as the appropriate *ethical substance* of a novel ethics of consumption. It is folly to ignore the role of pleasure and desire in the use of alcohol and other drugs (see O'Malley and Valverde 2004); better to render the 'use of pleasure' in more ethical terms in order to maximise 'good' or healthy encounters with drugs. Foucault's last writings would suggest that the moderation of the pleasures derived from consumption could serve both to intensify these pleasures in the less frequent instances in which use occurs, but also to minimise the harms potentially associated with it. One might, in this sense, subject oneself to the 'reason' of moderation in the cultivation of safer, healthier encounters with drugs. As I have noted, this *mode of subjection* will just as likely involve no use at all, as the more moderate use of substances in accordance with the dictates of practical reason, health and wellbeing. The *mode of asceticism* called for in the practice of such an ethics ought to concern the cultivation of an art of the encounter. Indeed, if it is the encounter with drugs which ultimately determines their health consequences – and if these encounters are just as likely to generate health, happiness, pleasure or an increase in one's power of acting, as they are to yield sadness, harm or danger – then an ethics of the drug assemblage would seem to be inevitably concerned with the *effects of the encounter* with drugs. As I noted in Chap. 6, individual bodies would seem best placed to assess these effects, either in the course of lived experience or with the advantage of the shared learning of one's cultural and affective endowment. An ethics of the drug assemblage must therefore, concern the effects of each encounter with drugs, articulated in the expression of an ascetics of moderation, and oriented in practice towards the achievement of controlled consumption. The *telos* of these varied efforts should, of course, concern the body's transition to the limit of its power of acting, in the full embrace of its health in life. Only then may one speak of healthy or safe drug use.

7.3 A New Empiricism for the Health and Social Sciences

Practised in reason, realised in the scope of a body's manifest activity, and yielding ultimately to the joys of freedom in life, Deleuze's ethics require that bodies become sensitive to the conditions of their encounters in real experience. An ethics of the assemblage must, in this regard, model itself on the *empirical study* of relations, bodies, milieus, signs, affects and events such that one may come to determine good from bad encounters, and so advance towards the limits of one's power of acting in life. This is another of the great virtues of Deleuze's empiricism, furnishing a mode of practical reason to guide an ethics of the assemblage capable of promoting health on a line of 'becoming well'. I should like to close this chapter, and this book, with some final reflections on the everyday practice of such an empiricism, and the prospects of its broader adoption across the health and social sciences.

If Deleuze's (1988: 123) ethics may be said to express a "zone of subjectivation" wherein one may become "master of one's speed . . . one's molecules and particular features", then it would seem vital to *posit a method* by which mastery of "life within the folds" may be achieved. This, I wager, is exactly what Deleuze's empiricism affords; a tool, method, art or technique for bending the forces of life in the formation and reformation of an assemblage of health. Transcendental empiricism exposes the virtual clamour of events, affects and relations as they manifest in the real experience of bodies in their encounters. It affords *a pedagogy of the sign* whereby bodies may become sensitive to the actualisations of life in its becomings. Such a pedagogy, and the practical learning it suggests, describes an "empirical study of bodies in order to know their relations, and how they are combined" (Deleuze 1992: 212). I have argued throughout this book that a body's health depends on this study, both in terms of the practical learning bodies accrue as they strive to manage their health, and in the formative processes by which cultures develop ways of knowing sufficient to ensure the continuity of health among a population of bodies. Such an empiricism empowers bodies to take control of their encounters in a novel practice of health, just as it requires a broader intelligence, a community of scholars thinking and acting together, to identify the collective activities that may effect some increment in a population's capacities. It is for these reasons that I would conclude that transcendental empiricism yields both a novel ethics of the encounter, and a discrete method to guide research innovation across the health and social sciences.

Turning first to consider the *real experience of health*, the empiricism demanded of this experience necessarily entails the assessment of affects, relations and events as they modify, promote or imperil the everyday maintenance of health. The goal is to identify the specific points, lines or zones whereby an assemblage of health may be established in practice. Adopting insights from Foucault's last writings, it is arguable that this project should further adhere to what Foucault (1984: 46) called the "historical ontology of ourselves", although, in accordance with Deleuze's ethics this ontology must be applied to the entire 'zone of subjectivation' wherein human life is modulated. The practical reason required of this expanded ontology puts (human) life "to the test of reality, of contemporary reality, both to grasp the points where change is possible and desirable, and to determine the precise form this change should take" (Foucault 1984: 46). Such is the test that 'life in the folds' must be subjected to. A test by which one may conjure an ethics from the work of identifying all that extends life to the limits of its power of acting (Dean 1994: 44–45). This is an ethics of joy elevated to a "grand and rare art"; an art of living well amidst a "free nature, wild, arbitrary, fantastic, confused and surprising" (Nietzsche 1974: 290). Chapter 2 offered a means of identifying the particular amplitude of relations, affects and events in an assemblage of forces, while the analysis presented here, and in Chap. 6, has sought to confirm how affects, relations and events may be modified in the practice of a novel health ethics. Just as health should be taken to be a product of forces that extend a body's power of acting, ethics too should assume as its primary focus the manipulation of these forces in a practice of becoming well.

Yet the learning that bodies accrue in their varied encounters and then apply to the maintenance of their health and wellbeing is equally subject to a 'formative process' in culture. Health is not merely the effect of agreeable encounters between bodies in other words, nor is it some kind of mystical outcome pursuant to a long, near hermetic period of personal reflection. As important as these processes may be for some people (Ramey 2012: 148–160), the learnings essential to the discrimination of good and bad encounters, and the subsequent promotion of a body to the limit of its power of acting, are among the most enduring objects of scholarly endeavour. In philosophy, art and science, knowledge has advanced in step with the promotion of this power of acting, establishing, in turn, something of the ways health may be promoted and suffering endured (Deleuze 1998: 4–6). For this reason, science, art and philosophy remain potent sources of criteria for distinguishing 'good' from 'bad' encounters in the practice of health. Each mode of thought avails lines of flight by which health may be promoted, provided it adheres to the distinction Deleuze (1994) draws between *real experience* and *possible experience* to describe a superior empiricism. Consistent with this distinction, philosophy, science and art contribute to the 'formative processes' necessary for the promotion of health whenever they reveal the actual circumstances in which bodies encounter one another in the promotion of health. Interest in the conditions of *possible experience* – such as one finds in most scientific analysis of practices, behaviours and factors that may increase the probability of harm or illness in a given population – offers some guidance in the conduct of healthy encounters, yet rarely as much guidance as is required to negotiate risks and opportunities in real experience (Lupton 1995: 84–89).

It must be said that the health and social sciences seem for the most part reluctant to encroach upon the *actual experience* of health and illness as it is lived. While, of course, lived experience is the principal object of research in medical anthropology and much contemporary sociology of health and illness (see Fox 2011; Turner 2008), this work is dwarfed by the focus on *possible experience* that characterises the vast majority of research in the health and social sciences. This tendency is especially evident in the preoccupation with populations, epidemics, social conditions and 'determinants' that describes most recent scholarship in these fields. Actual bodies all but disappear in this research in deference to the machinations of risk and its associated probabilities (Lupton 1995; Rose 2007). Without ignoring the obvious merits of this work, and its application in the design of more effective local responses to select health problems (see Baum 2008), the focus on populations, and the conditions in which illnesses are disseminated, mostly ignores the specificity of health as it is lived. Yet the main problem with this approach is that after a century and a half of dedicated scholarship in the health and social sciences, there appears to be nothing in possible experience that does not affect health in some way. Indeed, it is sometimes hard to know what is healthy anymore, given that even the most innocuous of activities now seem to carry at least some risk of harm (Lupton 1995; Metzl 2010). As such, the web of structural determinants of health and illness revealed in recent studies has arguably become so complex that is it increasingly unclear what the proper goals of health and social policy ought to be (Rhodes 2009). By focusing on the social determinants of health and illness, as much as their biological aspects, health and social scientists conjure a possible experience of health (or illness) in which an array of human, biological, organic, technological, social, structural, semiotic and affective forces may potentially (if not actually) mediate health. And so, for example, welfare policy, labour market fluctuations, gender, environmental conditions and migration trends may potentially mediate health outcomes, although their impact in real experience is more often assumed than demonstrated. As a result, scholars tend to say more about the epidemiology of health and illness than the particularities of health as it is lived (Law and Mol 2002).

Based on Deleuze's empiricism, I would argue in contrast for renewed attention to the real experience of health and illness, and renewed focus on the spaces, bodies, forces, affects and relations active in each event of health and illness. Real experience is forever conveyed in the relations, affects and events that comprise the flux of becoming; the virtual forces beneath the actual form of individuated life. These forces ought to constitute the primary focus of scholarly inquiry in the health and social sciences, such that life's becomings may be more readily accommodated in the study of health and illness. As I noted in Chap. 2, much existing work in the health and social sciences seeks to return thought to real experience, to the actual conditions of everyday life. Including the various *affective, spatial* and *relational* turns that have inspired so much recent activity in these sciences (see Anderson and Harrison 2010; Clough and Halley 2007), wider adoption of the concepts and methods presented in Deleuze's empiricism should reveal more of the "practices, actors, atmospheres and representations that generate new interactions" supportive of the health of bodies in their encounters (McFarlane 2011: 379). This is to plot a course by which the health and social sciences may be folded into assemblages of health in actual experience. It is to suggest another mechanism whereby the health and social sciences may contribute to the 'formative processes' necessary for distinguishing good from bad encounters in the real experience of health and illness.

In closing I would note that such an approach to research innovation in the health and social sciences ought to help resolve the three principal research problems I identified at the outset of this book. That is: the utility of articulating the substantive content of health as an object of thought and practice; the urgency of generating methodologies that are more sensitive to the imbrication of human and nonhuman forces in the modulations of health and illness; along with a novel method for studying the structural determinants of health that isn't content to allow complexity to proliferate at the cost of an adequate explanation of how structural processes actually impact the lived experience of health and illness. As I hope the intervening chapters have demonstrated, Deleuze's empiricism furnishes a compelling basis for responding to each of these challenges. All that remains is the patient labour of thought and practice in the ongoing articulation of a minor science of health.

7.4 Health, Ethology, Life

As much as I have been concerned throughout this book to contribute to a range of emerging debates in the health and social sciences, I have mainly been concerned to chart a course by which health may be promoted in everyday life. This is why I have emphasised the need for a more positive and substantive account of health capable of yielding diverse ethical principles for the restoration, maintenance and/or promotion of health in an assemblage of human and nonhuman forces. We live in an age in which health is manifest, pervasive and abundant and yet everywhere appears to be under threat. Perhaps human life has always been like this, although it seems important to stress that the resources available to support health and wellbeing have never been greater, despite their grossly uneven distribution. We are truly the beneficiaries of the 'health society', and even as this society adopts ever more effective instruments for the commodification of 'biovalue', health flourishes in the margins. This is why I find Deleuze's adaptation of Spinoza's ethics of joy, combined with his interest in Foucault's vision of 'life in the folds' and Bergson's discovery of the *elan vital*, to be so compelling. For this is Deleuze's great contribution; a *philosophy of joy* and the triumph of strength, reason and freedom over the tyranny of sad passions and all that separates us from our power of acting. The living of this philosophy calls for an ethology, an empiricism of everyday encounters, which I have here applied to the experience of health in order to determine how bodies may trace a line of becoming well in life. Health may, in this sense, be described as a process that draws bodies together in an assemblage of forces. Determining how bodies ought to combine, or affect one another, in the realisation of health gives rise to an ethics of rare utility. Determining how such an ethics ought to be practised in the promotion of life is surely in the very art of living.

References

Aldridge, J., F. Measham, and L. Williams. 2011. *Illegal leisure revisited: Changing patterns of alcohol and drug use in adolescents and young adults*. London: Routledge.

Anderson, B., and P. Harrison (eds.). 2010. *Taking place: Non-representational theories and geography*. London: Ashgate.

Ansell Pearson, K. 1999. *Germinal life: The difference and repetition of Gilles Deleuze*. London: Routledge.

Baum, F. 2008. *The new public health*, 3rd ed. Melbourne: Oxford University Press.

Buchanan, I. 1997. The problem of the body in Deleuze and Guattari, or, what can a body do? *Body & Society* 3(3): 73–91.

Cheung, N., and Y. Cheung. 2006. Is Hong Kong experiencing normalization of adolescent drug use? Some reflections on the normalization thesis. *Substance Use & Misuse* 41(14): 1967–1990.

Clough, P., and J. Halley (eds.). 2007. *The affective turn: Theorizing the social*. Durham: Duke University Press.

Davenport-Hines, R. 2002. *The pursuit of oblivion: A global history of narcotics*. London: WW Norton & Company.

Dean, M. 1994. *Critical and effective histories: Foucault's methods and historical sociology*. London: Routledge.

Decorte, T. 2001. Drug users' perceptions of 'controlled' and 'uncontrolled' use. *International Journal of Drug Policy* 12(4): 297–320.

Deleuze, G. 1988. *Foucault*. London: The Athlone Press.

Deleuze, G. 1992. *Expressionism in Philosophy: Spinoza* Trans. Martin Joughin. New York: Zone Books.

Deleuze, G. 1994. *Difference and repetition*. London: The Athlone Press.

Deleuze, G. 1998. *Essays Critical and Clinical*. Trans. Daniel W. Smith and Michael Greco. London: Verso.

Foucault, M. 1984. *The Foucault reader*, ed. Paul Rabinow. London: Penguin.

Foucault, M. 1985. *The history of sexuality. Vol. 2: The use of pleasure*. London: Penguin.

Foucault, M. 1991. Governmentality. In *The Foucault effect: Studies in governmentality*, ed. Burchell Graham, Gordon Colin, and Miller Peter. Chicago: University of Chicago Press.

Fox, N. 2002. Refracting 'health': Deleuze, Guattari and body-self. *Health* 6(3): 347–363.

Fox, N. 2011. The ill-health assemblage: Beyond the body-with-organs. *Health Sociology Review* 20(4): 434–446.

Fraser, S., and D. Moore. 2011. *The drug effect: Health, crime and society*. Melbourne: Cambridge University Press.

Greco, M. 2009. Thinking beyond polemics: Approaching the health society through Foucault. *Oesterreichische Zeitschrift fuer Soziologie* 34(2): 13–27.

Keane, H. 2002. *What's wrong with addiction?* Melbourne: Melbourne University Press.

Latour, B. 2005. *Reassembling the social: An introduction to actor-network theory*. Oxford: Oxford University Press.

Law, J. 2004. *After method: Mess in social science research*. London: Routledge.

Law, J., and A. Mol (eds.). 2002. *Complexities: Social studies of knowledge practices*. Durham: Duke University Press.

Leamy, M., V. Bird, C. Le Boutillier, J. Williams, and M. Slade. 2011. Conceptual framework for personal recovery in mental health: Systematic review and narrative synthesis. *British Journal of Psychiatry* 199: 445–452.

Lupton, D. 1995. *The imperative of health: Public health and the regulated body*. London: Sage.

Lupton, D., and J. Tulloch. 2002. Life would be Pretty Dull without risks: Voluntary risk-taking and its pleasures. *Health, Risk & Society* 4(2): 113–24.

Malbon, B. 1999. *Clubbing: Dancing, ecstasy and vitality*. London: Routledge.

McFarlane, C. 2011. On context: Assemblage, political economy and structure. *City* 14(3–4): 375–388.

Measham, F., and K. Brain. 2005. 'Binge' drinking, British alcohol policy and the new culture of intoxication. *Crime, Media, Culture* 1(3): 262–283.

Measham, F., J. Aldridge, and H. Parker. 2001. *Dancing on drugs: Risk, health and hedonism in the British club scene*. London: Free Association Books.

Metzl, J. 2010. Introduction: Why against health? In *Against health: How health became the new morality*, ed. J. Metzl and A. Kirkland. New York: New York University Press.

Mol, A. 2002. *The body multiple: Ontology in medical practice*. Durham: Duke University Press.

Moore, D. 1993. Social controls, harm reduction and interactive outreach: The public health implications of an ethnography of drug use. *Australian Journal of Public Health* 17(1): 58–67.

Nietzsche, F. 1974. *The gay science: With a prelude in rhymes and an appendix of songs*. London: Vintage.

O'Malley, P., and M. Valverde. 2004. Pleasure, freedom and drugs: The uses of pleasure in liberal governance of drug and alcohol consumption. *Sociology* 38(1): 25–42.

Parker, H. 2005. Normalization as a barometer: Recreational drug use and the consumption of leisure by younger Britons. *Addiction Research & Theory* 13(3): 205–215.

Parker, H., L. Williams, and J. Aldridge. 2002. The normalization of sensible recreational drug use: More evidence from the North West England Longitudinal Study. *Sociology* 36(4): 941–964.

Parr, H. 2007. Mental health, nature work, and social inclusion. *Environment and Planning D: Space and Society* 25: 537–561.

Pearson, G. 2001. Normal drug use: Ethnographic fieldwork among an adult network of recreational drug users in inner London. *Substance Use & Misuse* 36(1 & 2): 167–200.

Peterson, C., and M. Seligman. 2003. *Character strengths and virtues: A handbook and classification*. Oxford: Oxford University Press.

Race, K. 2008. The use of pleasure in harm reduction: Perspectives from the history of sexuality. *International Journal of Drug Policy* 19(5): 417–423.

Race, K. 2009. *Pleasure consuming medicine: The queer politics of drugs*. Durham: Duke University Press Books.

Ramey, J. 2012. *The hermetic Deleuze: Philosophy and spiritual ordeal*. Durham: Duke University Press.

Rhodes, T. 2009. Risk environments and drug harms: A social science for harm reduction approach. *International Journal of Drug Policy* 20: 193–201.

Rieff, P. 1966. *The triumph of the therapeutic: Uses of faith after Freud*. Chicago: The University of Chicago Press.

Rose, N. 2007. *The politics of life itself: Biomedicine, power, and subjectivity in the twenty-first century*. Princeton: Princeton University Press.

Sen, A. 1999. *Development as freedom*. Oxford: Oxford University Press.

Slavin, S. 2004. Drugs, space, and sociality in a gay nightclub in Sydney. *Journal of Contemporary Ethnography* 33(3): 265–295.

Southgate, E., and M. Hopwood. 2001. The role of folk pharmacology and lay experts in harm reduction: Sydney gay drug using networks. *International Journal of Drug Policy* 12(4): 321–335.

Tucker, I. 2010. Mental health service user territories: Enacting 'safe spaces' in the community. *Health* 14(4): 434–448.

Turner, B. 2008. *The body & society: Explorations in social theory*, 3rd ed. London: Sage.

Veyne, P. 1986. The final Foucault and his ethics. *Critical Inquiry* 20(1): 1–9.

Walton, S. 2002. *Out of it: A cultural history of intoxication*. London: Penguin.

Williams, L., and H. Parker. 2001. Alcohol, cannabis, ecstasy and cocaine: Drugs of reasoned choice amongst young adult recreational drug users in England. *International Journal of Drug Policy* 12(5): 397–413.

Wolfe, C. 2010. *What is posthumanism?* Minneapolis: University of Minnesota Press.

Wright, K. 2010. *The rise of the therapeutic society: Psychological knowledge and the contradictions of cultural change*. Washington, DC: New Academia Publishing.

Zammito, J. 2004. *A nice derangement of epistemes. Post-positivism in the study of science from Quine to Latour*. Chicago: The University of Chicago Press.

Zinberg, N. 1984. *Drug, set, setting: The basis for controlled intoxicant use*. New Haven: Yale University Press.

Bibliography

Anthony, W., M. Cohen, M. Farkas, and C. Gagne. 2006. *Psychiatric rehabilitation*, 2nd ed. Boston: Center for Psychiatric Rehabilitation.

Atkinson, S., S. Fuller, and J. Painter (eds.). 2012. *Wellbeing and place*. London: Ashgate.

Boothroyd, D. 2007. *Culture on drugs: Narco-cultural studies of high modernity*. Manchester: Manchester University Press.

Cockerham, W. (ed.). 2010. *The New Blackwell companion to medical sociology*. London: Wiley Blackwell.

Corrigan, P., and R. Ralph. 2005. Introduction: Recovery as consumer vision and research paradigm. In *Recovery in mental illness: Broadening our understanding of wellness*, ed. R. Ralph and P. Corrigan, 3–17. Washington, DC: American Psychological Association.

Crang, M., and N. Thrift (eds.). 2000. *Thinking space*. London: Routledge.

Crawford, R. 2006. Health as a meaningful social practice. *Health* 10(4): 401–420.

Diamond, I., K. Dovey, J. Fitzgerald, and Y. Choi. 2001. Safety becomes danger: Dilemmas of drug-use in public space. *Health & Place* 7(4): 319–331.

Fogel, A., B. King, and S. Shanker (eds.). 2008. *Human development in the twenty-first century: Visionary ideas from systems scientists*. Cambridge: Cambridge University Press.

Fox, N. 1999. *Beyond health: Postmodernism and embodiment*. London: Free Association Books.

Hansen, M. 2000. Becoming as creative involution?: Contextualizing Deleuze and Guattari's biophilosophy. *Postmodern Culture* 11(1): 1–18.

Harman, G. 2011. On the undermining of objects: Grant, Bruno, and radical philosophy. In *The speculative turn: Continental materialism and realism*, ed. L. Bryant, N. Srnicek, and G. Harman. Melbourne: Repress.

Hayden, P. 1998. *Multiplicity and becoming: The pluralist empiricism of Gilles Deleuze*. Indiana: Indiana University Press.

Heft, H. (ed.). 2001. *Ecological psychology in context: James Gibson, Roger Barker and the legacy of William James's radical empiricism*. New York: Lawrence Erlbaum Associates.

Hesse-Biber, S., and P. Leavy (eds.). 2010. *Handbook of emergent methods*. London: The Guildford Press.

Hickey-Moody, A., and P. Malins. 2008. *Deleuzian encounters: Studies in contemporary social issues*. London: Palgrave Macmillan.

Hooke, A. 1987. The order of others: Is Foucault's anti-humanism against human action? *Political Theory* 15(1): 38–61.

Jones, K., and M. Cready (eds.). 2008. *Health and human behaviour: An introduction*, 2nd ed. Oxford: Oxford University Press.

Jun, N., and D. Smith (eds.). 2011. *Deleuze and ethics*. Edinburgh: Edinburgh University Press.

Keane, H. 2004. Disorders of desire: Addiction and problems of intimacy. *Journal of Medical Humanities* 25(3): 189–204.

C. Duff, *Assemblages of Health: Deleuze's Empiricism and the Ethology of Life*,
DOI 10.1007/978-94-017-8893-9,

Kowalski, R., S. Limber, and P. Agatston. 2012. *Cyberbullying: Bullying in the digital age*. Oxford: Wiley-Blackwell.

Marmot, M., and R. Wilkinson (eds.). 2006. *Social determinants of health*, 2nd ed. Oxford: Oxford University Press.

Masny, D., and D. Cole (eds.). 2009. *Multiple literacies theory: A Deleuzian perspective*. Rotterdam: Sense Publishers.

Massumi, B. 1992. *A user's guide to capitalism and schizophrenia: Deviations from Deleuze and Guattari*. Cambridge: MIT Press.

Massumi, B. 2011. *Semblance and event: Activist philosophy and the occurrent arts*. Cambridge, MA: MIT Press.

Measham, F., and M. Shiner. 2009. The legacy of 'normalisation': The role of classical and contemporary criminological theory in understanding young people's drug use. *International Journal of Drug Policy* 20(6): 502–508.

Nestle, M. 2006. Food marketing and childhood obesity – A matter of policy. *New England Journal of Medicine* 354: 2527–2529.

Rabinow, P. 1996. *Essays on the anthropology of reason*. Princeton: Princeton University Press.

Robinson, K. 2010. Back to life: Deleuze, Whitehead and process. *Deleuze Studies* 4(1): 120–133.

Sabisch, P. 2011. *Choreographing relations: Practical philosophy and contemporary choreography*. Munich: Epodium.

Semetsky, I. 2006. *Deleuze, education and becoming*. Rotterdam: Sense Publishers.

Semetsky, I. 2009. Deleuze as a philosopher of education: Affective knowledge/effective learning. *The European Legacy* 14(4): 443–456.

Smith, D. 2007. The conditions of the new. *Deleuze Studies* 1(1): 1–21.

Travers, J. (ed.). 2005. *Handbook of human development for health care professionals*. New York: Jones & Bartlett Publishers.

Waldby, C. 2000. *The visible human project: Informatic bodies and posthuman medicine*. London: Routledge.

Waldby, C. 2002. Stem cells, tissue cultures and the production of biovalue. *Health* 6(3): 305–323.

Wilkinson, R., and Kate Pickett. 2010. *The spirit level: Why equality is better for everyone*. London: Penguin Books.

Williams, J. 2003. *Gilles Deleuze's difference and repetition: A critical introduction and guide*. Edinburgh: Edinburgh University Press.

Index

C. Duff, *Assemblages of Health: Deleuze's Empiricism and the Ethology of Life*, DOI 10.1007/978-94-017-8893-9, © Springer Science+Business Media Dordrecht 2014

The manufacturer's authorised representative in the EU is Springer Nature Customer Service Centre GmbH, Europaplatz 3, 69115 Heidelberg, Germany. If you have any concerns regarding our products, please contact ProductSafety@springernature.com

Printed and bound by CPI Group (UK) Ltd, Croydon, CR0 4YY
25/09/2026
02222896-0003